Functional
Adaptation
Mobility
Medications
Sleep/Rest
Emergency Situations

Physical
Skin Integrity
Nutrition
Elimination
Metabolic
Digestion
Sexual
Sensory/Communication

Psychosocial
Cognition/Perception
Self Image
Role Relationships

Spiritual
Guilt
Hope
Love and Relatedness
Meaning and Purpose

DECISION MAKING

IN

GERONTOLOGIC
NURSING

Clinical Decision Making Series

DECISION MAKING IN GERONTOLOGIC NURSING

Paula A. Loftis, MS, RN, CNS
Director, Department of Geriatrics
Parkland Memorial Hospital
Dallas, Texas

Adjunct Faculty, School of Nursing
The University of Texas at Arlington
Arlington, Texas

Clinical Associate Faculty, School of Nursing
Texas Woman's University
Dallas, Texas

Clinical Nurse Specialist, Zale-Lipshy University Hospital
The University of Texas Southwestern Medical Center
Dallas, Texas

Talar L. Glover, MS, RN, CNS
Quality Assurance and Education Coordinator
Baylor Center for Restorative Care
Dallas, Texas

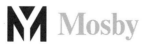
Mosby

St. Louis Baltimore Boston Chicago London Philadelphia Sydney Toronto

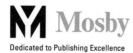

Executive Editor: Linda L. Duncan
Developmental Editor: Kathy Sartori
Production Editor: Vicki Hoenigke
Designer: Elizabeth Fett
Illustrations courtesy of JoAnn Elliott
Cover colors chosen by: Sandra Higgins Hanna

Printed in the United States of America

Mosby–Year Book, Inc.
11830 Westline Industrial Drive
St. Louis, Missouri 63146

ISBN 1-55664-186-9

93 94 95 96 97 CL/MV 9 8 7 6 5 4 3 2 1

CONTRIBUTORS

DEBORAH ANTAI-OTONG, M.S., R.N., C.S., A.N.P.
Psychiatric Clinical Nurse Specialist, Outpatient Psychiatry Triage Unit, Department of Veteran Affairs, Medical Center of Dallas, Dallas, Texas

CAROLYN SPENCER ARTHUR, B.S., R.N., C.N.A.
Quality Assurance/Resource Manager, Jerry L. Pettis VA Medical Center, Department of Veterans Affairs, Loma Linda, California

DONNA A. BACHAND, Ph.D.c, R.N., C.S.
Vice President, Clinical Services, Oncology Clinical Nurse Specialist, Y Medical Associates, Dallas, Texas

DENNIS M. BELLETT, R.N.
Staff Nurse, Outpatient Clinic, Parkland Memorial Hospital, Dallas, Texas

KAY BOLDING, B.S.N., R.N., C.C.R.N.
Practice Director of Cardiology and Cardiovascular Services, Presbyterian Hospital of Dallas, Dallas, Texas

SHERAL CADE, R.D., L.D.
Dietitian, Nutrition Clinic, Parkland Memorial Hospital, Dallas, Texas

OLIVIA CATOLICO, M.S., R.N.C.
Associate Chief, Nursing Service for Education, Jerry L. Pettis VA Medical Center, Department of Veterans Affairs, Loma Linda, California

CAROLYN COLE, M.S.N., A.R.N.P.
Advanced Registered Nurse Practitioner, Department of Veterans Affairs, Seattle, Washington

TOM EMANUELE, R.N.C., MsT
HIV Homecare Case Manager, AIDS Clinic, Parkland Memorial Hospital, Dallas, Texas

CONI FRANCIS, M.S., R.D., L.D.
Instructor, Department of Clinical Nutrition, The University of Texas Southwestern Medical Center at Dallas, Dallas, Texas

TALAR L. GLOVER, M.S., R.N., C.N.S.
Quality Assurance and Education Coordinator, Baylor Center for Restorative Care, Dallas, Texas

SUSAN GOAD, Ed.D., R.N.
Professor, Texas Woman's University, Dallas, Texas

PATRICIA GUIDA, B.S.N., R.N.
Staff Nurse, Medicine, Jerry L. Pettis VA Medical Center, Department of Veterans Affairs, Loma Linda, California

ETTA HALL, R.N.
Staff Nurse, Outpatient Clinic, Parkland Memorial Hospital, Dallas, Texas

CATHERINE A. HILL, B.S.N., R.N.
Nurse Manager, Humana Hospital Brandon, Tampa, Florida

LESLIE C. TRISCHANK HUSSEY, R.N., Ph.D.
Assistant Professor, Baylor University School of Nursing, Dallas, Texas

JANE H. KASS-WOLFF, M.S., R.N.C.
Faculty Associate, Women's Health Care Advanced Nurse Practitioner Program, The University of Texas Southwestern Medical Center at Dallas, Dallas, Texas

ESTELLE KINCAID, B.S.N., R.N.
Former Coordinator Uro-Radiology and Nursing Home Coordinator, Parkland Memorial Hospital, Dallas; Director of Nursing, OakBrook Health Care Center, Whitehouse, Texas

NINA A. KLEBANOFF, Ph.D.c, R.N., C.S.
Psychosocial Clinical Nurse Specialist Consultant, Horizon Mental Health Services, Dallas, Texas

PAULA A. LOFTIS, M.S., R.N., C.N.S.
Director, Department of Geriatrics, Parkland Memorial Hospital; Clinical Associate Faculty, School of Nursing, Texas Woman's University; Clinical Nurse Specialist, Zale-Lipshy University Hospital, The University of Texas Southwestern Medical Center, Dallas; Adjunct Faculty, School of Nursing, The University of Texas at Arlington, Arlington, Texas

ELIZABETH MACKRELLA, B.S.N., R.N.
Staff Nurse, Surgical Intensive Care, Jerry L. Pettis VA Medical Center, Department of Veterans Affairs, Loma Linda, California

SUE MILLER, M.S.N., R.N., C.S.
Geriatric Clinical Nurse Specialist, Department of Geriatrics, Parkland Memorial Hospital, Dallas, Texas

BETH GOODE MOFFETT, M.S.N., R.N.C., G.N.P.
Gerontological Nurse Practitioner, Dallas Home for the Jewish Aged, Dallas, Texas

SYLVIA MORENO, B.S.N., R.N.
AIDS Clinic Manager, Parkland Memorial Hospital, Dallas, Texas

BARBARA HARRISON NAUSS, M.S.N., R.N.C., F.N.P.
Nurse Practitioner, FHP Health Care, Fountain Valley, California

MARYBETH NAVAS, M.N., R.N., C.C.R.N.
Instructor, Critical Care, Jerry L. Pettis VA Medical Center, Department of Veterans Affairs, Loma Linda, California

PREFACE

In most practice settings, nurses are seeing more and more elderly. Just as children are not little adults, older adults differ from younger adults, and their nursing care can be a perplexing medley of

- declining function
- underreporting of problems
- atypical presentation
- multisystem involvement
- nonspecific complaints

requiring care and support from nurses, family, and caregivers.

The nursing decision-making process approaches complex problems in a systematic way that focuses *not* on medical diagnoses or body systems but rather on

- the functional abilities of the elderly
- relationships
- problem solving

The nursing decision-making process uses all facets of a nurse's ability to

- assess
- obtain a history
- observe
- listen
- plan
- integrate
- problem solve
- evaluate
- utilize appropriate resources

This book is designed to serve as a practical, easy-to-read, clinically relevant reference for both novice and advanced practice nurses to guide decision making in the nursing care of older adults in all practice settings:

- acute care
- primary care
- long term care
- outpatient care
- community health

The content presupposes a basic knowledge of nursing, anatomy, physiology, and pathophysiology and is not intended to replace textbooks on geriatric nursing.

The book is organized into four major units reflecting the nursing perspective. The chapter titles are *not* medical diagnoses, but rather chief complaints that might be expressed by a patient or caregiver. Each chapter is based on an algorithm that guides the decision making process. The algorithms contain letters that correspond to the chapter text. The correlating text begins with the letter from the tree and is written to explain points on the decision tree as well as guide the nurse in the decision making process. At the end of each section are relevant

- instruments or tools for assessment
- teaching aids
- reference materials

Illustrations are used to depict key concepts involved in caring for the older adult. To increase accessibility to the nurse in an active clinical setting liberal use has been made of

- illustrations
- tables
- boxes
- bulleted text

Although much thought and care has gone into selecting the contents of this book, topic exclusions are bound to occur. Reader comments and input are requested and will be gratefully received by either editor.

UNIT DESCRIPTIONS	
Unit	*Focus*
Functional	Independence Self-care abilities
Physical	Health-related issues
Psychosocial	Interpersonal relationships
Spiritual	Connections Beliefs

ACKNOWLEDGMENTS

In acknowledgment of Patricia Ann Shelton, who was of immeasurable assistance in the typing of this book and who was taken from us too soon. Special thanks go to the contributors for their considerable expertise and work in making this book possible.

**To our husbands,
who offered tremendous support
during this effort.**

CONTENTS

FUNCTIONAL

Adaptation

Tools:

Mobility

Tools:

Medication

Tools:

Sleep/Rest

Tool:

Emergency Situations

PHYSICAL

Skin Integrity

Sensory/Communication

Tool:

Nutrition

Tools:

Digestion

Tools:

Elimination

Tools:

Metabolic

Tools:

Sexual/Reproduction

PSYCHOSOCIAL

Cognition/Perception

Functional

ADAPTATION

BALANCE CHANGE

Pat Challis Sellards

Alterations in balance foster voluntary and involuntary decrease in mobility, gait changes, falls, and fractures, which may lead to death or institutionalization. Causes of balance change are listed in the box "Causes of Balance Change."

A. Ask about
- fear of falling
- falls (see p. 90)
  - circumstances in which fall occurred
  - time of day
  - relation to change in position
- dizziness or lightheadedness
- changes in ability to perform activities of daily living (ADL)
- use of assistive devices
- changes in mental status
- pain in joints and feet
- medications
  - psychoactive drugs
  - antihypertensives
  - vasodilators
  - alcohol intake
  - drug abuse
- chronic illnesses
  - diabetes
  - cardiovascular disease, hypertension
  - arthritis
- vision changes
- hearing changes

B. Measure
- blood pressure and pulse with patient lying and after standing 3 to 5 minutes
- visual acuity, accommodation, field of vision, and color perception
- hearing
- cognitive status (see the tools on pp. 268–273)
Observe
- gait (see Gait Disturbances, p. 42 and the tool *Balance and Gait,* p. 61)
- posture and muscular alignment
- coordination of motor activities
- position changes lying to sitting and sitting to standing
- footwear
- foot deformities (see Foot Deformities, p. 54)
Perform neuromuscular assessment
- strength
- flexibility and range of motion
- reaction time
- vibratory sense
- position sense and stability (see the box "Ways to Test Position Sense and Stability")
Obtain laboratory studies
- blood chemistries, including electrolytes and blood urea nitrogen
- hemoglobin, hematocrit
- therapeutic drug levels
Consider ambulatory cardiac rhythm monitoring if transient arrhythmia or heart block is suspected.

C. Safety measures include
- review of the environment for
  - proper lighting
  - unsafe throw rugs
  - nonskid mats in the bathtub
  - grab bars or rails near the toilet or bath and on stairs
  - clutter
  - unstable chairs
  - access to outdoors
- assessment of assistive devices for stability, state of repair
- review of medication regimen to determine compliance
- nurturing self-confidence with familiar surroundings

Causes of Balance Change

Orthostatic hypotension
Muscular weakness in lower extremity, decreased range of motion, or pain
Sensory impairment: vision, hearing, proprioception, sensation
Postural instability
Decreased reaction time
Pharmacologic agents
Vertebrobasilar syndrome
Loss of self-confidence

Ways to Test Position Sense and Stability

Proprioception test—Have patient walk with eyes closed to assess if conflicts between visual cues and sensations from the feet occur.

Sway test—Have patient stand with feet apart and eyes open, and observe sway pattern. Next, have patient close eyes and observe if pattern changes. Greater sway means greater instability.

Vertebrobasilar testing—Have patient rotate and extend neck while lying down and determine if nausea, dizziness, or nystagmus develops.

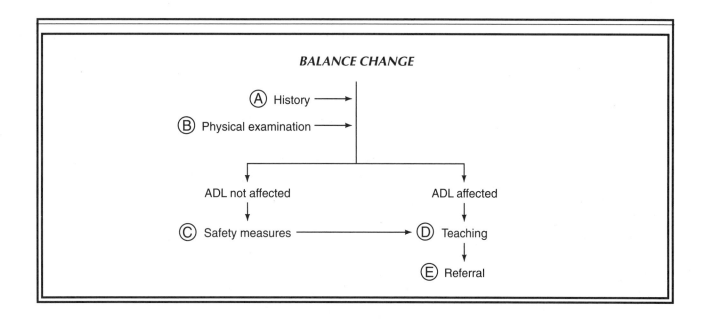

BALANCE CHANGE

(A) History →
(B) Physical examination →

ADL not affected   ADL affected

(C) Safety measures → (D) Teaching

(E) Referral

D. If orthostatic hypotension is mild, teach the patient to
    • get up slowly
    • dangle on side of bed before rising
    • stand still for 1 to 2 minutes before walking
    • consider use of support stockings such as TEDs
    If muscle weakness or tightness is discovered, stretching and strengthening exercises may improve balance and coordination. Rocking has been shown to improve balance by increasing muscle tone and stimulating the vestibular system. Teach the patient techniques for getting up after a fall.

E. Referral may be made for
    • correction of sensory impairments
    • treatment of foot deformities
    • change or evaluation of medication regimens
    • home health services to maintain the patient in familiar surroundings and assess and manipulate the environment
    • physical or occupational therapy
    • gait training
    • muscle strengthening
    • fitting of assistive devices
    • adaptive behavior education

References

Lewis CB. Improving mobility in older persons: A manual for geriatric specialists. Rockville, MD: Aspen Publications, 1989.

Lewis CB, Campanelli LC. Improving balance. Health promotion and exercise for older adults: An instructor's guide. Rockville, MD: Aspen Publications, 1990.

COORDINATION CHANGE

Patricia Guida

Proper integration of the nervous and musculoskeletal systems is coordinated and controlled by the cerebellum, auditory nerve, and cerebral cortex. Changes that occur with aging include increased reaction time and dulled reflexes.

A.   History taking should ask about changes in
   • coordination
   • sensation, including loss of feeling and tingling
   • sensory organ function
   • mental status: thought processes, memory, personality (see section Cognition/Perception, pp. 250–266)
   • ability to perform activities of daily living (ADL)
   • neuromuscular status: spasms, tremors, rigidity, tics
   Elicit information about
   • medication history, including over-the-counter drugs
   • personal medical history or family history, particularly
     • neuromuscular disorders
     • hypertension
     • stroke
     • diabetes
     • epilepsy
     • mental disorders
     • blood dyscrasias
   • falls (see p. 90)
   Ask questions to
   • sequence signs and symptoms of described changes
   • determine onset and duration of problems
   • assess support systems
   • explore history of alcohol and recreational drug use
   • review treatments tried and outcomes experienced

B.   Observe
   • posture and balance
   • gait (see Gait Disturbances, p. 42)
   • ability to sense position change
   • smoothness of movements and ataxia
   • signs of obvious injury
   • ability to follow commands
   • appropriateness of response
   • mental status, affect, and facies
   Measure
   • range of motion
   • muscle strength (see the tool, *Muscle Strength Testing*, p. 67)
   • reflexes
   • cranial nerve function, particularly nerves II through VIII
   Ask the patient to walk heel to toe (tandem). Perform a Romberg test (see the tool, *Romberg Test*, p. 63).

Evaluate fine muscle activity by asking the patient to rapidly supinate and pronate the hands or touch each finger to the thumb on the same hand. Establish the patient's orientation to person, place, and time. Is communication logical and to the point? Assess short- and long-term memory using tools on pp. 268–273. Laboratory studies obtained rule out metabolic disease or drug effect
   • thyroid profile and/or thyroid-stimulating hormone
   • therapeutic drug levels
   • serum chemistries, electrolytes, calcium/magnesium ratio
   • complete blood count

C.   Safety measures can help prevent injury from accidents
   • minimize clutter in the home
   • encourage adequate lighting, using at least 100-watt bulbs
   • ensure that support or safety devices are in working order:
     • rails and grab bars for stairs and bath
     • nonskid tub surfaces, shower wands
     • hearing aids, glasses
     • canes, walkers, shower chairs
   • encourage exercise to
     • enhance eye-hand coordination
     • improve muscle strength
   • discourage use of alcohol and tobacco
   • encourage good nutrition
   • encourage maximum safe independence
   • teach patient and caregiver that
     • haste plus inattention plus coordination change can mean injury
     • loss of independence may cause personality changes

D.   Referral to the primary physician is necessary for testing to exclude neuromuscular or musculoskeletal disease
   • radiographs or CT scans
   • electroencephalogram (EEG)
   • cerebroangiogram
   Medical intervention may also be necessary if polypharmacy (see Polypharmacy, p. 72) or drug interaction is suspected. Other referrals may be made for home care to
   • assess the living situation
   • provide housekeeping services
   • provide home-delivered meals
   Counseling, support groups, or respite services may be helpful for the caregiver.

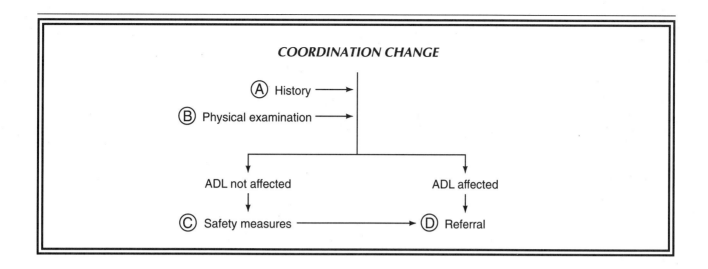

COORDINATION CHANGE

Ⓐ History

Ⓑ Physical examination

ADL not affected   ADL affected

Ⓒ Safety measures ⟶ Ⓓ Referral

References

Biggs A. Family caregiver versus nursing assessments of elderly self-care abilities. J Gerontol Nurs 1990; 16:11.

Eliopoulos C. Gerontological nursing. 2nd ed. Philadelphia: JB Lippincott, 1987:248.

Wright B, Aizenstein S, Vogler G, et al: Frequent fallers. Leading group to identify psychological factors. J Gerontol Nurs 1990; 16:15.

INABILITY TO PERFORM ACTIVITIES OF DAILY LIVING

Earla Parillo
Talar L. Glover

Activities of daily living (ADL) can be classified as basic or instrumental (see Katz Index of ADL, p. 28). Maintenance of independence for the elderly requires more than the ability to toilet and dress. Physical, cognitive, and affective skills are required for cooking, eating, grocery shopping, laundry, cleaning, and attending social functions such as church.

A. Information collected in the history should include
   - skills the patient is able to perform
   - skills the patient is unable to perform
   - onset of difficulties
   - precipitating factors
   - previous level of functioning
   - support systems and services currently available
   - presence or absence of
     - pain
     - weakness
     - sensory changes
   - medical history
   - current medications
   - recent illness or injuries
   - psychological/emotional crisis (e.g., loss of a job, hobby, loved one)
   - socioeconomic status and recent changes
   - nutrition/fluid intake history
   During history taking, pay careful attention to
   - patient affect
   - patient ability to organize answers to questions
   - interactions with the caregiver or support person
   It is important to confirm the performance of ADL by proxy (family or friend) whenever possible.

B. Physical examination is performed not only to rule out injury or illness as a precipitating factor but also to evaluate the patient's functional level. General observations to make include
   - appearance
   - symmetry of extremities
   - gait (see Gait Disturbances, p. 42)
   - position
   - use of mobility aids
   Neurologic assessment can reveal
   - disorientation or confusion
   - ability to perform fine muscle movements
   - hand-eye coordination
   - strength, including proximal versus distal weakness
   - ability to move all extremities
   - balance
   Laboratory evaluation is performed to rule out undiagnosed or iatrogenic physical problems. Electrolyte imbalance, undiagnosed diabetes, infection, anemia, hypothyroidism, even leukemia can affect function by altering energy level, oxygen exchange, or normal cellular function. In the elderly a thyroid stimulating hormone (TSH) level may be more indicative of hypothyroidism than a thyroid profile. Obtain a vitamin B_{12} level to differentiate treatable peripheral neuropathy.

C. Physiologic causes of inability to perform ADL may be classified as acute or chronic. An acute alteration in ability to perform ADL may result from an injury or illness from which there is an expectation of recovery to previous functional levels (e.g., fractures, uncontrolled diabetes). Chronic inability to perform ADL due to cognitive or nonreversible physical changes can be much more devastating. Chronic conditions (e.g., cerebrovascular accident with residual neurologic deficits) can trigger a loss of independence as well as a feeling of isolation. Progressive loss of self-care ability is identifiable with dementia, commonly Alzheimer's disease. The initial deficit may be an instrumental ADL problem such as loss of driving skills that over time extends to basic ADL task impairment.

D. Psychosocial causes of inability to perform ADL include
   - fear of falling
   - changes in cognition (see Confusion/Cognitive Changes/Dementia, p. 254)
   - depression/grief
   - decreased self-esteem
   - hopelessness (see Loss of Hope, p. 310)
   - social isolation
   - lack of social support
   - loss of motivation
   Psychosocial causes often combine to create a domino effect that isolates the patient and increases feelings of helplessness and hopelessness (see Depression, p. 282).

E. Evaluation of functional level requires synthesis of the data collected during the history and physical examination. Analyze basic and instrumental ADL (see the tool *Scale for Instrumental Activities of Daily Living* [IADL], p. 30) related to
   - the amount of assistance needed to perform
   - the type of assistance needed to perform, differentiating the use of assistive devices and need for physical assistance
   - the energy level needed to perform
   - the time needed to perform
   - whether the problem is temporary or permanent
   For example, does eating breakfast require 2 hours of

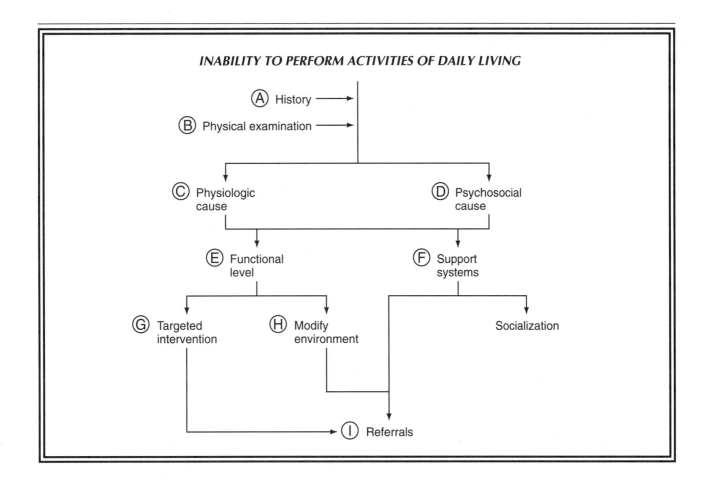

INABILITY TO PERFORM ACTIVITIES OF DAILY LIVING

(A) History

(B) Physical examination

(C) Physiologic cause

(D) Psychosocial cause

(E) Functional level

(F) Support systems

(G) Targeted intervention

(H) Modify environment

Socialization

(I) Referrals

constant cuing? or can the patient no longer use the stove?

F. Support systems are a major consideration when formulating a plan of care for patients with inability to perform ADL. Investigate
    • who the caregivers/helpers are
    • when caregivers/helpers are available
    • what caregiver/helper capabilities are
    • how healthy caregivers/helpers are
    • what financial resources are available
    Be sure to consider the complexity and duration of help needed when evaluating support systems. Long-term situations can lead to caregiver burnout (see Caregiver Stress, p. 292) or the potential for neglect or abuse (see Neglect, p. 290, and Abuse, p. 300).

G. Interventions can target
    • treatment or correction of physiologic causes
    • knowledge deficits of the patient or caregiver/helper
    • the need for assistive devices
    • strengthening
    • retraining

H. It may be possible to modify the environment. Usually a home visit will determine safety hazards. The environment provides many clues to the cognitively impaired patient for initiating ADL tasks. Therefore the design and accessibility of the setting cannot be underestimated.

I. Referrals are based on the patient's functional level and the availability of or need for support. Consider using physical medicine and rehabilitation services for assessment and intervention. Physical and occupational therapy for assistive devices, ADL training, and adaptive equipment can be of considerable value in maintaining the patient in the least restrictive environment. A physician order is indicated for home health care. Home-delivered meals may be arranged for someone who cannot prepare a meal while the caregiver is absent. Other in-home care services include homemaker, chore services, and home health aide assistance.

References

Applegate WB. Use of assessment instruments in clinical settings. J Am Geriatr Soc 1987; 35:45.

Chenitz WC, Stone JT, Salisbury SA. Clinical gerontological nursing: A guide to advanced practice. Philadelphia: WB Saunders, 1991.

Katz S, Downs TD, Cash HR, et al. Progress in development of the index of ADL. Gerontologist 1970; 10:20.

Kuriansky J, Gurland B. Performance of activities of daily living. Int J Aging Hum Devel 1976; 7:343.

Pinholt EM, Kroenke K, Hanley JF, et al. Functional assessment of the elderly: A comparison of standard instruments with clinical judgment. Arch Intern Med 1987; 147:484.

LIMITED RANGE OF MOTION

Carolyn Spencer Arthur

Range of motion refers to the movement of joints or bones by muscles in relation to body planes, and is measured in degrees. Range of motion can be limited by
• injury
• degenerative processes
• pain
• inactivity
• lack of exercise (deconditioning)
Limitations in range of motion can be defined as
• full (joint able to move 90–100% of expected)
• limited (joint able to move >50% of expected)
• severely limited (joint able to move <50% of expected)
Limited range of motion in one joint places added stress on other joints, both ipsilateral and contralateral. It also affects
• ability to perform activities of daily living (ADL)
• social roles
• self-image/concept

A. Ask questions to elicit information about the neuro-logic and musculoskeletal systems, such as
  • pain
    • muscles
    • joints
    • along dermatomes
  • swelling
  • changes in function or strength
    • weakness
    • numbness
    • tingling
  • injury
    • fracture
    • sprain
    • dislocation
    • fall
    • other traumatic injury
  • congenital musculoskeletal conditions
  • chronic or acute problems
    • arthritis
    • seizures (see p. 94)
    • tremors (see p. 48)
  • sleep pattern disturbances
  • use of orthopedic devices
  • cognitive/perceptual problems
    • loss of consciousness
    • confusion
    • forgetfulness
  • previous coping patterns
    • use/abuse of alcohol and drugs
    • anxiety
  • current medication/alcohol use
  Obtain a history of the range of motion limitation, including
    • joint(s) involved
    • onset
    • duration
    • level of involvement
    • interference with ADL and instrumental ADL (see Inability to Perform Activities of Daily Living, p. 6)

B. Proceed from general to specific when performing a physical examination, covering
  • general appearance
    • posture
  • motor function
    • movement
    • gait (see Gait Disturbances, p. 42)
    • balance (see p. 2)
    • coordination (see p. 4)
  • joint function
    • range of motion in degrees
    • muscle strength (see the tool *Muscle Strength Testing*, p. 67)
    • deep tendon reflexes
  • neurologic factors
    • proprioception
    • position sense
    • speech
    • sensory
    • cognition
    • affect
    • perception
  Laboratory tests that may be helpful include
  • sedimentation rate
  • antinuclear antibodies (ANA)

C. Education should focus on optimizing range of motion to prevent complications or injury and maintain function and independence. Both patient and care-giver can be taught
  • use of proper body mechanics
  • positioning to maintain body alignment
  • range of motion exercises to strengthen and limber muscles
  • specific exercise to prevent further deconditioning
  • how to take medications prescribed
  • use of heat, if not contraindicated by neuropathy

D. A safe environment must be provided if mobility is decreased (see Falls, p. 90). Consider
  • furniture placement
  • use of area rugs
  • use of assistive devices
  • safe clothing
    • supportive shoes with nonskid soles
    • easily manipulated, nonrestrictive clothing

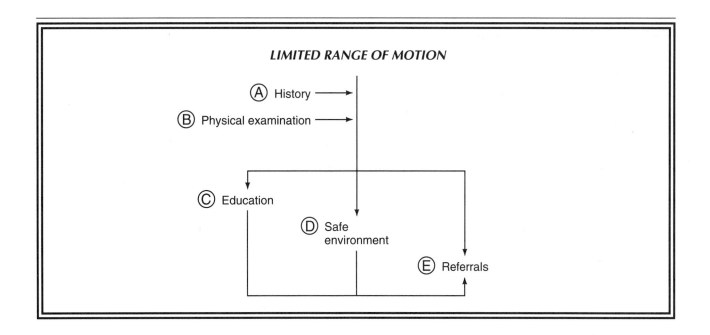

LIMITED RANGE OF MOTION

(A) History

(B) Physical examination

(C) Education

(D) Safe environment

(E) Referrals

E. Referrals are made on the basis of physical findings and interference with ADL to the following
    • physician (radiographs, medications)
    • social worker (social/family assessment, financial assistance, community referrals)
    • occupational therapist (to evaluate the functional level)
    • physical therapist (therapy to increase mobility and ability to perform ADL, and for assistive devices and home environment assessment)
    • psychologist (behavioral and psychological testing and evaluation)
    • dietitian (nutritional assessment and counseling)

References

Brown M. Selected physical performance changes with aging. Top Geriatr Rehabil 1987; 2:68.

Dittmar S. Rehabilitation nursing: Process and application. Baltimore: CV Mosby, 1989.

Kaufman T. Posture and age. Top Geriatr Rehabil 1987; 2:13.

Koltke FT, Stiwell GK, Lehmann JF, eds. Krusen's handbook of physical medicine and rehabilitation. 3rd ed. Philadelphia: WB Saunders, 1982.

Sine RD, Holcomb JD, Roush RE, et al. Basic rehabilitation techniques: A self-instructional guide. Rockville, MD: Aspen, 1981.

EDEMA

Marybeth Navas

Edema can result from decreased coronary blood flow, increased coronary work load, impaired myocardial function, or increased vascular load. Generalized edema is the result of hepatic, cardiac, renal, or nutritional disorders. Edema can cause skin changes, fibrosis, and changes in the lymphatic system that may lead to skin ulceration.

A. Ask about
   - history of edema
      - where it occurs
      - whether onset was gradual or sudden
      - how long it has been going on
      - when it developed
      - when it is most severe
      - when it is least severe
      - what improves it
      - what aggravates it
         - foods high in sodium
         - low-protein diet
         - prolonged standing or sitting
   - associated symptoms
      - shortness of breath
      - aching legs with prolonged standing
      - paroxysmal nocturnal dyspnea
      - change in mental status
      - lower extremity ulcer
      - dyspnea on exertion
      - orthopnea
      - fatigue
      - dry, hacking cough
      - frothy sputum
   - prior treatment such as support hose, elevation, or drugs
   - significant medical history
      - phlebitis or vascular occlusion
      - cardiovascular disease
      - varicose veins
      - hypertension
      - renal failure
      - vena caval interruption device
      - surgeries that may result in obstruction of veins or lymphatics
      - anemia
      - infections
   - nutrition history
   - medication or drug history

B. Physical examination evaluates
   - vital signs for arrhythmias, heart rate
   - pulmonary status
   - abdomen for palpable liver
   - edema and skin, specifically

TABLE 1 Grading of Edema

Grade	Impression	Description
0	0 mm	No edema
1+	1 mm	Slight; impression disappears in less than 10 seconds
2+	2 mm	Noticeable; impression disappears in 10 to 15 seconds
3+	3 mm	Deep; impression disappears in 1 to 2 minutes
4+	4 mm	Marked; impression disappears in greater than 5 minutes

   - grade (Table 1)
   - location
   - circulation, including
      - presence or appearance of lesions
      - peripheral pulses
      - venous distention or enlargement
      - presence or absence of hair
      - color
      - temperature
      - pain
      - capillary refill

Laboratory data may include
   - complete blood count
   - therapeutic drug levels
   - culture of lesions with signs of infection
   - serum protein/albumin
   - PT/PTT if on anticoagulant therapy
   - urinalysis to screen for infection or protein
   - electrolytes/glucose
   - blood urea nitrogen/creatinine
   - lipid profile
   - thyroid function
   - arterial blood gases

Pulse oximetry is a noninvasive procedure that can be used instead of blood gases to determine extent of oxygenation. Oxygen-carrying capacity of the blood (anemia) must be considered in evaluating results.

C. Specific interventions strive to minimize edema, maintain nutrition and fluid balance, prevent or treat skin ulceration, and ensure appropriate follow-up (see box "Interventions for Edema"). Interventions may require patient or caregiver education.

D. Referrals are made based on patient or caregiver need and response to interventions and may include the disciplines and activities listed in the box "Referrals for Edema."

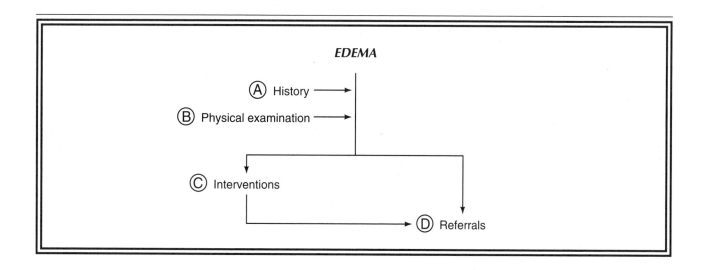

EDEMA

Ⓐ History →

Ⓑ Physical examination →

Ⓒ Interventions

Ⓓ Referrals

Interventions for Edema	
Goal	*Intervention*
Reduce edema	Planned rest periods Elevation of legs when sitting Fitted support stockings: proper application, wearing schedule Avoidance of restrictive clothing Appropriate and safe use of mobility aids
Maintain nutrition and fluid balance	Monitoring of intake and output Daily weight Providing adequate protein and calories Supplementation with appropriate vitamins and minerals Sodium or fluid restriction if indicated
Prevent or treat skin ulceration	Pressure reduction devices Frequent position changes Skin care • keep clean and use moisturizer • assess for changes • avoid trauma to skin Wound care • cleanliness of wound • dressing changes • topical or systemic medication use • signs of infection • splinting • care of occlusive dressings, total contact cast or Dome paste bandages
Ensure appropriate follow-up	Regularly scheduled monitoring of ordered medications, such as PT/PTT Instructions on when to call between regularly scheduled follow-up • increased pain • dyspnea • signs of infection • increased edema • skin breakdown

Referrals for Edema	
Discipline	*Activity*
Physician	Wound care Change in medication Referral to physical medicine services Surgical intervention
Physical or occupational therapy	Energy conservation program Hydrotherapy Splinting Assistive devices
Dietitian	Nutrition Dietary restrictions

References

Baum PL. Taking the P.V.D. patient's history. Nursing 1986; 16:30.

Doenges ME, Moorhouse MF. Nursing diagnosis with interventions. Philadelphia: FA Davis, 1992:47.

Herman JA. Treatment modalities in peripheral vascular disease. Nurs Clin North Am 1986; 21:241.

Wagner MM. Pathophysiology related to peripheral vascular disease. Nurs Clin North Am 1986; 21:195.

INFLAMMATION

Donna A. Bachand

Inflammation is a health response generated by the immune system. Normal immune function declines with age, predisposing the elderly to systemic infection after tissue injury. When tissue injury occurs, multiple substances are released into the injured area and cause local inflammation. One of the first results of the inflammatory process is to "wall off" the area of injury to protect the remaining tissues from invasion.

A. History taking should determine
   - onset
   - duration
   - trauma
   - exposure to infection
   - foreign debris or substance involved
   - chemical contact
   - thermal exposure
   - insect bite
   - medical illness
     - cardiovascular
     - impaired immune system
     - diabetes mellitus
     - cancer
   - medications, specifically
     - corticosteroids
     - nonsteroidal anti-inflammatory agents
     - cancer chemotherapy
   - allergies
   - self-applied relief measures that may mask infection or worsen local symptoms
     - heat or cold
     - topical steroid creams
     - oral analgesics
     - other home remedies

B. Physical assessment ascertains
   - signs and symptoms of infection
     - temperature
     - localized area of
       - induration (measure in millimeters)
       - swelling
       - pain
       - heat
       - redness
     - purulent drainage

Pus formation is a healthy response to bacterial invasion. However, an elderly person may lack sufficient neutrophils and macrophages to make up the pus that destroys bacteria. If the organism migrates out of the area of inflammation, a systemic infection will occur. An allergic response is signified by
- urticaria
- pruritus
- shortness of breath or bronchospasm
- hypotension
- serosanguineous drainage

Concomitant bronchospasm or hypotension warrants immediate medical intervention. Obtain a CBC with differential and culture any colored drainage from the area. Consider radiography for gross deformity or impairment of motion.

C. Fever indicates systemic infection and requires medical intervention. Cellulitis or inflammation of cellular or connective tissue warrants medical evaluation and management.

D. The most effective means of alleviating distressing symptoms associated with inflammation is to remove the causative factor, but this may not always be possible. Application of cold may not halt the inflammatory process but will palliate the symptoms. Antihistamines slow histamine release into the tissues and may lessen edema. Nonsteroidal anti-inflammatory analgesics are recommended for pain unless contraindicated. Elevation of the area may also help.

E. Follow-up aims to
   - evaluate resolution of symptoms
   - ascertain compliance with the treatment plan
   - reinforce avoidance of causative factors

References

Gioiella EC, Bevil CW. Nursing care of the aging client: Promoting healthy adaptation. Norwalk, CT: Appleton-Century-Crofts, 1985.

Yurick AG, Spier BE, Robb SS, Ebert SS. The aged person and the nursing process. Norwalk, CT: Appleton-Century-Crofts, 1984.

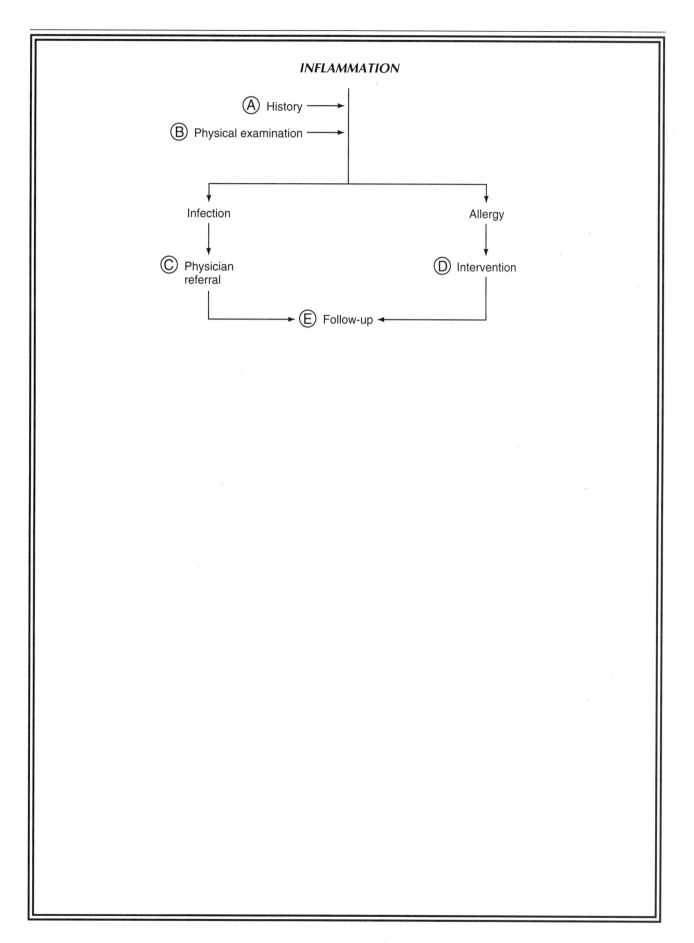

FATIGUE

Susan Goad
Lana Ralston

Fatigue, an abnormal state of exhaustion after physical, emotional, or mental activity, is a widely accepted symptom of aging. Approximately 70% of all older patients report they experience fatigue, and of that number 59% experience it often. Fatigue, a self-recognized phenomenon, often goes unreported and can interfere with activities of daily living (ADL). Acute fatigue, unlike chronic fatigue, responds to rest or correction of deficiencies, such as with nutritional supplements (see the box "Causes of Acute Versus Chronic Fatigue").

A. Ask questions about
   - onset
   - nutritional or diet habits
   - alcohol and tobacco use
   - tiredness in the morning
   - stress
   - presence of chronic illness
   - ability to perform ADL
   - precipitating factors
   - medication history
   - hours of sleep or rest per day
   - exercise tolerance
   - recent losses
   - past or present coping strategies
   - snoring or sleep apnea
   Elicit information from family or caregiver as well as the patient.

B. Observe
   - general appearance
   - facial expression
   - personal grooming
   - decision-making ability
   - color
   - posture
   - level of alertness
   - ability to concentrate
   Examine patient to determine
   - muscle strength and tone
   - cardiovascular status: blood pressure, pulse rate response to activity, presence of edema
   - respiratory status: respiratory rate, signs of exertional dyspnea
   Physiologic studies that may prove helpful include
   - complete blood count
   - blood glucose
   - thyroid function studies
   - iron studies, including total iron-binding capacity
   - chest radiography
   - therapeutic drug levels
   - ferritin
   - electrolytes
   - electrocardiogram

Causes of Acute Versus Chronic Fatigue	
Acute	*Chronic*
Intense physical exertion	Anemia, thyroid disorders
Emotional stress	Cardiac disease
Inadequate sleep or rest	Diabetes mellitus
Improper diet	Cancer
Insufficient exercise	Neuromuscular deficits
Drug therapies	Nutritional deficiencies
Anxiety	Midbrain dysfunction
	Fibromyalgia syndrome
	Chronic fatigue syndrome
	Metabolic changes
	Aging
	Drug therapies
	Tuberculosis

Findings to Refer to a Physician	
Assessment Parameter	*Finding*
Medication	Polypharmacy
	Drug interactions
Previously diagnosed chronic illness	Poorly controlled
	New complication
Complete blood count	Anemia
Total iron-binding capacity/ vitamin B$_{12}$	Pernicious anemia
	Vitamin B$_{12}$ deficiency
Thyroid profile/thyroid-stimulating hormone	Hypothyroidism
Electrolytes/glucose	Hyperglycemia
	Abnormal electrolytes
Chest radiography	Infiltrates
	Mass
Electrocardiogram	New arrhythmia

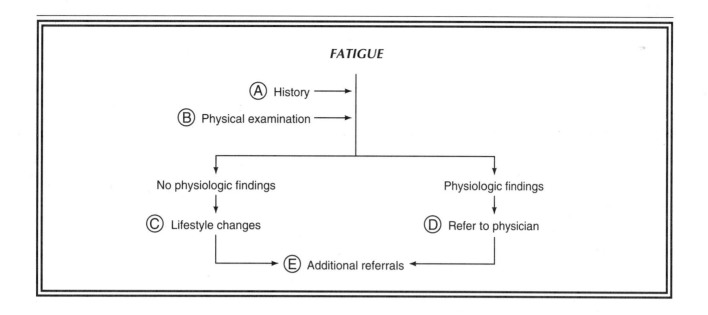

FATIGUE

A ⃝ History

B ⃝ Physical examination

No physiologic findings

C ⃝ Lifestyle changes

Physiologic findings

D ⃝ Refer to physician

E ⃝ Additional referrals

C. If no physiologic cause is found for fatigue, a psychosocial etiology must be considered. Interventions that facilitate lifestyle changes, increase the patient's sense of control, and help to change fatigue-inducing habits may be
- smoking cessation
- scheduling exercise or rest periods
- problem-solving exercises
- starting an exercise program
- arranging household items for ease in utilization
- scheduling activities at times of day when energy is high
- additional teaching about chronic illness routines or medications
- nutrition counseling
- stress reduction techniques
- increasing socialization
- energy conservation

D. When a physiologic or iatrogenic cause is suspected, referral to a primary care physician may be warranted. Medical work-up may include computed tomography scan (see the box "Findings to Refer to Physician").

E. Additional referrals may be in order. Depending on the practice setting, a physician order may be required for
- occupational therapy to set up an energy conservation program
- home-delivered meals
- home health aide or homemaker service

References

Brody EM, Kleban MH. Day to day mental and physical health symptoms of older people: A report on health logs. Gerontologist 1983; 23:75.

Gueldner SH, Spradly J. Outdoor walking lowers fatigue. J Gerontol Nurs 1988; 14:6.

Mitchell CA. Generalized chronic fatigue in the elderly: Assessment and intervention. J Gerontol Nurs 1986; 12:19.

Tally J. Geriatric depression: Avoiding the pitfalls of primary care. Geriatrics 1987; 42:53.

MALAISE

Lana Ralston
Susan Goad

Malaise is defined as a vague feeling of uneasiness, indisposition, bodily weakness, or discomfort. Patients complain of feeling tired and weak, and of an inability to accomplish desired tasks. Malaise may mark the onset of disease and should not be considered interchangeable with fatigue (see box below).

A. History questions should focus on
  • acute illness
  • chronic medical problems
  • emotional stress
  • depression screening (see the tool *Geriatric Depression Scale or Mood Assessment Scale*, p. 266)
  • medications
  • therapies, particularly radiation or chemotherapy

B. Physical examination is performed to rule out infection or other physiologic disorders. A complete neurologic examination is necessary. Laboratory studies that may prove helpful are
  • CBC
  • urinalysis
  • serum electrolytes
  • blood glucose
  • dexamethasone suppression test

In approximately 50% of patients with chronic depression or melancholia, suppression of plasma cortisol does not occur.

C. Lifestyle modification focuses on teaching and counseling. Areas of concern include
  • stress management
  • exercise
  • rest
  • adequate nutrition
  Patients should also be taught about concurrent physical problems and medication regimens.

D. Psychosocial interventions are particularly important if malaise is depression induced, because of the risk of suicide and the damage that depression inflicts on the patient and caregivers. (See Depression, p. 282.) Specific interventions are:
  • manipulation of the environment
  • cognitive therapy
  • group activities
  • resocialization
  • exercise programs

E. Referral to a physician is warranted. The possibility of an insidious illness necessitates a diagnostic evaluation. Positive response to antidepressant therapy may relieve malaise. Modification of radiation or chemotherapy may be indicated.

Diseases Related to Malaise	
Acute	*Chronic*
Infection	Depression
Electrolyte imbalance	Radiation therapy
Mononucleosis	Chemotherapy
Gastroenteritis	Physical deterioration
Urinary tract infection	Metabolic changes
Muscle discomfort	Emotional stress
Physical exhaustion	Drug therapies
	Cancer

References

Kobashi-Schoot J, Ans M, Hanewald Gerrit JFP, et al. Assessment of malaise in cancer patients treated with radiotherapy. Cancer Nurs Dec 1985; 8:306.

Talley J. Geriatric depression: Avoiding the pitfalls of primary care. Geriatrics 1987; 42:53.

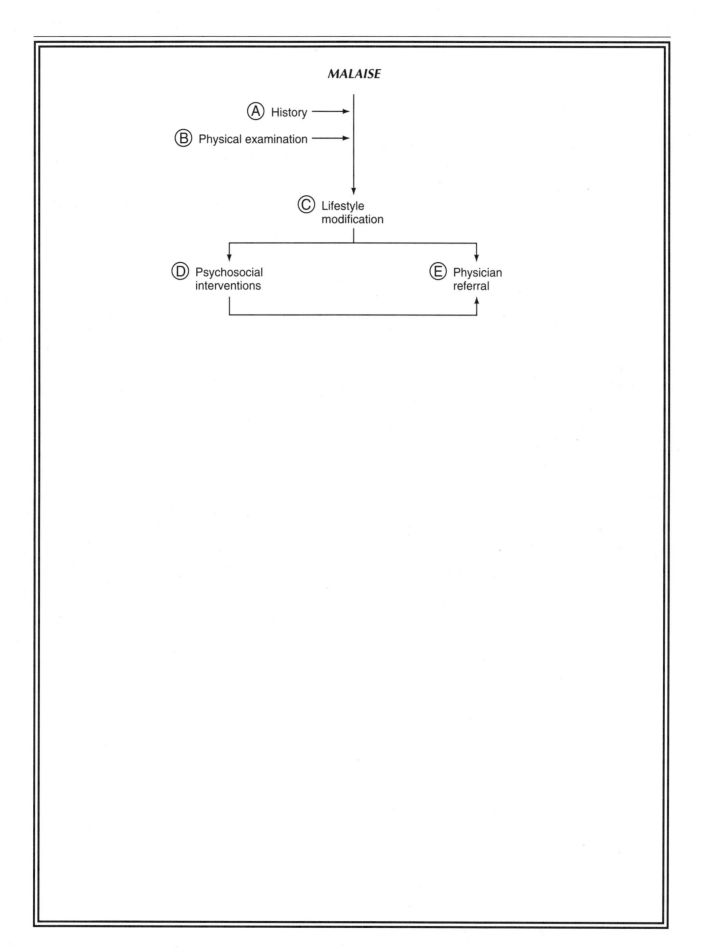

MALAISE

Ⓐ History

Ⓑ Physical examination

Ⓒ Lifestyle modification

Ⓓ Psychosocial interventions

Ⓔ Physician referral

WEAKNESS

Olivia Catolico

Weakness is defined as
- a lack of strength, physical vigor, or energy
- decreased capacity for physical or mental work
- inability to sustain or exert much weight, pressure, or strain

Weakness may present as a generalized, vague complaint or as a symptom of some other physiologic or psychological problem.

A. History taking should explore such subjective and objective symptoms as
- onset
- duration
- interference with activities of daily living (ADL)
- ability to concentrate
- need for additional energy to accomplish routine tasks
- current stressors
- losses
  - family, spouse, significant others
  - support system
  - moving/relocation
  - diminished income
- retirement
- chronic illnesses
- current medications, prescription and over the counter

B. Physical examination is made to rule out pathophysiologic causes of weakness (see box). Neuromuscular examination should evaluate muscle strength and endurance (see the tool *Measuring Muscle Strength*, p. 66).
Laboratory studies to perform include
- CBC
- electrolytes and glucose
- serum protein and albumin

C. Intervention should focus on physiologic or psychosocial/emotional factors involving both patient and caregivers, such as
- identifying activity patterns that require increased exertion
- planning activities to conserve the patient's energy
- providing uninterrupted rest/sleep periods
- assisting with ADL
- involving the patient in graduated exercise/activity as tolerated
- checking for proper fit and use of assistive devices
- assessing environmental factors for patient comfort and safety
- explaining the medication regimen
- helping the patient to identify personal priorities through active listening
- encouraging caregiver support

D. Referrals may be made on the basis of physical findings. A referral to a primary physician or specialist may be appropriate if pathophysiology is found. Community resources that may be beneficial include
- homemaker services
- home-delivered meals
- consumer support groups through the American Cancer Society, American Heart Association, American Diabetes Association, local hospitals, or health departments
- senior citizen or nutrition centers
- social services for financial referrals
- physical and/or occupational therapy for energy-conservation programs

Pathophysiologic States Associated with Weakness

System	Condition
Neuromuscular	Gait disorders Parkinson's disease Arthritis Multiple sclerosis Myasthenia gravis Cerebrovascular accident
Cardiopulmonary	Congestive heart failure Chronic obstructive pulmonary disease Peripheral vascular disease Valvular disorders Myocardial infarction Hypertension Anemia Pneumonia
Endocrine/metabolic	Diabetes mellitus Hypothyroidism Hyperparathyroidism Pituitary disorders Addison's disease Fever
GI/nutritional	Crohn's disease Malabsorption syndrome Hepatitis Malnutrition
Renal	Acute renal failure End-stage renal disease Hypertension
Immune/infectious	AIDS Pancreatitis Acute infections Malignancy/cancer
Psychiatric	Alcoholism Depression

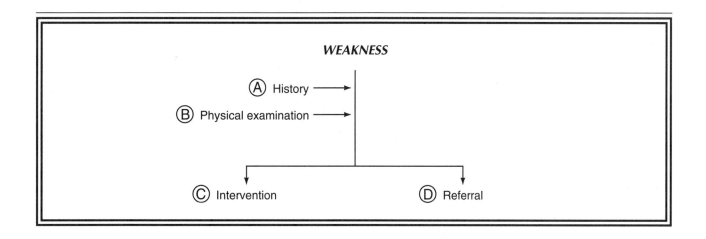

References

Calvani DL, et al. Functional assessment: A holistic approach to rehabilitation of the geriatric client. Rehab Nurs 1991; 16:330.

Milner-Brown HS, et al. Increased muscular fatigue in patients with neurogenic muscle weakness: Quantification and pathophysiology. Arch Phys Med Rehab 1989; 70:361.

Simmons SJ. Staff nurses promote wellness. Am Nurse 1991; 23:12.

Stoto MA, et al. National health objectives for the year 2000: The demographic impact of health promotion and disease prevention. Am J Public Health 1991; 81:1456.

Walker SN. Health promotion and aging: The time is now. I Gerontol Nurs 1991; 17:4.

HEAT EXHAUSTION

Leslie C. Trischank Hussey

Heat exhaustion occurs as a result of the body trying to maintain a normal body temperature in a hot environment. It is also called heat prostration or collapse. The box below lists risk factors for heat-related illness. Heat exhaustion is characterized by
- normal or slightly elevated core body temperature (not >103°F or 39.5°C)
- dehydration or volume depletion

If the condition is recognized quickly the prognosis is good, although improvement may take several days.

A. Ask about specific symptoms
- profuse sweating
- lightheadedness
- weakness
- muscle cramps
- faintness
- nausea
- vomiting
- headache
- postural hypotension
- loss of consciousness

Do not mistake these symptoms for influenza.

B. Take vital signs. The only way to differentiate between heat exhaustion and heat stroke is to determine core body temperature either rectally or with a tympanic thermometer. Check for hypotension and tachycardia. Assess the skin. Initially, skin will be cool, pale, and moist; it will feel dry if the patient is significantly dehydrated. Observe the level of consciousness. Unless the patient is significantly dehydrated, laboratory values will be unchanged and laboratory tests may not be indicated.

Risk Factors for Developing Heat-Related Illness

- diarrhea
- skin diseases
- chronic conditions
  - arteriosclerosis
  - hypertension
  - cerebrovascular accident
  - Parkinson's disease
  - diabetes mellitus
  - cardiovascular disease
- obesity or overweight
- alcoholism and other drug use (especially amphetamines and cocaine)
- conditions or situations that reduce the capacity to sweat
  - use of antipyretics
  - burns

C. Immediate treatment includes
- moving the patient to a cooler environment
- repletion of fluids
  - use electrolyte-containing fluids orally if the patient is alert
  - hypotonic or normotonic IV solutions may be indicated if the patient is unable to take oral fluids
- cool water sponge baths

Treatment of heat exhaustion does not require hospitalization unless the patient
- suffers from an altered level of consciousness
- does not respond to therapy, indicating
  - severe dehydration
  - electrolyte imbalance
  - rhabdomyolysis

D. Prevention is the best treatment for heat exhaustion. Instruct the patient or caregiver to take the following precautions when the environmental temperatures rise above 90°F:
- increase fluid intake
  - the amount should be 1.5 times that which quenches thirst
  - do not use alcohol
  - avoid sugary drinks
  - avoid caffeine
- do not use salt tablets unless approved by the physician
- eat a diet high in potassium
- move to a cooler environment
- get air moving to increase evaporative cooling
- limit physical activity
- have a regular contact person to monitor
  - patient condition
  - patient ability to respond appropriately to environmental changes
- avoid safety hazards (e.g., nailing windows shut) that would prevent air circulation

E. Referrals can be made for
- utility bill assistance
- community-provided fans or air conditioners
- a senior citizen center

References

Birrer R. Heat stroke: Don't wait for the classic signs. Emerg Med 1988; 20:8.
Knochel JP. Update in summer heat syndromes. Patient Care 1989; 23: 15:78.

HEAT EXHAUSTION

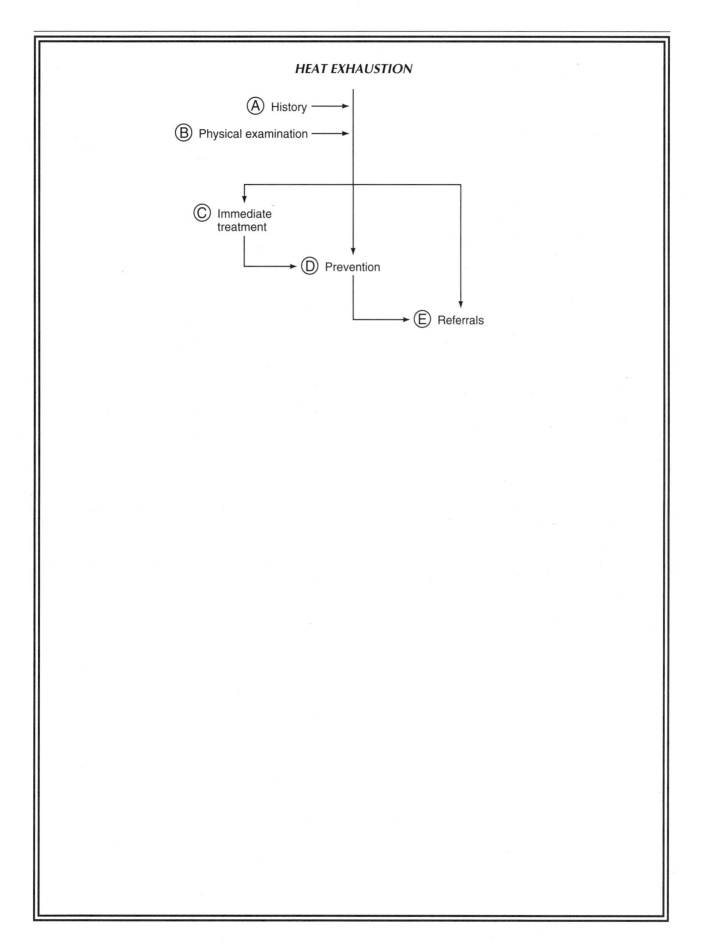

HEAT STROKE

Leslie C. Trischank Hussey

Heat stroke is a condition caused by prolonged exposure to excessive heat. It is a serious medical emergency that affects the elderly more often than any other part of the population. Death occurs in almost 80% of heat stroke cases in persons over 65 and is especially lethal in women. Exertional heat stroke is usually seen in young athletes and is characterized by a high temperature and mental status abnormalities. Nonexertional or classic heat stroke is a syndrome of acute failure of thermoregulation when the environmental temperature rises over a short time to about 95°F (35°C) or humidity reaches 75%. It is characterized by
- failure of homeostatic mechanisms such as perspiration and evaporation
- core temperature >105°F (40.5°C)
- CNS abnormalities

Aging changes that may promote heat stroke consist of
- increased sweat threshold
- decreased water content of the body
- chronic medical problems or medications that
  - promote dehydration
  - reduce the ability to sweat
  - interfere with hypothalamic thermoregulatory systems
  - interfere with normal cardiovascular responses to heat

A. Ask about specific symptoms of heat stroke, such as
- dry skin
- vertigo
- headache
- thirst
- dizziness
- faintness
- fatigue
- nausea
- muscle cramps
- shortness of breath

Question patients about temperature perception and whether they normally perspire. Determine the presence of contributing factors, such as
- cardiovascular disease
- congestive heart failure
- medications, particularly
  - diuretics
  - beta blockers
  - antiparkinsonian drugs
  - antidepressants
  - anticholinergics
  - major tranquilizers
- diabetes mellitus
- obesity
- chronic obstructive pulmonary disease
- central nervous system disease, such as stroke

B. Check vital signs immediately. Take temperatures rectally or on the tympanic membrane to reflect the true core temperature. Determine whether the patient is hypotensive or has a rapid, irregular pulse or flushed skin. The skin is usually hot and dry in heat stroke. Observe for confusion and altered level of consciousness. Laboratory tests evaluate the extent of electrolyte imbalance and/or dehydration. Obtain
- CBC
- arterial blood gases
- electrolytes
- BUN, serum creatinine
- serum phosphorus, magnesium, and calcium

Look for
- elevated WBC
- hematocrit consistent with dehydration
- hypokalemia
- hyponatremia
- azotemia
- decreased levels of phosphorus, magnesium, and calcium
- respiratory alkalosis.

The ECG will frequently show some type of arrhythmia.

C. Emergency treatment provides immediate cooling either by evaporation or by direct immersion. The more rapidly and effectively the patient is cooled, the more likely is the recovery. Ice packs or ice water immersion are the treatments of choice. Fluid replacement is essential. Electrolytes and minerals must also be replaced to decrease the potential for lethal arrhythmias. Take care to prevent the development of congestive heart failure during repletion.

D. Prevent heat stroke by teaching patients how to avoid precipitating factors when possible and making referrals for needed human services. Teach precautions to take when temperatures rise to >90°F, instructing patients to
- increase the amount of fluid intake (water, fruit and vegetable juice)
- avoid alcohol
- eat a diet high in potassium
- move to a cooler environment, or go to a library, store, or movie theater during the hottest hours
- keep air moving to promote evaporative cooling
- limit physical activity
- take cool baths or showers
- avoid strenuous activity
- stay out of direct sunlight
- apply cool towels to the body
- wear lightweight, loose-fitting, light-colored clothing, preferably cotton

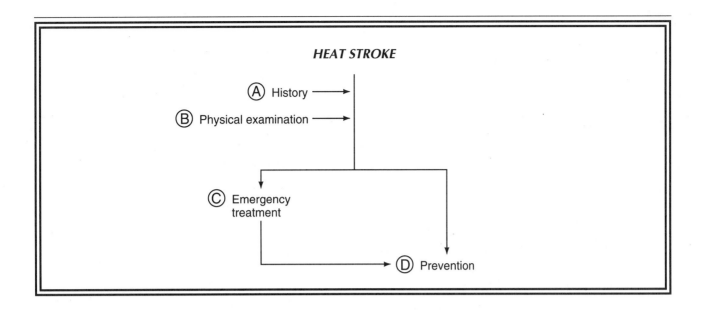

HEAT STROKE

Ⓐ History

Ⓑ Physical examination

Ⓒ Emergency treatment

Ⓓ Prevention

Referrals can be made for
• utility bill assistance
• community-provided fans or air conditioners
• a senior citizen center
In high crime neighborhoods, instruct the patient and family to avoid safety hazards such as nailing windows shut.

References

Birrer R. Heat stroke: Don't wait for the classic signs. Emerg Med 1988; 20:8.

Halle A, Repasy A. Classic heatstroke: A serious challenge for the elderly. Hosp Pract 1987; 22:26.

HYPOTHERMIA

Leslie C. Trischank Hussey
Donna A. Bachand

Hypothermia is defined as a core body temperature below 35° C (95° F). Physiologic changes that place elderly persons at risk for hypothermia are decreased heat production, decreased cold perception, and impaired neurovascular response to cold. Many other conditions may be more evident such as injuries, pneumonia, and inadequate hydration or nutrition, so the diagnosis of hypothermia may be delayed.

A. Ascertain the presence of risk factors, including
   • exposure to cold
   • alcohol use
   • activity level
   • medications, specifically hypnotics, phenothiazines, barbiturates, anesthetics, and benzodiazepines
   • activity tolerance in cold weather
   • poor nutritional intake
   • inadequate fluid intake
   Risk data to be obtained for surgically induced hypothermia include
   • response to anesthesia
   • intraoperative fluid loss
   • blood, fluid, drug administration
   • any drop in temperature
   Socioeconomic and environmental factors to determine include
   • ability to see or adjust thermostat
   • availability of hot and cold water
   • finances to purchase adequate clothing
   • type and source of heat
   • ability to pay utilities

B. Physical examination includes
   • initial and serial vital signs
   • skin temperature
   • neurologic assessment
   • cardiovascular status
   • physical appearance
   • mental status
   • musculoskeletal function
   When temperature registers ≤36° C (96.8° F), a core temperature must be obtained. Devices are available to measure core temperature by several routes: rectal, esophageal, tympanic, and urethral. Findings on physical examination differ depending on core body temperature (Table 1). Routine blood work should be drawn, including complete blood count, electrolytes, glucose, blood urea nitrogen, creatinine, amylase, and arterial blood gases. A chest radiograph is

TABLE 1 Physical Findings of Hypothermia

Parameter	Temperature		
	33°–35° C	<33° C >30° C	<30° C
Mental state	Confusion Disorientation	Amnesia	Unresponsiveness
Reflexes/ neurologic	Weakness	Decreased coordination Slurred speech Dilated pupils	Absent reflexes Fixed pupils
Musculo-skeletal	Shivering	Muscle rigidity	Muscle flaccidity
Cardio-vascular	Bradycardia	Arrhythmias Hypotension	Little or no pulse
Skin	Cool	Cold	Very cold

essential because pneumonia and atelectasis are common complications. An electrocardiogram detects arrhythmias such as the characteristic J wave, a positive deflection at the junction of the QRS and ST segments that occurs in approximately 33% of hypothermic patients.

C. Patients with a core temperature of >35° C (95° F) require measures to bring the temperature back to normal (37° C, 98.6° F):
   • Provide a warm environment, adjusted on the basis of core body temperature rather than perceived temperature. Remove cold or wet clothing.
   • Offer warm fluids by mouth. Avoid the use of caffeine-containing fluids, which cause vasodilation.
   • Apply external warmth. Use warmed blankets next to the skin. Heat can be carefully applied with a heating pad or hot water bottle in some instances.

D. Passive rewarming is the treatment of choice if body temperature has been no lower than 32° C and cardiopulmonary status is adequate. The core temperature must be raised slowly with conservation of body heat, prevention of further heat loss, and a warm environment. Warm blankets and a room temperature above 21° C (69.8° F) are used to raise the core temperature at a rate of approximately 0.5° C per hour. If the temperature rises much faster, hypotension and dangerous arrhythmias can occur.

HYPOTHERMIA

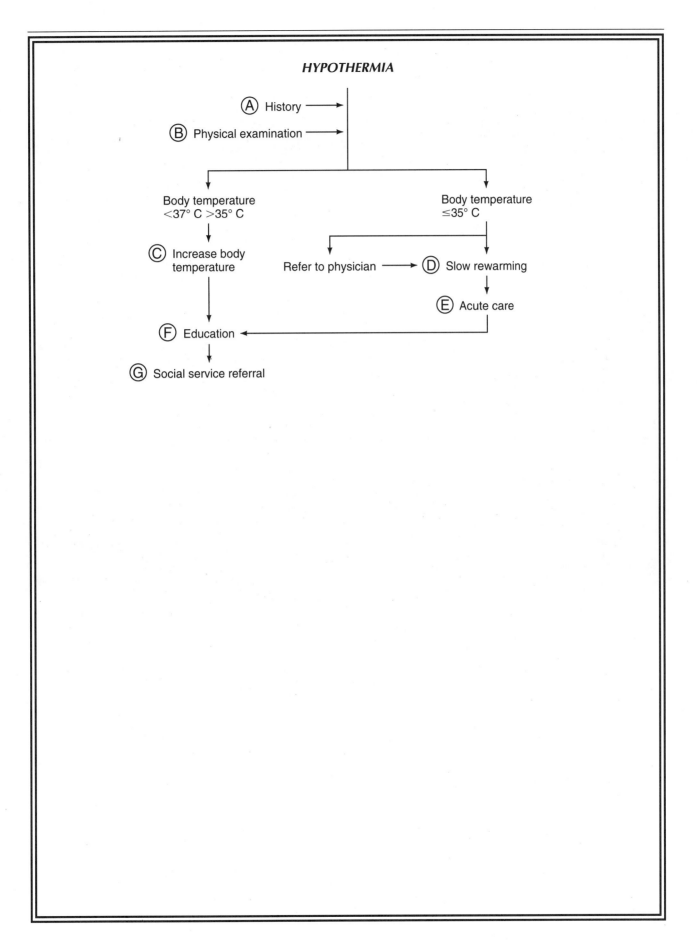

A. History

B. Physical examination

Body temperature
<37° C >35° C

Body temperature
≤35° C

C. Increase body temperature

Refer to physician → D. Slow rewarming

E. Acute care

F. Education

G. Social service referral

E. A core temperature <32° C (89.6° F) will necessitate mechanical ventilation and cardiopulmonary resuscitation. If these measures are inadequate, the next step is rapid core rewarming using cardiac bypass technique. Three major factors predisposing to hypothermia in the operating room are a cool temperature, the type of anesthesia administered, and the positioning and cleansing of the operative site. Specific operating room care includes
- raising ambient room temperature
- warming surgical instruments
- using warming mattresses
- administering inhalation anesthesia via heated humidifier
- using warm blankets before surgery
- using blood and fluid warmer
- covering patient's head

Measures in the recovery room to help decrease heat loss are use of
- humidified oxygen
- warmed fluids for infusion
- warm blankets and mattresses
- radiant heating lamps

During the rewarming period, shivering occurs. Shivering stresses the body by increasing oxygen demand, which an elderly patient may not be able to meet. A hypothermic patient with limited cardiopulmonary reserve may be at high risk for developing heart failure, cardiac arrhythmias, and myocardial infarction. Prolonged anesthesia and a cool surgical environment can cause peripheral vasoconstriction, which reduces blood flow to the extremities, thus increasing the risk of peripheral venous thrombosis. The rewarming process is ended when the patient's temperature reaches a level that is 1 to 2 degrees below normal. Always keep in mind that postoperative complications can occur very quickly in elderly patients and advance rapidly to life-threatening situations.

F. Education should focus on preventing hypothermia or recurrence of hypothermic episodes and increasing awareness of environmental hazards (Table 2).

G. Referral to social services to ameliorate the cause of hypothermia is warranted. Some state governments forbid utility companies to discontinue gas and electric services and/or have mandated a reduction in utility costs to elderly and disabled persons living on limited incomes. Patients unable to pay utility costs should be informed of legislation or community resources available to assist them. Relocation to appropriate housing and use of available support services may be indicated.

TABLE 2 Hypothermia Prevention and Risk Assessment

Environmental	Behavioral	Functional
Keep plenty of blankets on bed	Wear clothes in layers, with lighter garments next to skin to trap body heat, heavy or waterproof layers outermost	Ability to obtain and prepare food and fluids
Wear socks, nightcap, and long underwear		Ability to control thermostat or heat
Use flannel sheets and a wool or sheepskin mattress cover	Avoid alcohol, especially near bedtime	
	Choose warm liquids	Finances to pay utilities and obtain clothing
Keep room temperature at no less than 70° F; if unable to afford to heat entire dwelling, heat two rooms, including the bedroom, and spend most of the time there	Increase physical activity to promote circulation and heat production	Awareness of self-care needs and safety precautions
	If living alone, ask someone to look in once a day	
Avoid exposure to extreme temperatures		
	Medication or drug abuse	
Hot and cold water availability		

References

Burkle NL. Inadvertent hypothermia. J Gerontol Nurs 1988;
14:26.

Gioiella EC, Bevil CW. Nursing care of the aged client:
Promoting healthy adaptation. Norwalk, CT: Appleton-
Century-Crofts, 1985.

Magnussen MH. Body protection in the aged. In: Yurick AG,
ed. The aged person and the nursing process. 2nd ed.
Norwalk, CT: Appleton-Century-Crofts, 1984:500.

Matz R. Hypothermia: Mechanisms and countermeasures.
Hosp Pract [Off] 1986; 21:45.

KATZ INDEX OF ACTIVITIES OF DAILY LIVING EVALUATION FORM

Name _____ Date of Evaluation _____

Independence means without supervision, direction, or active personal assistance, except as specifically noted below. This is based on actual status and not ability. A patient who refuses to perform a function is considered as not performing the function, even though he or she is deemed able.

For each area of functioning listed below, circle description that applies (the word "assistance" means supervision, direction, or personal assistance)

Bathing—either sponge bath, tub bath, or shower

Receives no assistance (gets in and out of tub by self if tub is usual means of bathing)	Receives assistance in bathing only one part of body (such as back or a leg)	Receives assistance bathing more than one part of body (or does not bathe self)

Dressing—gets clothes from drawers; puts on clothes, including underclothes, outer garments; manages fasteners (including braces, if worn)

Gets clothes and gets completely dressed without assistance	Gets clothes and gets dressed without assistance except for tying shoes	Receives assistance in getting clothes or in getting dressed or stays partly or completely undressed

Toileting—going to the "toilet room" for bowel and urine elimination; cleaning self after elimination and arranging clothes

Goes to "toilet room," cleans self, and arranges clothes without assistance (may use object for support such as cane, walker, or wheelchair and may manage night bedpan or commode, emptying same in morning)	Receives assistance in going to "toilet room" or in cleaning self or in arranging clothes after elimination or in use of night bedpan or commode	Does not go to room termed "toilet" for the elimination process

Transfer

Moves in and out of bed and in and out of chair without assistance (may use objects for support such as cane or walker)	Moves in or out of bed with assistance	Does not get out of bed

Continence

Controls urination and bowel movement completely by self	Has occasional "accidents"	Supervision helps keep urine or bowel control; catheter is used or is incontinent

Feeding

Feeds self without assistance	Feeds self except for getting assistance in cutting meat or buttering bread	Receives assistance in feeding or is fed partly or completely by tubes or intravenous fluids

From Katz S, et al. Studies of illness in the aged. The index of ADL: A standardized measure of biological and psychological function. JAMA 1963; 185:94. Copyright 1963, American Medical Association; with permission.

Barthel Index with Corresponding Values for Independent Performance of Tasks

Index	"Can Do by Myself"	"Can Do with Help of Someone Else"	"Cannot Do at All"
Self-Care Index			
1. Drinking from a cup	4	0	0
2. Eating	6	0	0
3. Dressing upper body	5	3	0
4. Dressing lower body	7	4	0
5. Putting on brace or artificial limb	0	−2	0 (not applicable)
6. Grooming	5	0	0
7. Washing or bathing	6	0	0
8. Controlling urination	10	5 (accidents)	0 (incontinent)
9. Controlling bowel movements	10	5 (accidents)	0 (incontinent)
Mobility Index			
10. Getting in and out of chair	15	7	0
11. Getting on and off toilet	6	3	0
12. Getting in and out of tub or shower	1	0	0
13. Walking 50 yards on the level	15	10	0
14. Walking up/down one flight of stairs	10	5	0
15. If not walking: propelling or pushing wheelchair	5	0	0 (not applicable)

Rating: Highest level of performance 100
Lowest level of performance   0

From Granger CV, et al. Outcome of comprehensive medical rehabilitation: Measures of PULSES profile and the Barthel index. Arch Phys Med Rehabil 1979; 60:145; with permission.

Scale for Instrumental Activities of Daily Living (IADL)

Male score		Female score
	A. Ability to use telephone	
1	1. Operates telephone on own initiative; looks up and dials and so on	1
1	2. Dials a few well-known numbers	1
1	3. Answers telephone but does not dial	1
0	4. Does not use telephone at all	0
	B. Shopping	
1	1. Takes care of all shopping needs independently	1
0	2. Shops independently for small purchases	0
0	3. Needs to be accompanied on any shopping trip	0
0	4. Completely unable to shop	0
	C. Food preparation	
	1. Plans, prepares, and serves adequate meals independently	1
	2. Prepares adequate meals if supplied with ingredients	0
	3. Hosts and serves prepared meals, or prepares meals but does not maintain adequate diet	0
	4. Needs to have meals prepared and served	0
	D. Housekeeping	
	1. Maintains house alone or with occasional assistance (e.g., heavy-work domestic help)	1
	2. Performs light daily tasks such as dish washing and bed making	1
	3. Performs light daily tasks but cannot maintain acceptable level of cleanliness	1
	4. Needs help with all home maintenance tasks	1
	5. Does not participate in any housekeeping tasks	0
	E. Laundry	
	1. Does personal laundry completely	1
	2. Launders small items; rinses socks, stockings, and so on	1
	3. All laundry must be done by others	0
	F. Mode of transportation	
1	1. Travels independently on public transportation or drives own car	1
1	2. Arranges own travel via taxi, but does not otherwise use public transportation	1
0	3. Travels on public transportation when assisted or accompanied by another	1
0	4. Travel limited to taxi or automobile, with assistance of another	0
0	5. Does not travel at all	0
	G. Responsibility for own medication	
1	1. Is responsible for taking medication in correct dosages at correct time	1
0	2. Takes responsibility if medication is prepared in advance in separate dosages	0
0	3. Is not capable of dispensing own medication	0
	H. Ability to handle finances	
1	1. Manages financial matters independently (budgets, writes checks, pays rent and bills, goes to bank); collects and keeps track of income	1
1	2. Manages day-to-day purchases, but needs help with bank for major purchases and so on	1
0	3. Incapable of handling money	0

From Lawton HP, Brody EM. Assessment of older people: Self-maintaining and instrumental activities of daily living. Gerontologist 1969; 9:179; with permission.

Functional Independence Measure
(FIM)

L E V E L S	7 Complete Independence (Timely, Safely) 6 Modified Independence (Device)	NO HELPER
	Modified Dependence 　5 Supervision 　4 Minimal Assist (Subject = 75%+) 　3 Moderate Assist (Subject = 50%+) Complete Dependence 　2 Maximal Assist (Subject = 25%+) 　1 Total Assist (Subject = 0%+)	HELPER

Self-Care   ADMIT   DISCHG   FOL- UP

A. Feeding
B. Grooming
C. Bathing
D. Dressing–Upper Body
E. Dressing–Lower Body
F. Toileting

Sphincter Control

G. Bladder Management
H. Bowel Management

Mobility

Transfer:
　I. Bed, Chair, W/Chair
　J. Toilet
　K. Tub, Shower

Locomotion

L. Walk/wheelChair   w c
M. Stairs

Communication

N. Comprehension   a v v n
O. Expression

Social Cognition

P. Social Interaction
Q. Problem Solving
R. Memory

Total

Note: If stem is not testable, enter level 1.

Copyright 1987 Research Foundation–State University of New York

NOTE: Training in tool utilization is necessary.

From: Granger CV, Hamilton BB, Keith RA, et al. Advances in functional assessment for medical rehabilitation. Topics in Geriatric Rehabilitation 1986; 1:59; with permission. Copyright 1987, Research Foundation—State University of New York, Brooklyn, New York.

MOBILITY

DECREASED MUSCLE STRENGTH

Donna A. Bachand

Decreased muscle strength as a result of prolonged immobility or muscle changes that normally occur in the elderly may lead to loss of muscle mass owing to a decrease in the number and diameter of muscle fibers. Lost muscle tissue is replaced by fibrous tissue, leading to diminished strength and endurance. Muscle strength is related to muscle size and tone, which are directly affected by activity. Acute insult or chronic disease affecting neuronal, hormonal, and vasomotor interactions may result in loss of muscle strength. High levels of activity retard the degenerative process.

A. Determine the patient's usual and safe level of activity in a 24-hour day. Focus on the time of day for peak energy levels, frequency and duration of fatigue, and specific activities that precipitate weakness. Ask about changes in functional level or ability to perform activities of daily living (ADL). Elicit a smoking history. Smoking causes vasoconstriction and impaired oxygen transport to the muscles, exacerbating weakness, and is a risk factor for the development of osteoporosis. Ask whether there are precipitating factors or events that affect muscle strength.

B. Assess strength by observing the muscles' ability to overcome resistance. (See the tool *Muscle Strength Testing*, p 67.) Muscle strength should be greater on the dominant side. Assess range of motion of spine, neck, and extremities. Palpate the neck by having the patient turn the head side to side against resistance. Note any weakness or pain. Assess the patient's ability to grasp and push against resistance with extremities. Baseline measurements of muscle size are useful in the future assessment of muscle loss.

C. Individualize exercise programs according to the patient's ability, current functional level, and previous exercise patterns. Any exercise program should allow a gradual increase in activity as strength and tolerance improve. Individuals with muscle atrophy may begin with active or passive exercises, although passive exercises do not enhance size or strength of muscles. For the elderly, three nonconsecutive exercise sessions per week are ideal. Once the patient is conditioned, each session should include a 5-minute warm-up, 10–20 minutes of rhythmic muscle activity, and a 5-minute cool-down. Walking is an excellent exercise because it requires minimal equipment, is a known skill, and encourages weight bearing on long bones. Remember, benefits from exercise persist only as long as the activity continues. Older adults may be encouraged to join group activities; social interaction may reinforce regular exercise patterns.

D. If the patient displays a disruption in ability to perform activities of daily living or a decrease in functional level, a referral for physical therapy (PT) and/or occupational therapy (OT) evaluation is appropriate. Such intervention may require a physician's order. Specific exercises may be designed by a licensed therapist for each patient based on their needs and abilities, the characteristics of each activity performed, the amount of effort and specific body movements required, and the patient's preferences. Occupational therapy may be particularly helpful in reclaiming lost activities of daily living.

References

Carotenuto R, Bullock J. Physical assessment of the gerontologic client. Philadelphia: FA Davis, 1980.

Yurick AG, Spier BE, Robb SS, Ebert NJ. The aged person and the nursing process. 2nd ed. Norwalk, CT: Appleton-Century-Crofts, 1984.

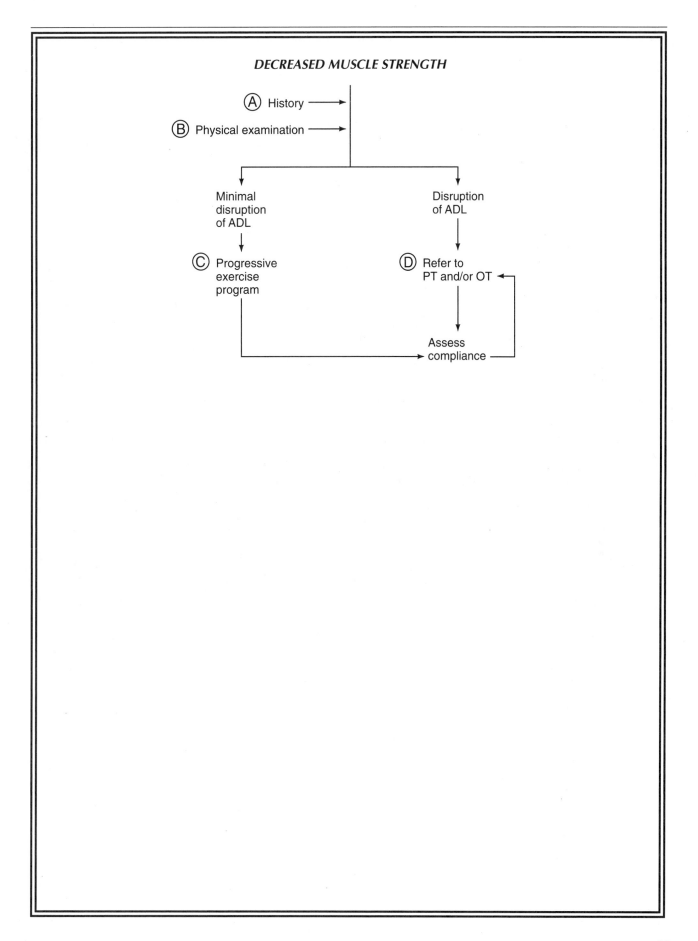

DECREASED MUSCLE STRENGTH

Ⓐ History

Ⓑ Physical examination

Minimal disruption of ADL

Disruption of ADL

Ⓒ Progressive exercise program

Ⓓ Refer to PT and/or OT

Assess compliance

MUSCLE PAIN

Donna A. Bachand

Muscle pain often accompanies a variety of chronic illnesses. Any acute or chronic condition that causes an individual to restrict use of a muscle group can ultimately result in pain secondary to overuse of complementary or contralateral muscles. Severe muscle cramps, usually in the calf, may occur at night as a result of poor circulation, fatigue, or mineral loss. Muscle pain may produce serious consequences for the elderly, who have fewer energy reserves and are less adaptable to stress. In addition, physiologic consequences of aging result in muscle atrophy. The most deleterious response to pain is immobility.

A. History taking can reveal the type, onset, and duration of pain. Acute pain lasts from minutes to days and occurs as a result of tissue damage. Chronic pain lasts for months to years and follows a course of exacerbations and remissions. Muscular pain, whether acute or chronic, usually has an organic component, although the elderly may have difficulty pinpointing the exact location and quality of the pain. Direct questions about the site, radiation, quality, and intensity of pain are useful in obtaining accurate data. It may be helpful to suggest words to describe intensity (mild, moderate, severe; tolerable, agonizing) and quality (sharp, dull, stabbing, burning) or to use a rating tool such as the McGill-Melzack pain perception tool. Ask about precipitating factors or events. Determine whether there is a history of fractures, musculoskeletal surgery, or occupational or recreational injuries. Physical characteristics to be identified are
   • swelling
   • redness
   • numbness
   Elicit the factors that make the pain better or worse, such as
   • environmental (heat or cold)
   • activity
   • psychosocial factors
   • positioning
   • weight bearing
   Determine whether the pain interferes with activities of daily living, work, or recreation.

B. During the physical examination, ask two questions: (1) Can the pain be localized? (2) Are there contralateral symptoms? Note any redness or swelling. Observe the position in which the painful area is placed while the patient is moving and at rest. If pain changes after elevation, consider vascular involvement. If pain increases with movement, consider muscular, connective tissue, or bony injury. Observe weight bearing and ambulation. Watch for guarding, limp, or other symptoms of complementary muscle use. Look for symmetry between contralateral structures as well as involuntary or abnormal body movements. Note any atrophy. It may be necessary to measure bilateral extremity circumference. Palpate for sensitivity to touch, heat, spasm, or atrophy. Compare findings of corresponding body parts when possible. Electrolyte determination can identify chemical causes of muscle pain. The erythrocyte sedimentation rate is usually elevated when inflammation is present. Thyroid disease should be ruled out. Attempt range of motion if no obvious injury or limitation of movement is seen. Test muscle strength of contralateral muscle groups. Light tapping of a muscle group may elicit mechanical irritability. When there is swelling, pain, or redness, assess Homan's sign to differentiate deep vein thrombosis. Always consider infection when there is pain, induration, or redness.

C. The most effective way to alleviate muscle pain is to remove the causative stress, but if the pain is chronic in nature this may not be possible. Patient teaching focuses on the hazards of immobility and safe ways to progressively increase activity, such as
   • turning
   • coughing
   • deep breathing
   • range of motion
   • repositioning
   • adequate nutrition and fluids
   • gradual increase in activity
   • body mechanics
   • use of assistive devices

D. Behavioral techniques that decrease muscle tension may be used to treat both acute and chronic pain; even something as simple as deep breathing may be useful. More sophisticated relaxation techniques that can be successful are numerous. Meditation or imagery may be used to decrease muscle tension and gain control over pain. Distraction techniques redirect attention from the painful body part, thus temporarily reducing the perception of pain. The pain will recur when the distraction is removed. Exercise has multiple beneficial effects when treating pain. It can
   • reduce tension
   • provide distraction
   • improve flexibility
   • increase muscle strength
   • enhance the sense of well-being
   Remember, the benefits of exercise are maintained only as long as the activity continues.

E. Referral to the primary physician is important when dealing with acute pain to determine whether bony injury has occurred or, with chronic pain, to rule out malignancy. Medical evaluation may include labora-

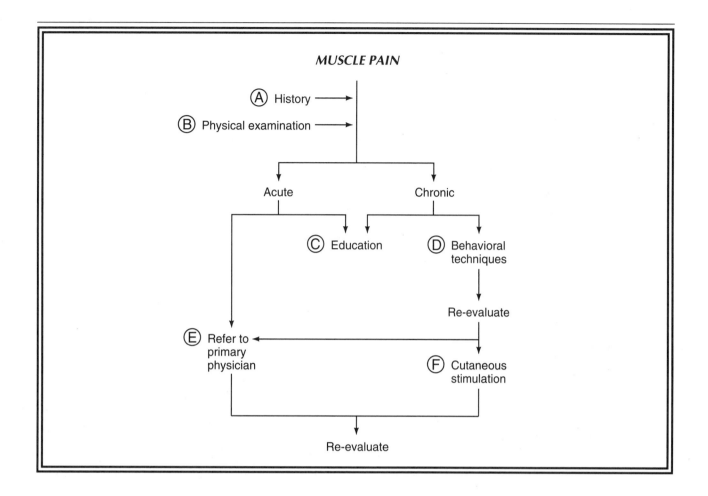

MUSCLE PAIN

(A) History →
(B) Physical examination →

Acute   Chronic

(C) Education   (D) Behavioral techniques

Re-evaluate

(E) Refer to primary physician ←   (F) Cutaneous stimulation

Re-evaluate

tory interpretation for underlying metabolic disorders or an inflammatory process, radiologic assessment for injury, and pharmacologic treatment. Medications may include nonsteroidal anti-inflammatory agents or analgesics, as tolerated.

F. Cutaneous stimulation effectively reduces muscle pain and may facilitate muscle mobility. Massage reduces tension while increasing circulation. Application of heat increases circulation to the affected muscle; cold reduces the sensation of pain. Menthol rubs decrease pain by providing a distracting sensation. If an area is too sensitive to touch or inaccessible because of casts

or splints, stimulation to the contralateral muscle group may be effective.

References

Breitung JC. Care of the older adult. New York: Tiresias Press, 1981.

Gioiella EC, Bevil CW. Nursing care of the aging client: Promoting healthy adaptation. Norwalk, CT: Appleton-Century-Crofts, 1985.

Melzack R. The McGill pain questionnaire: Major properties and scoring methods. Pain 1975; 1:277.

JOINT PAIN

Elizabeth Mackrella

In the aging process, joints lose their normal functioning capacity, becoming drier, more fibrinous (due to increased collagen and decreased elastin), less resilient, and therefore stiffer. Movements of joints are impaired, predisposing the elderly to aches and pains. Major joint disorders evident in the elderly include osteoarthritis, rheumatoid arthritis, and gout. Elderly patients may have impaired mobility due to degenerative changes in joint functioning. These changes may affect a wide range of function: movement, balance, motion stability, agility, endurance, and coordination.

A. History taking should elicit biophysical information such as
  • onset
  • medical history, especially chronic illnesses
  • current medications: prescription and over the counter
  • usual body weight
  • activity and rest patterns
  • nutrition assessment (see p. 90)
  • previous injuries and illnesses
    • treatment
    • residual effects
  • falls (see Falls, p. 90)
  • trauma (see Trauma, p. 96)
  • functional level
Ask about psychosocial aspects such as
  • perception of dysfunction
  • acceptance of dysfunction
  • effect of disability on patient lifestyle
  • support systems
    • caregiver involvement
    • caregiver commitment
  • adherence to prescribed therapy
  • past and current methods for coping with pain
Be an active listener and do not assume that aches and pains are an expected part of the aging process.

B. Physical examination should include assessment of
  • height and weight
  • appearance
  • stature
  • posture
  • body alignment
  • range of motion of all joints
  • gait (see Gait Disturbances, p. 42)
  • balance (see Balance and Coordination Change, p. 2, 4)
  • joint swelling or effusion
  • muscle pain
  • symmetric involvement
Inspect, palpate, and auscultate for crepitation during movement of affected joints. Assess function of the musculoskeletal system for
  • ability to perform activities of daily living
  • evidence of injury
  • use of assistive devices (see Gait Disturbances, p. 42)
Laboratory tests may include
  • CBC with differential
  • electrolytes
  • rheumatoid arthritis (RA) factor
  • antinuclear antibody
  • synovial fluid analysis, including Gram's stain and culture
  • sedimentation rate
False-positive tests may result when connective tissue disease is present. The RA factor may be negative while the clinical picture is positive. Radiography of affected joints assists the differential diagnosis.

C. Acute joint pain may occur as a result of acute gouty arthritis, a hereditary metabolic disease marked by inflammation and excessive urate deposits in the joint. This acute form of arthritis often occurs after excessive or long-term diuretic use. Gout characteristically affects the big toe, but in older people may also affect joints of fingers, hands, wrists, and less often joints in the instep or ankle. Joints may appear hot, tender, inflamed, dusky red, or cyanotic.

D. Chronic joint pain may occur as a result of osteoarthritis or RA, the most common degenerative joint conditions affecting older persons. Osteoarthritis is often a chronic, progressive, noninflammatory disorder that causes degeneration and abrasive insult to the joint cartilage, primarily in the weight-bearing joints (knees, hips, hands, and lower back). Limited motion and bony overgrowth (spurs) caused by the disorder may produce nerve impingement, manifested by pain and numbness or tingling in the involved joint.

E. Referral to the primary physician is indicated if a degenerative joint, arthritis, or gout is suspected. If these conditions remain untreated, pain and stiffness may discourage movement of affected joints and cause permanent limitations in joint immobility due to atrophy of structures around the joint, eventually leading to contractures. Prescriptions for anti-inflammatory, antispasmodic, or analgesic medicines may also be written. Low-dose anti-inflammatory agents interspersed with acetaminophen can be helpful. Systemic steroids are not used to treat osteoarthritis in the elderly. Surgery for correction of deformity and pain relief may be required. Referral for physical or occupational therapy will yield guidance and recommendations for preventive measures, and exercise programs to promote maintenance of function and retraining in activities of daily living. Assistive or orthotic devices may also be provided.

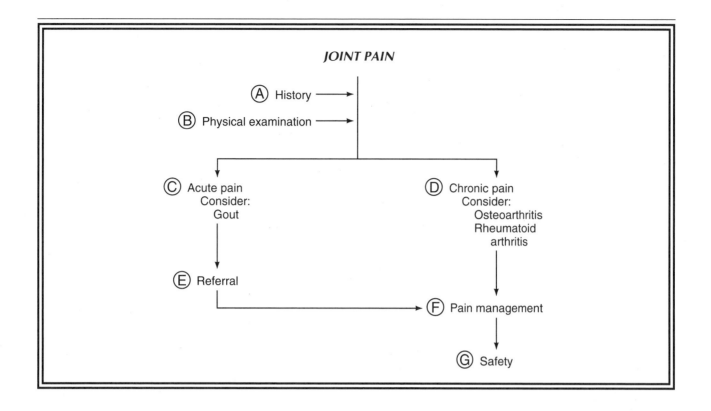

JOINT PAIN

Ⓐ History

Ⓑ Physical examination

Ⓒ Acute pain
Consider:
Gout

Ⓓ Chronic pain
Consider:
Osteoarthritis
Rheumatoid
arthritis

Ⓔ Referral

Ⓕ Pain management

Ⓖ Safety

F. Pain management focuses on pain reduction and the patient's response to pain. Teach
- activity/rest regimens
- weight reduction programs
- how to take prescribed medications
- comfort measures
  - warm bath or shower at bedtime and upon arising
  - gentle massage
Promote
- previous constructive methods for coping with pain
- use of relaxation techniques
  - imagery
  - progressive relaxation
  - cutaneous stimulation

G. Safety measures should involve both patient and caregiver to
1. promote optimal mobility and prevent deformity
   - use assistive devices correctly (braces, splints, wheelchair, cane, handrails, walker)
   - wear appropriate clothing
     - shoe selection (see the tool *Foot Care,* p. 60)
     - avoiding long, flowing garments
   - perform prescribed exercises depending on the level of fitness and ability
     - passive exercise
     - range of motion

- flexion and stretching
- maintain activity-rest regimens
2. prevent injury
   - modify the environment
     - use of stair rails, ramps, or bathroom aids
     - adequate lighting
     - avoid unsecured throw rugs and extension cords across pathways
     - arrange furniture to maximize clear pathways
   - avoid moving heavy objects
   - do not climb on unstable surfaces
   - demonstrate proper body mechanics and body alignment
   - use constant surveillance to guard against accidents

References

Esberger K, Hughes S. Nursing care of the aged. Norwalk, CT: Appleton & Lange, 1989.

Gioiella E, Bevil C. Nursing care of the aging client. Promoting health adaptation. Norwalk, CT: Appleton-Century Crofts, 1985.

Matteson M, McConnell E. Gerontological nursing. Philadelphia: WB Saunders, 1988.

Reich ML. Arthritis: Avoiding diagnostic pitfalls. Geriatrics 1982; 37:46.

LOW BACK PAIN

Carol Spencer Arthur

Back problems seriously limit activity, present difficulties in pain management, and affect psychosocial functioning. Disability is now regarded as the most reliable indicator of the severity of back pain. Acute and chronic low back pain are familiar complaints in all societies, affecting 60–80% of adults at some point in their lives. Low back pain is an affliction often accepted by the geriatric population as inevitable.

A. History taking includes
- present illness
  - onset
  - association with trauma such as
    - lifting
    - twisting
    - falling
- systems review
- previous and current medical history
- socioeconomic background
- family profile, specifically
  - physical health of parents, grandparents, and siblings
  - patterns of illness

A complete pain history includes
- circumstances in which pain occur
- review of factors that increase or lessen pain
- effect of activity levels on the pain
- presence of numbness or paresthesia
- assessing the pain (see box below)
  - onset
  - nature
  - intensity
  - site of origin
  - areas of radiation

Pain Assessment	
Method	*Technique*
Grade	Ask patient to rate pain on scale of 1–10 1–absence of pain 2–least intense pain 10–most intense pain
Pain drawing	Use a drawing of the body Ask patient to indicate areas of • abnormal sensation • pain
Graded pain drawing	Use a drawing of the body Ask patient to • indicate areas of pain • write a grade of 1–10 at each pain area
Description	Ask patient to describe pain Note adjectives used

B. Physical examination focuses on
- vital signs
  - increase in blood pressure, heart rate, or respiratory rate may be indicative of pain
- musculoskeletal system
  - changes in strength
  - muscle tone
  - flexibility
  - range of motion
  - body posture
- neurologic factors
  - localized weakness
  - reflex changes
  - sensory loss

Observe for
- physical and emotional responses to
  - interviewing process
  - perception of illness
- nonorganic components of the patient's illness that may indicate heightened emotional response
  - excessive facies
  - inappropriate facies
  - groaning
  - grimacing

Assess for signs and symptoms of
- acute disc herniation
- endocrine or systemic disease
- bone disease or malignancy
- infection of the disc space or vertebrae
- spinal cord tumors
- referred pain from other areas

Laboratory evaluation may include
- CBC with differential
- sedimentation rate
- serum calcium
- TSH and/or thyroid profile
- blood sugar and/or glycohemoglobin

C. There are numerous scales that look at functional performance of activities of daily living (ADL) (see the tools *Katz Index of Activities of Daily Living (ADL) Evaluation Form*, p. 28; *Scale for Instrumental Activities of Daily Living (IADL)*, p. 30; and *Barthel Index with Corresponding Values for Independent Performance of Tasks*, p. 29). The degree of disability relative to activities in the home, in a leisure setting, or in the workplace is helpful.

D. Acute disruption in activities of daily living generally requires a referral to the primary physician. Radiography of the back can evaluate
- fracture
- osteoporosis
- misalignment
- disc integrity

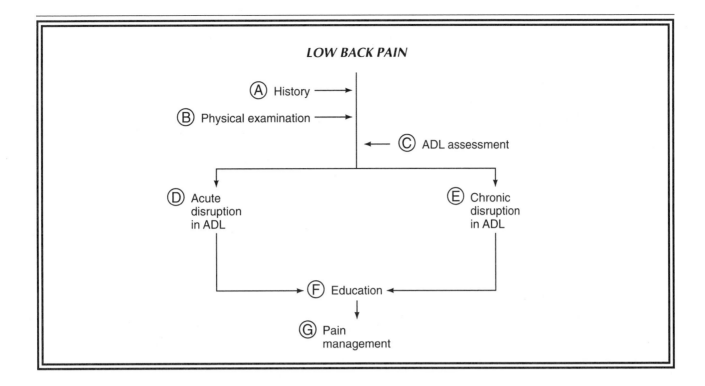

LOW BACK PAIN

- (A) History
- (B) Physical examination
- (C) ADL assessment
- (D) Acute disruption in ADL
- (E) Chronic disruption in ADL
- (F) Education
- (G) Pain management

Be aware that many patients seek chiropractic evaluation and treatment for low back pain. Initial medical treatment may include
- local injection of trigger points with hydrocortisone/lidocaine
- bed rest
- muscle relaxants

Progressive symptoms or lack of improvement may cause the physician to further evaluate the patient, using
- myelography
- electromyography (EMG)
- bone scan
- CT scan
- MRI

or to refer the patient to a neurologist, orthopedist, or back specialist. Surgery may be considered after all conservative measures have failed.

E. Chronic disruption in ADL can precipitate feelings of isolation, depression, and dependency. Encourage the patient to
- take an active role in pain management
- maintain an interest in avocations
- socialize
- develop stress relief measures
- maintain sound spiritual health

Consider referrals for evaluation and intervention by other therapies, including
- neurology
- physical therapy
- occupational therapy
- social work
- orthotist
- psychosocial counseling

F. Patient education is vital to successful treatment of low back pain and includes
- body mechanics
- exercise to
  - improve strength and endurance
  - improve flexibility and mobility
  - prevent recurrence of acute episodes
- application of supports or braces
- pain management techniques
- nutrition counseling
- attaining and maintaining ideal body weight

Modification of old behaviors may be necessary (see the box "Back Pain Education Guidelines"). Caution patients to discontinue exercise if pain increases.

G. Pain is a subjective experience and its assessment and management can be difficult (see the box "Pain Management"). Attitudes of caregivers concerning pain can complicate care. Factors that may influence pain management include
- the patient's perception of pain
- the patient's personal attitudes toward pain
- the severity of the original injury or condition

Both acute and chronic low back pain require patient education and a focus on behavior modification. The goal in acute pain management is relief of pain while healing takes place. The goal in chronic pain management cannot always be pain relief, but rather controlling pain so that it does not interfere with ADL. Re-evaluate pain perception, using the same tool or tools (see the box "Pain Assessment"), at each visit, when the patient's condition changes, or weekly. Note changes in affect. Medication usage also needs to be followed.

Text continued on page 40.

Back Pain Education Guidelines

1. Maintain proper alignment when sitting, standing, lifting, or resting:
   - maintain a straight spine
   - flex the knees and hips when stooping
   - lift with the load close to the body
   - lift with the legs, avoiding twisting
   - avoid lifting above waist level or reaching up for prolonged periods
   - use a firm mattress and avoid sleeping prone
2. Keep active and moving, but alternate periods of rest and activity:
   - rest at short intervals (fatigue precipitates muscle spasm)
   - avoid prolonged sitting, standing, or driving (pressure on intervertebral discs is increased)
   - sit in a straight-back chair with the knees higher than the hips (use a footstool)
   - sit with the buttocks tucked under to flatten the hollow of the back
   - avoid knee and hip extension (when driving, use a back support and keep the seat forward)
3. Emphasize prevention:
   - identify and practice positive coping skills
   - limit stress, which enhances pain
   - daily exercise is vital in preventing recurrence
   - do prescribed exercises twice daily, unhurriedly
   - walking is a preferred exercise (increase pace and distance)
   - keep weight within normal range
4. Provide medication education:
   - avoid prolonged use of pain medication
   - know the action, interaction, and side effects of both prescribed and over-the-counter medications

Pain Management

Acute	Chronic

• bed rest
  • on a firm mattress
  • pillow between flexed knees while lying on the side
• analgesics
• muscle relaxants
• heat application
• distraction
	• analgesics or nonsteroidal anti-inflammatory agents
	• weight and nutrition maintenance
	• ice/heat application
	• exercise program
	• back support
	• relaxation techniques
	• socialization
	• biofeedback
	• TENS

References

Adjei-Boachie O. Conservative management of low back pain. Postgrad Med 1988; 84:127.

Adjei-Boachie O. Evaluation of the patient with low back pain. Postgrad Med 1988; 84:110.

Frymoyer JW, Cats-Baril WL. An overview of the incidences and costs of low back pain. Orthop Clin North Am 1991; 22:263.

Patenaude SS, Sommer M. Low back pain, etiology and prevention. AORN J 1987; 46:472.

Shotkin JD, Bolt B, Norton DA. Teaching program for patients with low back pain. J Neurosci Nurs 19:240.

GAIT DISTURBANCES

Paula A. Loftis

The ability to ambulate can become a problem with age. Evaluation of the elderly should include routine testing of gait and posture. Gait involves proprioception, the awareness of the external environment and the position of the body within space as well as receipt of stimuli from the surroundings. In addition, visual perception and information from the vestibular system contribute to mobility. Gait disturbances can lead to instability and the risk of falls or injury (see Falls, p. 90). Mobility is also important in maintaining independence and self-confidence.

A. History focuses on
   • falls or near-falls (see Falls, p. 90)
   • unsteadiness in walking
   • ear or hearing problems
   • visual impairment or difficulty seeing in the dark
   • chronic diseases, including cardiovascular, osteoarthritis, diabetes mellitus, and neurologic disorders, including Parkinson's disease and cerebrovascular disease
   • dizziness and lightheadedness when walking
   • alcohol use
   • pernicious anemia, vitamin B_{12} deficiency
   • activities of daily living (ADL) or instrumental activities of daily living (IADL) impairment by self-report and collaborative sources
   • prescription and nonprescription medications, including
      • medications that promote orthostatic hypotension
         • sedatives
         • hypnotics
      • medications that impair vestibular function
         • aspirin, large doses
         • quinine

B. Physical examination should concentrate on gait and posture. Specific tests and evaluation data include
   • vital signs: blood pressure—lying, sitting, and standing with concomitant change in pulse to assess for orthostatic hypotension
   • Romberg's test (see p. 63)
   • nudge test (see p. 61)
   • comprehensive gait and balance evaluation (see p. 61)
   • tandem gait: walking heel to toe, which remains intact in the normal elderly
   • standing on one leg: frequently impaired
   • Get Up and Go Test (see p. 62)
   • visual acuity (see Decreased Vision, p. 118)
   • ability to focus on a fixed target while moving and on a moving object while stationary
   • hearing screen (see Hearing Loss, p. 122)
   • ear inspection, including cerumen impaction
   • range of motion: head and neck, shoulders, elbows, wrists, hands, hips, knees, ankles, and back

   • muscle strength
   • vibratory sense
   • examination of feet (see Corns, Calluses, Toenail Deformities, p. 52, and Foot Deformities, p. 54)
   • neurologic examination
   • cognitive evaluation (see tool on p. 60 and Confusion/Cognitive Changes/Dementia, p. 254)
   Laboratory analysis includes electrolytes, CBC, thyroid function tests, serum glucose, blood urea nitrogen, and vitamin B_{12} and folate levels. A rheumatoid factor, antinuclear antibodies, and alkaline phosphatase evaluation may be warranted with joint complaints. A chest film and electrocardiogram may be indicated to evaluate cardiovascular or pulmonary disease. When there are findings of cerebellar dysfunction or focal neurologic findings, a CT scan or MRI may be indicated. Electroencephalograms are reserved for suspected seizure disorder. Differential evaluation includes normal pressure hydrocephalus and intracranial lesion. Specific gait disorders are identified in Table 1.

C. Aims of follow-up and patient education are
   • prevention of falls
   • maintenance of independence
   • reassurance
   • safety
   Target areas for maintaining the patient's functional ability include
   • environmental adaptation (see Falls, p. 90)
   • vision and hearing correction
   • chronic disease management and treatment

D. Physician orders may be necessary for physical and occupational therapy, depending on the state of residency, or direct access to therapy may be available. Appropriate management and treatment for gait disturbances focus on
   • recommendations for appropriate adaptive equipment and assistive devices
   • gait training
   • improving posture
   • muscle strengthening
   • establishing a home exercise program
   • maneuvering on various floor surfaces
   • negotiating stairs
   • lifestyle and mobility adjustment, including
      • slow position changes
      • learning methods to regain footing after a fall
      • balance techniques

E. Assistive devices and/or adaptive equipment may provide the necessary support and reduce the sensation of unsteadiness. Good muscle strength is required in the elbow extensors and shoulder depressors to

Text continued on page 44.

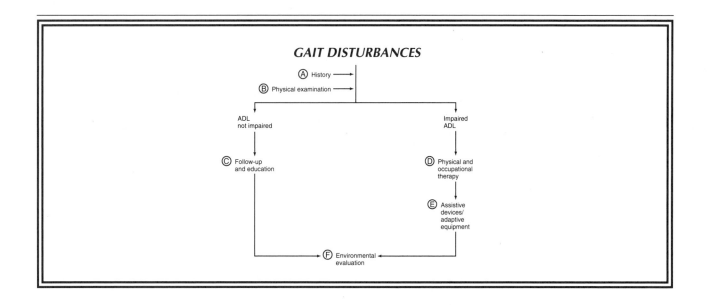

GAIT DISTURBANCES

(A) History

(B) Physical examination

ADL not impaired

Impaired ADL

(C) Follow-up and education

(D) Physical and occupational therapy

(E) Assistive devices/ adaptive equipment

(F) Environmental evaluation

TABLE 1 Common Gait Disorders

Type	Characteristics
Parkinson's dyskinesia	Flexion of knees, hips, trunk, neck, and elbows on standing Forward shift in center of gravity Arms close to body Short, shuffling steps Difficulty in initiating ambulation Stiff, forward-leaning walk Festinating gait seen with accelerating steps once walking is initiated Retropulsion tendency
Normal-pressure hydrocephalus	Ataxia (with concomitant dementia and urinary incontinence) Unsteady, short, and clumsy steps
Sensory ataxia, associated with peripheral neuropathy secondary to diabetes mellitus vitamin B_{12} deficiency alcoholism thyroid problems	Disturbed proprioception Difficulty standing and walking Wide-based gait Irregular, high, slapping steps Conscious observation of feet/legs in relation to floor Impaired vibratory sense
Frontal lobe syndrome	Body flexed forward Wide-based stance On initiating walking, foot appears stuck to floor and difficult to move Slight sway
Idiopathic gait disorder	Impaired balance, movement, and rapidity of walk Wide-based stance and gait Short steps
Arthritic gait disturbance	With hip pain: Tilt of body toward painful joint Shift in center of gravity With knee pain: Flexion and internal rotation of knee Foot flexion Walking on toes With foot pain: Various gaits to avoid weight bearing on painful sites
Hemiplegia	Lateral, arc swinging, or circumduction of affected side Spastic Stiff-legged
Footdrop	Toe touch first instead of heel (no active dorsiflexion) Tendency to bring knee up high followed by foot slap
Paraparesis	Scissoring

TABLE 2 Ambulation Assistive Devices

Type	Indication	Measuring/Features	Instructions
Canes Single-tipped cane Three-point cane Quad or four-point cane	With fair balance Primarily used for support, not to decrease weight bearing Poor control or weakness of one side of body Three-point and four-point cane: increased support more difficult to move than single-tipped cane	Grip of cane aligns with wrist or grip of cane level with hip (see p. 64)	Stand erect; look ahead and not down at feet Held on stronger or uninvolved side of body Held 6–10 inches to side of foot *On walking:* Advance cane first when walking Move cane forward 12 inches Weaker leg moved forward even with cane Stronger leg brought forward and ahead of cane and weaker leg
Walkers Standard	Impaired balance Disability, weakness, or inability to weight bear on one or both legs More support than cane Need for more security than cane	Walker grips at wrist 30-degree elbow angle Proper height to avoid stooping (see p. 65)	Avoid carrying walker Place all four walker legs on floor at same time Pick up and move forward about 6 inches or with back legs just in front of toes Step with weaker leg first Step halfway into walker Both feet should be even inside walker
Rolling walker	Inability to lift standard walker		Lean forward on walker without body touching front of walker Do not use on stairs Attachments such as baskets or bag carriers are useful
Crutches	Good balance necessary Weight-bearing limitations	Stand upright, feet slightly apart Wear consistent shoe type and heel height Underarm support 2 inches below axilla Shoulders should be level 30-degree bend at elbow for appropriate handgrip placement Adequate padding on underarm supports and handgrips Intact rubber tips	Leave space wide enough to fit body through Two- and three-point gaits, depending on weight-bearing ability Training by therapist in proper walking gait may be indicated Weight is carried on handgrips, not underarm supports (pressure on axillas can result in brachial plexus damage)
Braces and splints	Support weak extremity or back Restrict joint movement Decrease pain Prevent deformity	Customized by therapist or orthotist	Protect skin and bony prominences Individualized training in use

walk with assistive devices. Patients should wear nonskid shoes, walk on nonskid surfaces, and avoid walking in stockings or bootees. Appropriate choice and use of equipment are imperative to avoid exacerbating safety and mobility problems (Table 2). Gait patterns with assistive devices vary in safety, speed, and the amount of energy expended (Table 3). Sensory adaptation such as visual aids and hearing amplification devices may also help maintain self-care and ADL independence.

F.   Environmental evaluation ascertains
   • adaptive equipment needs such as
     • elevated toilet seat
     • tub and stair rails
     • tub seat
   • safety hazards (see Falls, p. 90)

TABLE 3 Gait Patterns with Assistive Devices

Pattern	Characteristics
Four-point	Safest pattern Most stable pattern Slow Used with 　muscle weakness 　poor balance 　poor coordination
Three-point, non–weight bearing	Normal use of trunk, upper extremities, and one leg More rapid than four-point Requires strength and balance Commonly used with 　orthopedic patients 　unilateral amputees
Three-point, partial–weight bearing	Requires less balance than non–weight bearing Physician specification needed on allowable weight bearing for involved extremity
Two-point	Rapid gait Requires balance Resembles normal walking
Cane gait	Supportive Commonly used with hemiplegic patients

References

Bortz WM. Disuse and aging. JAMA 1982; 248:1203.

Burrage RL. Physical assessment: Musculoskeletal and nervous systems. In: Chenitz WC, Stone JT, Salisbury SA, eds. Clinical gerontological nursing. Philadelphia: WB Saunders, 1991:71.

Caranasos GJ, Israel R. Gait disorders in the elderly. Hosp Pract 1991; 26:67.

Hough JC, McHenry MP, Kammer LM. Gait disorders in the elderly. Am Fam Physician 1988; 43:33.

Imms FJ, Edholm OG. Studies of gait and mobility in the elderly. Age Ageing 1981; 10:147.

RIGIDITY

Patricia Guida

Rigidity, defined as stiffness or an inability to bend or be bent, can be the result of disuse caused by disease or pain. Half of the population 65 years of age experience some form of mobility discomfort. Some loss of agility occurs through the natural decline of bone and muscle mass, but this loss can be exacerbated by a disease process or as an accommodation to pain. Rigidity can be related to four areas: muscle, bone, joint, or skin. Atrophy or disuse of muscle can directly influence joint movement or function leading to contracture. Abnormal bone density and reabsorption can cause overt deformities and limit mobility. The skin influences rigidity by providing a barrier to movement.

A. History taking should collect data concerning
  • current/past musculoskeletal problems requiring medical treatment
    • treatment regimen
    • outcome of treatment
  • recent/old fractures, pain at fracture site
  • current medications
  • self-care practices for maintaining muscle/joint mobility
    • chiropractor
    • adaptive devices
    • analgesics
    • exercise
    • home remedies
  • chronic and acute illnesses
    • neoplasm
    • metabolic disease
    • Parkinson's disease
  • weight and height changes
  • back pain
  • diet
  • ill-fitting dentures
  • family history of musculoskeletal disease
  • ability to perform activities of daily living (ADL) and instrumental ADL (IADL)
  • change in ability to enjoy and perform hobbies
  Use a pain scale to assess
    • the patient's perception of pain
    • changes in functional status due to pain

B. Physical examination looks at skin, joints, and musculoskeletal function. Observe
  • gait pattern (see Gait Disturbances, p. 42, and the tool *Balance and Gait*, p. 61)
  • height
  • posture
    • scoliosis
    • kyphosis
  • overt deformities
  • muscle wasting
  • contractures
  • guarding of an area

• response to movement that might indicate pain
  • grimacing
  • hesitance
  • decreased range of motion
• smoothness of joint movement
• intention tremor
• balance (see p. 2)
Inspect
• the skin for
  • trauma
  • keloids
  • hypertrophied scars
  • scleroderma
  • dermatomyositis, which may indicate muscle involvement
• the muscles for
  • wasting
  • flaccidity
• the bone for deformity
• the joint for
  • edema
  • deformity
Palpate bone, muscle, and joints for
• pain
• tenderness
• crepitus
• temperature
Assess joint movement in supination, pronation, flexion, extension, abduction, adduction, rotation, circumduction, eversion, inversion, protraction, and retraction. Perform both active and passive range of motion (ROM). Use a goniometer to measure active angle movement the patient can maintain without assistance. Measure muscle strength and endurance (see Decreased Muscle Strength, p. 32, and the tools *Measuring Muscle Strength or Endurance*, p. 66, *Muscle Strength Testing*, p. 67). It is important not to be overzealous in the application of force or to allow the patient to be injured. Laboratory analysis includes
• CBC
• electrolytes, creatinine
• sedimentation rate

C. Referral to the primary physician is warranted to rule out bony injury or malignancies. Additional diagnostic studies may include
• radiographic spinal cord/neural evaluation
• electromyography (EMG)
• bone scan
Pharmacologic interventions, including analgesic or anti-inflammatory agents, may be recommended, depending on the clinical findings. Referrals to neurology, physical medicine and rehabilitation, rheumatology, or mineral metabolism may be indicated. Physical and occupational therapy can be extremely

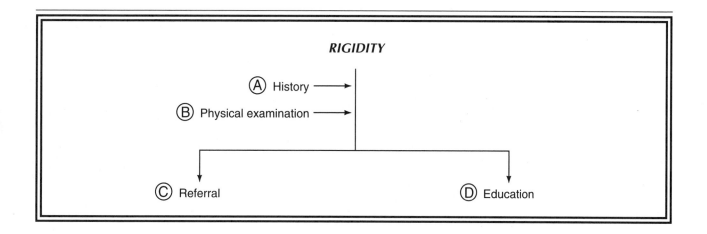

RIGIDITY

(A) History →

(B) Physical examination →

(C) Referral

(D) Education

beneficial. Consider referral to home health care services, home-delivered meals, or other community supports.

D. Patient and caregiver education should be individualized and encompass
- daily passive and active ROM exercise for each joint
- massage
  - in a circular motion over joints
  - avoiding acutely inflamed joints
- application of heat
  - avoid excessive amounts or intense degree of heat to reduce the potential for injury
- patient/caregiver commitment to resolve or minimize rigidity
- adequate diet
- proper use of supportive devices such as walkers, braces, canes, graspers
- accurate use and knowledge of medication regimen
- need for follow-up to assess
  - ROM

- muscle strength
- ADL/IADL performance
- ambulatory aids and supportive devices
- support of family/caregivers
- caregiver burden
- medication usage and drug levels as indicated

References

Bockman R, Bone H, Scopelitis E. Joints in metabolic bone disease. Patient Care 1990; 24:53.

Conn V. Joint self-care by older adults. Rehab Nurs 1990; 15:182.

Eliopoulos C. Gerontological nursing. 2nd ed. Philadelphia: JB Lippincott, 1987:224.

James B, Parker A. Active and passive mobility of lower limb joints in elderly men and women. Am J Phys Med Rehab 1989; 68:162.

TREMOR

Kathy B. Wright

Tremor is defined as rhythmic, purposeless, quivering movement resulting from involuntary, alternating contraction and relaxation of opposing groups of skeletal muscles. Tremors usually involve the distal limbs; the head, tongue, or jaw; and (rarely) the trunk. Often several different tremors exist in the same patient and must be treated individually. Classifications of tremors may vary. Table 1 offers common tremor classifications and subcategories.

A. History will address
- medical problems including
  - Parkinson's disease
  - liver disease
  - thyroid disorder
  - cardiac disease
  - pulmonary insufficiency
  - renal failure
  - diabetes mellitus
  - psychiatric or emotional disorders
  - head injury
- family background of
  - neurologic disease
  - tremor
- past or present exposure to industrial wastes, heavy metals, or environmental toxins
- medications, prescription and over the counter
- chronic alcohol or barbiturate use
- nutritional intake
- tremor specifics
  - body parts involved
  - activity that elicits tremor such as
    - exercise
    - precision movements
    - resting
  - question family/caregivers regarding the presence of the following during sleep
    - muscular fasciculations (flickering muscle movements of calves, hands, feet, and eyelids)
    - clonus
    - seizure activity
- impairment of ADL
- emotional disturbance and embarrassment caused by tremor

B. Physical assessment includes observation for
- resting tremor in the head, face, arms, hands, trunk, legs, and feet
- nystagmus
- tremor
  - frequency/rate (number per second: average is 3–6 beats/sec but faster rates occur)
  - amplitude
    - coarse?
    - fine?
  - speed
    - rapid?
    - slow?
  - occurrence with physical movements while patient distracted, such as during disrobing or dressing
- neurologic examination includes
  - asking patient to touch the nose and alternate with touching the examiner's finger with accelerating speed
  - having patient run the heel down the opposite shin
  - asking patient to stand with arms outstretched in front of the body at a 90-degree angle with a piece of paper resting on the fingers
  - request patient to write or draw
  - gait assessment (see Gait Disturbances, p. 42)
- listening to the patient's voice for vocal tremor
- palpating for fine movements of muscles
- ADL evaluation (see pp. 28, 30)
Laboratory testing may encompass
- CBC
- serum electrolytes
- vitamin B_{12} level
- folate
- liver panel
- renal function tests
- thyroid profile
- serum ceruloplasmin level (rule out Wilson's disease)
- drug levels
- toxicology screen
Additional procedures for diagnostic work-up include
- electrocardiography and chest film if cardiopulmonary dysfunction is suspected
- head CT scan to rule out lesion if focal neurologic signs are present
- electroencephalography to distinguish between lesion, toxicity, or metabolic disorders
- referral to a sleep laboratory to observe tremor state during sleep
- a tremorometer, available in some sleep laboratories, for tremor measurement

C. In the presence of focal neurologic findings, impairment of activities of daily living (ADL), or new-onset or previously undiagnosed tremor, referral to a primary care physician or neurologist is indicated for further neurologic evaluation and medical intervention. Medical intervention is dictated by the etiology of the tremor. Tremors may be exaggerated by increased levels of catecholamines in the bloodstream and may be suppressed by drugs, such as propranolol, that block beta-adrenergic receptors. Medication therapy, including beta-adrenoreceptor antagonists or drugs are used to treat Parkinson's disease. Physical medicine and rehabilitation and neurosurgery are possible treatment modalities for tremors.

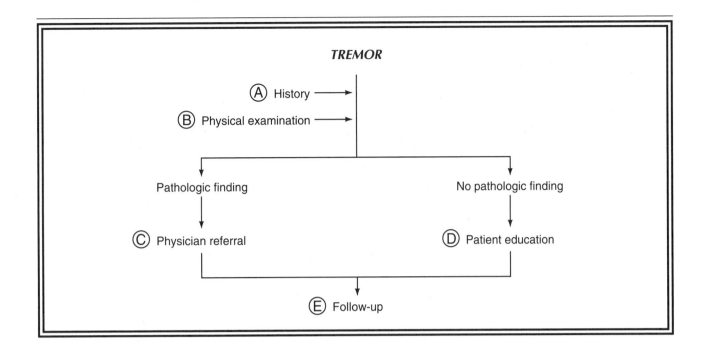

TREMOR

Ⓐ History ⟶

Ⓑ Physical examination ⟶

Pathologic finding — No pathologic finding

Ⓒ Physician referral — Ⓓ Patient education

Ⓔ Follow-up

D. Intervention for patients with tremor is aimed at treating the underlying cause and minimizing the effects of tremor on psychosocial well-being and ADL. Patient/family education focuses on
   • regular activity and an exercise program
   • medication education
   • balanced nutritional intake
   Supportive care and options include
   • active listening and reassurance
   • referral to a substance abuse program
   • physical and/or occupational therapy consultations
   • encouragement of effective coping mechanisms
   • community involvement and referrals for assistance in ADL

   • linkage to community organizations such as
     • local and national Parkinson's groups
     • International Tremor Foundation (360 West Superior, Chicago, IL 60610, 213-664-2344)
     • senior citizen's program and nutrition sites
     • recreational facilities

E. Provide periodic follow-up to determine and monitor
   • stability or progression of tremors
   • lifestyle adaptation
   • ability to perform ADL
   • safety concerns
   • tolerance and efficacy of medications
   • symptomatic relief

TABLE 1   Types of Tremors, Causes, and Characteristics

Type	Causes	Characteristics
1. Resting or static a. Parkinsonian, physiologic	Extrapyramidal system pathology (e.g., Parkinson's disease) Systemic illness Graves' disease Hypoglycemia Metabolic disorders Electrolyte imbalance Nutritional deficits Pheochromocytoma Exercise Fatigue Deconditioning, loss of muscle strength and function Wilson's disease	Fine, quick, regular, rhythmic, and continuous tremor; sometimes disappears with purposeful movements Often localized in one or both hands; occasionally in jaws, tongue, or lower extremities Disappears during sleep May be enhanced during stress No improvement with alcohol Present when walking Usually occurs at rest Can be unilateral or bilateral
b. Pill rolling	Parkinson's disease	Index finger flexes and extends in contact with thumb
c. Chemical	Bronchodilators and other beta agonists Peripheral metabolites of levodopa Amphetamines Theophylline Terbutaline Valproic acid Tricyclic antidepressants Xanthines in tea or coffee Lithium therapy Glucocorticoid therapy Caffeine	
2. Action	Iatrogenic etiology Numerous medical, neurologic, and psychiatric diseases or emotional conditions Advanced Parkinson's disease Experienced by normal individuals, or patients with essential familial tremor or Parkinson's disease	Irregular movement of active extremities occurring 6–8 per sec, slower in elderly Disappears with relaxation More difficult to interpret than resting or static tremor Involves outstretched hand, head, and (less often) lips and tongue

a. Hyperadrenergic (exaggerated physiologic)	Catecholamine excess
	  Intense anxiety
	  Excitement
	  Stage fright
	Thyrotoxicosis
	Hypoglycemia
		Mild form occurs in normal patients
		Exaggerated form may require medical treatment

b. Toxic	Alcohol or opiate withdrawal Hyperthyroidism Manganese poisoning Carbon monoxide poisoning Heavy metal poisoning Prescribed sympathomimetic drugs Caffeine Barbiturates Theophyllines Levodopa Antidepressants Industrial wastes Methyl bromide	Usually less rhythmic movement Can affect lips

TABLE 1 Types of Tremors, Causes, and Characteristics—*continued*

Type	Causes	Characteristics
c. Essential (senile, familial, or idiopathic)	Positive family tremor history may be present (familial) No specific pathologic lesion identified Cause unknown	Most common of all neurologic conditions Fine, quick movements, especially of upper extremities, with rhythmic head nodding Sporadic More rapid than parkinsonian Increased trembling during purposeful movements; interrupts ADL Intensified by anxiety, excitement, fatigue, or self-consciousness Never associated with parkinsonian symptoms of bradykinesia, rigidity, or loss of postural reflexes May begin in childhood but usually later in life, persisting throughout adulthood Most evident during voluntary movement with hands postured Speech quivering and distortion common Appearance of nervousness Can affect head alone, causing patient to constantly appear to be nodding "yes" or "no" Temporarily abolished by one or two drinks of alcoholic beverage, but becomes worse after alcohol dissipates
d. Intention or ataxic	Cerebellar dysfunction Advanced multiple sclerosis Severe Parkinson's disease Vascular lesions of subthalamus and midbrain Trauma Tumor Liver encephalopathy	Increases with performance of specific, goal-directed, voluntary, and precise movements With exacting tasks, movements become jerky Absent with limbs at rest and on initial movement May seriously impair ADL Intensity increases as target is approached

References

Delgado JM, Billo JM. Care of the patient with Parkinson's disease: Surgical and nursing interventions. J Neurosci Nurs 1988; 20:142.

Gillespie MM. Tremor. J Neurosci Nurs 1991; 23:170.

Growdon JH, Fink JS. Paralysis and movement disorders. In: Wilson JD, et al, eds. Harrison's principles of internal medicine. 12th ed. New York: McGraw-Hill, 1991:166.

Koller WC. Evaluation of tremor disorders. Hosp Pract 1990; 25:23.

Malasanos LJ. Tremors: Associations and assessment. J Neurosurg Nurs 1982; 14:290.

Mathews W. Evaluation of tremor in adults. Physician Assistant 1986; 10:47.

Mosby's medical, nursing, and allied health dictionary. 3rd ed. St. Louis: Mosby–Year Book 1990:1191.

Rodnitzky RL. Tremor: Different origins mandate different therapies. Consultant 1985; 25:87, 96.

CORNS, CALLUSES, TOENAIL DEFORMITIES

M. Elise Tidwell-Bissell

Corns and calluses are thickened areas of skin caused by friction or pressure from underlying bone. Corns are generally small, hard areas occurring over the dorsum of the fifth toe, between toes, and over bony prominences; they may be painful. Calluses may be related to fat pad atrophy on the plantar surface of the foot and are usually broader and less painful than corns. Toenail deformities include thickening of nails or ingrown toenails. Thickening is often caused by fungal growth within the nail. Ingrown toenails result from wearing tight, short shoes; congenital malalignment; or overcurvature of the nail plate.

A. History taking should include questions about
   * onset
   * duration
   * pain
   * foot care practices
   * shoe selection practices
   * use of foot care products
   * previous foot treatment
   * presence of chronic medical illness

B. Physical examination should focus on
   * appearance of the feet
     * location of the corn, callus, or toenail deformity
     * color of skin around the corn, callus, or toenail
     * presence of lesions
   * appearance of toenails
     * length
     * color
     * hypertrophy
   * footwear
     * toe box
     * areas of wear
     * heel fit
     * cushion
   * presence of vascular insufficiency or neuropathy
     * capillary refill
     * hair growth/loss on the feet or toes
     * skin temperature
     * sensation
     * vibratory sense

C. Patient education focuses on (see the tool *Foot Care*, p. 60)
   * selection of shoes
   * basic foot care
   * care of specific foot problems (Table 1)

D. Referral to a foot care professional is essential if there are signs of infection. Paring of corns or calluses should initially be done by a professional in most cases, and always when there is evidence of problems with peripheral circulation or neuropathy.

TABLE 1   Care of Specific Foot Problems

Type	Prevention	Treatment
Corns	Padding 　Lamb's wool 　Soft sponge 　Shoes with wide toe 　　box	Paring*
Calluses	Padding insoles to 　equalize weight 　bearing Shoes with wide 　toe box and thick 　soles	Paring* Metatarsal head pads
Toenail deformities	Shoes with wide toe 　box of adequate 　length	Trimming Oral antifungal agent*
Ingrown toenails		Trim straight across Place tuft of cotton under ingrown edge

*Requires referral to a foot care professional.

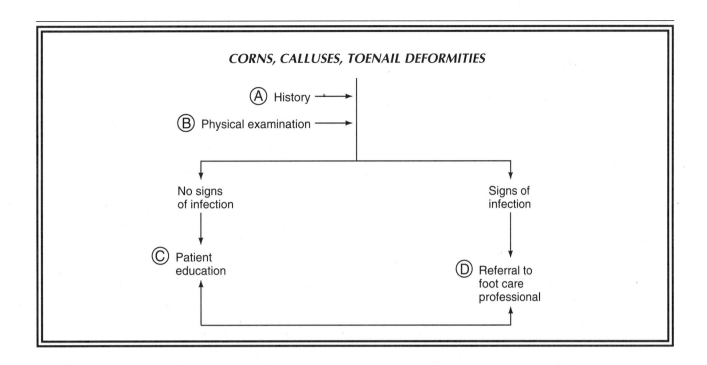

CORNS, CALLUSES, TOENAIL DEFORMITIES

(A) History

(B) Physical examination

No signs of infection

Signs of infection

(C) Patient education

(D) Referral to foot care professional

References

Brenner MA, ed. Management of the diabetic foot. Baltimore: Williams & Wilkins, 1987.

Evanski PM. Disorders of the foot. Philadelphia: WB Saunders, 1982.

Gould JS. The foot book. Baltimore: Williams & Wilkins, 1988.

Kozak GP, Hoar CS, Rowbotham JL, et al. Management of diabetic foot problems. Philadelphia: WB Saunders, 1984.

Levin ME, O'Neal LW. The diabetic foot. 4th ed. St. Louis: Mosby—Year Book, 1988.

Miller RA, Evans WE. Nurse and patient: Allies preventing amputation. RN July 1988; 51(6):38—43.

FOOT DEFORMITIES

M. Elise Tidwell-Bissell

The elderly commonly experience musculosketetal foot deformities as a result of age-associated degeneration of muscles, tendons, ligaments, and joints. Foot deformities have many causes: arthritis, congenital deformities, hallux valgus (bunions), diabetes. Others include hammertoes, clawtoes, overlapping toes, and deformities associated with amputation (Table 1).

A. During history taking, ask questions about
    • onset and duration of foot problems
    • previous foot treatment or surgeries
    • pain
    • chronic medical illnesses

B. During the physical examination, observe the patient walking and determine whether
    • there is a limp
    • one foot is "favored"
    Examine the foot for
    • deviations of the toes
    • swelling
    • pressure areas
    • corns or calluses
    • hygiene

Ask to inspect commonly used footwear (see the tool *Foot Care*, p. 60).

C. Footwear is the first line of defense against foot injury. Appropriate footwear can decrease pressure on foot deformities and prevent corn or callus development. Footwear features include
    • soft leather or material
    • adequate depth and width of forefoot
    • snug heel

D. Referral to a physician or podiatrist is essential if the patient's mobility is affected. The treatment ordered will depend on the deformity (Table 1).

E. Instruct in proper foot care (see the tool *Foot Care*, p. 60):
    • hygiene
    • nail care
    • footwear
    Provide written instructions on daily care to reinforce patient education. Caregiver and family involvement may be essential to avoid neglect of feet and maintain the patient's ambulation, function, and stability.

TABLE 1 Foot Deformities

Deformity	Appearance	Causes	Interventions
Hallux valgus (bunion)	Great toe deviates laterally Bony prominence appears over head of metatarsal	Congenital Prolonged wearing of tight-toed shoes Pronated flat foot Degenerative arthritis	Bunionectomy Custom footwear
Hammertoes	Toe contracted at one or more joints Clawlike appearance Callus build-up at weight-bearing distal tip of toe	Mechanical pressure of too short a shoe with elevated heel that pushes toes forward into toe box Intrinsic muscle atrophy Neuropathy Diabetes Flat-footedness Trauma	Hammertoe surgery Callus management
Charcot's joint	Bony deterioration of foot Red, warm, swollen tarsal joints Abnormal gait	Severe diabetic neuropathy Painless injury to ligament or fracture of small bone	Immobilization Non–weight bearing Molded shoes Orthopedic appliances: leg braces, walking casts, ambulatory assistive devices Surgery, rarely indicated except for chronic ulceration and infection

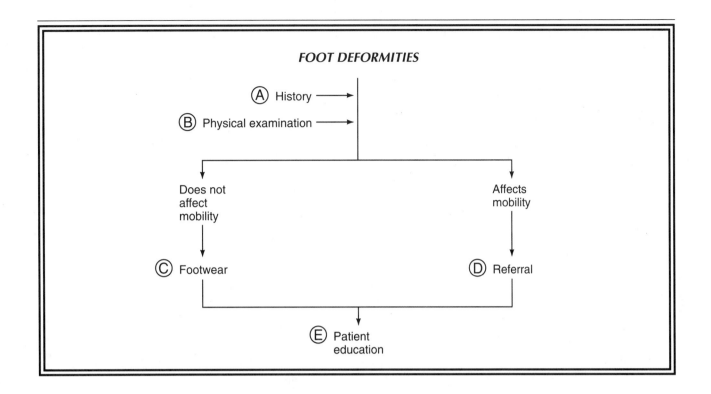

FOOT DEFORMITIES

(A) History

(B) Physical examination

Does not affect mobility

(C) Footwear

Affects mobility

(D) Referral

(E) Patient education

References

Brenner MA, ed. Management of the diabetic foot. Baltimore: Williams & Wilkins, 1987.

Gould JS. The foot book. Baltimore: Williams & Wilkins, 1988.

Kozak GP, Hoar CS, Rowbotham JL, et al. Management of diabetic foot problems. Philadelphia: WB Saunders, 1984.

Levin ME, O'Neal LW. The diabetic foot. 4th ed. St. Louis: Mosby–Year Book, 1988.

Miller RA, Evans WE. Nurse and patient: Allies preventing amputation. RN July 1988; 51(6):38–43.

FOOT LESIONS

M. Elise Tidwell-Bissell

Foot lesions are classified as either neuropathic or ischemic (Table 1). Neuropathic lesions are a result of pressure on insensate feet. Heavy callus build-up can cause the tissue beneath to degenerate, allowing the skin to crack. Ischemic foot lesions are a result of inadequate blood supply to lower extremities; because they are related to vascular compromise, they are difficult to heal.

A. Ask about chronic illnesses that predispose patients to neuropathy or vascular compromise, such as
   • hypertension
   • diabetes mellitus
   • peripheral vascular disease
   • neurologic disorders
   • alcoholism
   • obesity
   Obtain a smoking history. Try to determine the location, onset, and duration of
   • change or loss of sensation
   • numbness
   • corns or calluses
   • skin temperature changes
   • pain
     • at rest
     • relieved by walking
     • relieved by elevation
   Ask what exacerbates or alleviates these symptoms.

B. Check the vascular supply to the feet:
   • pedal pulse
   • posterior tibial pulse
   • capillary refill
   • skin color and character
   • loss of hair on the legs or toes
   • skin temperature with line of demarcation
   A Doppler may be needed to determine the presence of pulses. Perform a peripheral neurologic examination (see Foot Pain/Numbness, p. 58) to check for
   • vibratory sense
   • pinch
   • two-point discrimination
   • prick
   • reflexes, particularly patellar and Achilles tendons
   • temperature sense
   Carefully examine the lesion
   • measure
   • stage
   • location
   • signs of infection
     • erythema
     • warmth
     • purulent drainage
     • foul-smelling odor
     • fever
     • chills
   Obtain a wound culture. Radiography is recommended for stage III or IV foot lesions to determine the presence of underlying osteomyelitis. Be sure to examine footwear. Are the shoes tight or worn? Is there an adequate toe box?

C. Patient education includes
   • adequate fluids/water of 8 cups (2 L) per day
   • elevation of affected extremities
   • foot hygiene (see the tool *Foot Care*, p. 60)
   • technique for daily inspections of skin and lesion
   • signs and symptoms of infection
   • proper application of Ace wrap or support stockings
   • wound care
   • proper sock and footwear (see p. 60)
   • trauma prevention
   • changes to report to the physician
   Even with the most vigorous management, foot ulcers take months to heal. Scar tissue under a healed neuropathic ulcer is not flexible, is susceptible to the stress of walking, and is at high risk for recurrence. Instruct patients to walk slowly, taking short steps when the ulcer is healed.

D. Local wound management requires cleaning and packing the wound to maintain cleanliness as healing occurs. Dressing changes are recommended at least twice daily and more often are based on the amount and character of drainage. Initial treatment may be

TABLE 1 Comparison of Neuropathic and Ischemic Lesions

Type	Location	Characteristics
Neuropathic	Plantar surface of foot Over bony prominence	Deep Surrounded by hyperkeratotic corn or callus Circulation usually not compromised Little or no sensation
Ischemic/vascular	Foot or ankle Below knee	Painful Evidence of decreased circulation "Punched-out," necrotic center with sharp margins

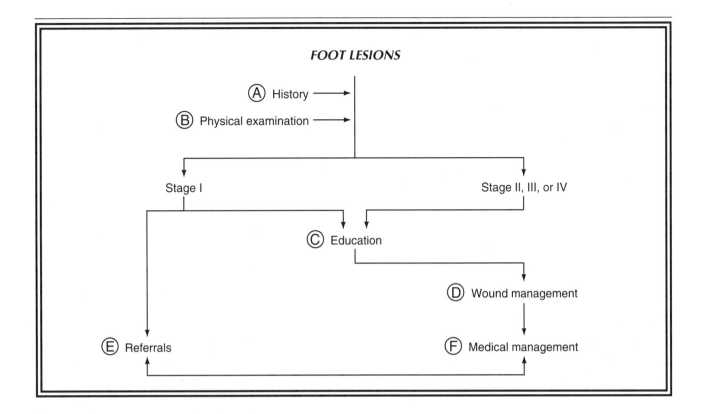

FOOT LESIONS

(A) History

(B) Physical examination

Stage I Stage II, III, or IV

(C) Education

(D) Wound management

(E) Referrals (F) Medical management

with mild soap and water followed by saline-soaked packing. Other types of cleansing agents or packing may be ordered, depending on physician preference or the results of wound cultures. The most important factor in healing a neuropathic lesion is to limit pressure to the area, usually weight-bearing. When possible, total bed rest is recommended. Therapeutic footwear or assistive devices to decrease pressure from walking may be used when bed rest is not possible. For ischemic lesions an Ace wrap or support stocking may help improve circulation. Care must be taken that such devices are not too tight or allowed to wrinkle, causing pressure or ulceration.

E. Consider referrals for any foot lesion. In most instances a physician or podiatrist order is required for other health care disciplines to be involved. Physical or occupational therapists can often manufacture a therapeutic sandal or insert to relieve pressure. Debridement of wounds can be done by physical therapists or skin/foot care practitioners. Social services may help the patient with funding for therapeutic shoes.

F. Medical management of antibiotic therapy is required in most settings. Surgical intervention, including incision and drainage as well as vascular bypass surgery, may also be necessary. Total contact casting provides a way to immobilize the foot and ankle movement in order to decrease the pressure on the ulcer, allowing ambulation while promoting healing.

References

Evanski PM. Disorders of the foot. Philadelphia: WB Saunders, 1982.

Gould JS. The foot book. Baltimore: Williams & Wilkins, 1988.

Miller RA, Evans WE. Nurse and patient: Allies preventing amputation. RN July 1988; 51(6):38−43.

FOOT PAIN/NUMBNESS

M. Elise Tidwell-Bissell

After the age of 65 years, three of every four adults complain of foot pain. Pain and numbness in the feet and legs may be caused by one or a combination of the following:
- peripheral vascular disease
- peripheral neuropathy
- malignancy
- spinal disorders

Peripheral vascular disease limits the blood supply to the lower extremities, producing leg and foot pain and prolonging wound healing. Neurologic deficits may affect sensory or motor function, often bilaterally and symmetrically.

A. Obtain information about the health history, such as
- chronic illnesses
  - diabetes
  - alcoholism
  - cancer
- circulatory problems
- medications
- hygiene habits
- restless leg syndrome

Try to determine the onset, duration, location, and when pain or numbness is experienced: at rest, when active, at night? Ask about
- symptoms of peripheral vascular disease
  - intermittent claudication
  - cold feet
  - nocturnal pain
- symptoms of peripheral neuropathy
  - tingling
  - burning
  - numbness
  - pain at rest

B. Observe the general appearance of the extremities with the patient's shoes and socks off, looking for
- shiny skin
- change in skin texture
- hair loss over the lower extremities
- deep red color when the feet are dependent
- edema
- changes in skin temperature
- areas of redness, pressure, or breakdown
- burns
- long, protruding toenails
- improperly trimmed nails, corns, or calluses

Check the pulses. A Doppler may be needed. Watch for color changes when the legs are elevated.

With a tuning fork, cotton ball, safety pin, and reflex hammer, test the sense of
- position
- vibration
- light touch
- pain
- temperature

Perform a neurologic examination to evaluate
- gait
- reflexes of knee and ankle

Examine shoes and socks for
- improper fit
- foreign objects
- curled threads in the socks

C. Surgical management is necessary for
- debridement of open wounds
- skin grafting or closure
- restoration of circulation, using vascular bypass

Determination of the cause of skin breakdown, whether vascular or neuropathic, will help guide the physician's course of action. Vascular compromise may not support healing in some cases and amputation may be the treatment selected. See Foot Lesions, p. 56, for alternative methods of treatment.

D. Prevention of skin breakdown requires
- patient/caregiver education
  - smoking cessation
  - weight reduction
  - foot care (see p. 60)
  - elimination of stockings or garters that impede circulation
- management of chronic illness
  - blood sugar control
  - alcohol abstinence
  - blood pressure control

E. Referrals may be made depending on the patient's need. Consider a podiatrist for patients who have poor eyesight, who cannot reach their feet, or who have severe neuropathy. Social services may be needed to facilitate the purchase of therapeutic footwear. A physician may be consulted when pain is so severe that it interferes with activities of daily living. Specific antidepressants are being tested for efficacy in treating neuropathic pain. Drugs may also be prescribed to enhance blood flow.

References

Kozak GP, Hoar CS, Rowbotham JL, et al. Management of diabetic foot problems. Philadelphia: WB Saunders, 1984.

Miller RA, Evans WE. Nurse and patient: Allies preventing amputation. RN July 1988; 51(6):38–43.

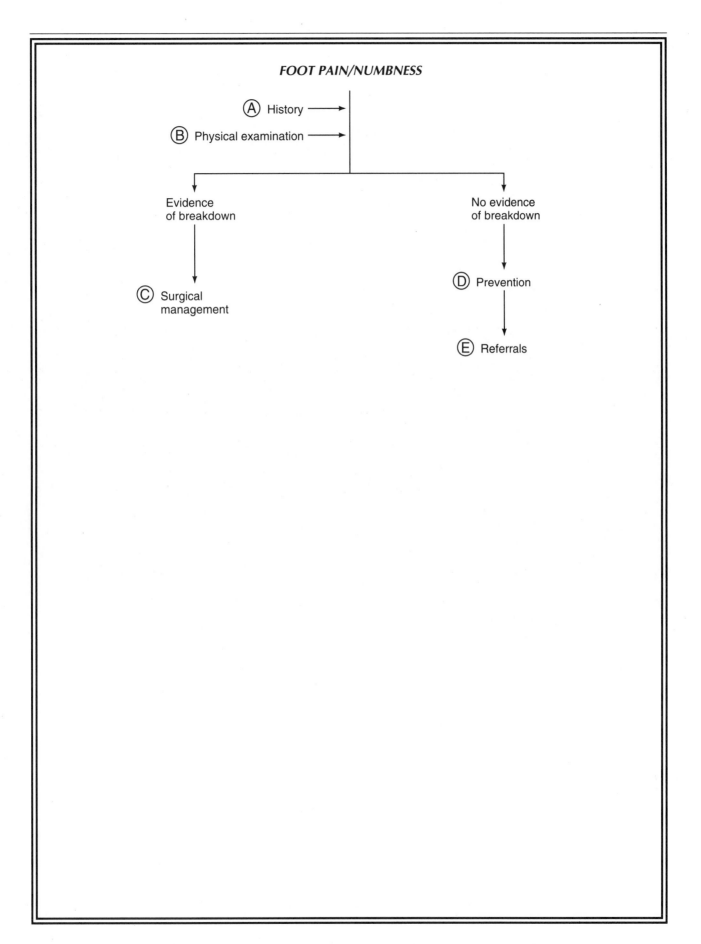

Foot Care

Topic	Content
Hygiene	1. Have someone with good eyesight check feet daily for redness, cuts, breakdown 2. Use warm, not hot water when washing feet (check temperature of water with hand or elbow) 3. Dry carefully between toes 4. Apply lotion to dry skin but not between toes 5. Use a pumice stone or emery board on corns or calluses after washing feet

Nail/foot care	1. Trim toenails straight across and even with tips of toes
	2. Have a professional treat corns and calluses
	3. Avoid
	  • razors
	  • salicylic acid pads
	  • over-the-counter corn and callus removers

General	1. Never walk barefoot 2. Avoid heating pads, hot water bottles, and heat lamps 3. Do not smoke 4. Avoid extreme cold 5. Avoid garters, tight or constricting stockings, knotting or use of elastic bands on stockings 6. Avoid getting a severe sunburn

Footwear and socks	1. Wear cotton socks whenever possible
	2. Change stockings or socks daily
	3. Wear socks inside out so seams cannot rub skin
	4. Check inside shoes visually and with fingers for rough spots or foreign bodies
	5. Buy shoes at end of day when feet may be swollen
	6. Test shoes on a hard surface as well as carpet
	7. Shoe characteristics
	  • wide, deep toe box
	  • leather or cloth that breathes
	  • soft, pliable shoe
	  • gridded or nonslip sole
	  • snug heels
	  • cushioning for comfort and shock absorption
	  • comfortable arch support

Balance and Gait

Maneuver	Instructions	Maneuver	Instructions

Patient is seated in hard armless chair.

1. Sitting balance
   - leans or slides in chair
   - steady, safe
2. Arise
   - unable without help
   - able but uses arms to help
   - able without use of arms
3. Attempts to arise
   - unable without help
   - able but requires more than one attempt
   - able to arise with one attempt

Attempt to get up with arms folded; patient should fold arms and then get up from chair; note the number of attempts

4. Immediate standing balance (first 5 seconds)
   - unsteady (staggers, moves feet, marked trunk sway)
   - steady but uses walker or cane, or grabs other object for support
   - steady without walker or cane or other support

With arms folded, the patient should rise and stand

5. Standing balance
   - unsteady
   - steady, but wide stance (medial heels more than 4" apart) or uses cane, walker, or other support
   - narrow stance without support

Give patient a chance to gain balance while standing and then instruct him or her to put feet as close together as possible

6. Nudge (patient at maximum position with feet as close together as possible; examiner pushes lightly on patient's sternum with palm of hand 3 times)
   - begins to fall
   - begins to fall, staggers, grabs, but catches self
   - steady

Instruct patient to stand with feet as close together as possible, then lightly push for about 2 seconds over the sternum; do not use sudden jerky motions

7. Neck (document exact symptoms)
   - symptoms or staggering with lateral movement or extension
   - marked decreased ROM but without symptoms or staggering
   - at least moderate ROM and steady

Instruct patient to turn head from side to side as far as possible and look up as far as possible

8. Eyes closed
   - unsteady
   - steady
9. Turn 360 degrees
   - discontinuous steps
   - continuous
   - unsteady (grabs, staggers)
   - steady

Self-explanatory

10. Able to stand on one leg for 5 seconds
    - symptoms or staggering with lateral movement or extension
    - marked decreased ROM but without symptoms or staggering
    - at least moderate ROM and steady

Instruct patient to turn head from side to side as far as possible and look up as far as possible

11. Back extension (let patient alone)
    - refuses to try, no extension, or uses walker while doing it
    - tries but little extension
    - good extension

Instruct patients to extend backward as far as possible

12. Reaching up (have patient reach to a high shelf)
    - unable or unstable, needs to hold on to steady self
    - able to reach up and is stable

Have patient take something down from a high shelf

13. Bending over (place pen on floor and ask patient to pick it up)
    - unable or is unsteady
    - able and is steady

Self-explanatory

14. Sit down
    - unsafe (misjudges distance, falls into chair)
    - uses chair
    - uses arms or not a smooth motion
    - safe, smooth motion

Self-explanatory

15. Turning
    - staggers, unsteady
    - discontinuous but no staggering, or uses walker or cane
    - steady, continuous
16. Able to pick up walking speed (tell patient to walk as fast as he or she can—a pace at which he or she feels *safe*)
    - None
    - Some
    - Marked
17. Is walking aid used appropriately?
    - No
    - Yes
    - Not applicable
18. Trunk
    - Asymmetric
    - Symmetric

Maneuvers are used as a structured evaluation of gait and balance. From Tinetti ME, Ginter SF. Identifying mobility dysfunctions in elderly patients: Standard neuromuscular examination or direct assessment? JAMA 1988, 259:1190; Copyright 1988, American Medical Association; with permission.

Get Up and Go Test

Purpose:
Measures risk of falling by assessing balance and sway during performance of specific tasks

Steps:
Instruct the patient to do the following:
1. Sit in a straight-backed chair with a firm, high seat, 10 feet from and facing a wall
2. Get up, stand still for a moment
3. Walk toward the wall; turn without touching the wall
4. Walk back to the chair
5. Turn around
6. Sit down

Rating:
1 = normal (indicates no risk of a fall)
2 = very slightly abnormal   ⎫ Correlates with incremental potential for a fall, with observation on
3 = mildly abnormal   ⎬ testing of slowness, gait disturbances, difficulty initiating movement,
4 = moderately abnormal   ⎭ or balance problems.
5 = severely abnormal   (indicates a high risk of falling observed during performance of the test)

From Mathias S, Nayak USL, Isaacs B. Balance in elderly patients: The "get up and go" test. Arch Phys Med Rehabil 1986; 67:387; with permission.

Romberg Test

Purpose:
To assess proprioception

Steps:
Instruct patient in the following procedure:
1. Stand, feet together, without support
   - the clinician should stand near the patient, with arms encompassing but not touching, ready to prevent a fall
2. Keep the eyes open, then close them
   - the clinician observes the patient's ability to maintain balance

Rating:
Normal = only slight swaying

Cerebellar ataxia = difficulty standing with eyes open and closed

Impaired proprioception or a positive Romberg test = standing position is maintained with the eyes open; balance is lost when the eyes are closed.

Proper Sizing of Canes

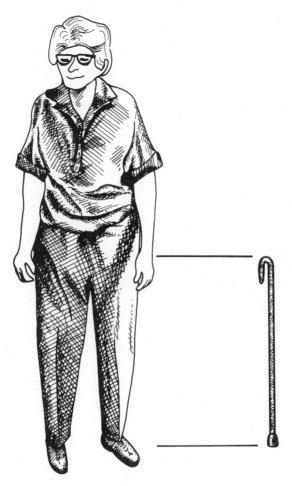

Proper Sizing and Use of Standard Walker

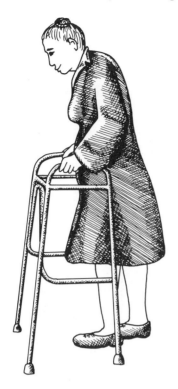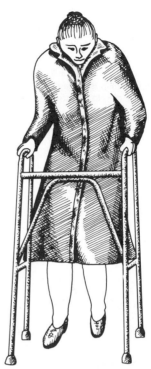

Measuring Muscle Strength or Endurance

Test	Technique	Grading/Scoring	Comments
Muscle strength	Have patient resist movement of a joint (see the tool *Muscle Strength Testing*, on facing page)	0 = paralysis/inability to resist gravity	Tests resistance to movement
		1 = muscle tightens but cannot resist movement	
Hand strength (grip)	Have patient squeeze examiner's crossed fingers	2 = muscle tightens and provides minimal resistance	
		3 = muscle provides initial resistance but not able to sustain for 10 sec	
		4 = muscle provides resistance but not able to sustain for 10 sec	
		5 = muscle able to resist movement for 15–30 sec	
Endurance	Have patient perform arm or leg lifts while in a comfortable position	Record number of repetitions done	Be alert to possibility of fatigue-related fall or injury
		Compare left to right side scores	Consider how cardiovascular or metabolic problems may affect endurance

Muscle Strength Testing

(⇐ indicates pressure from examiner)

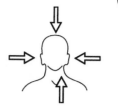

Neck

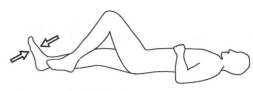

Ankle/Foot

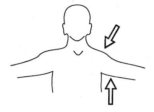

Shoulder

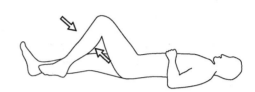

Knee

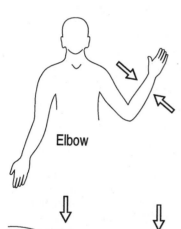

Elbow

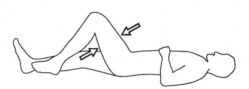

Hip/Abdomen

Side | Front

Hand

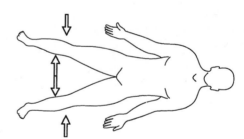

Hip abduction/adduction

MEDICATION

ADVERSE DRUG REACTIONS

Linda Tarkowski

An adverse drug reaction (ADR) is defined as any noxious or unintended response to a medication. ADRs are characterized by severity (mild, moderate, severe) and by mechanism (type A—dose dependent, predictable, preventable—and type B—idiosyncratic, not dose dependent, and not related to a drug's pharmacologic characteristics). Elderly patients are at increased risk for ADRs because of
- multiple disease states and medications
- age-related physiologic changes
- impaired kidney function
- altered receptor sensitivity

Drugs or drug classes most often associated with adverse effects in elderly persons include
- digoxin
- anticholinergics
- benzodiazepines
- systemic steroids
- nonsteroidal anti-inflammatory drugs
- antihypertensives (e.g., beta-blockers, calcium channel blockers)
- psychotropics

(See the tool *Common Medications and Side Effects*, p. 76).

A. Determine relationship between symptoms and a specific medication. Inquire about
- rash or pruritus
- chest pain or palpitations
- nausea, vomiting, abdominal pain
- constipation, diarrhea
- change in appetite
- symptoms of depression, sleep disorders
- visual changes, dry mouth
- blood in stool or urine
- urinary retention
- orthostatic hypotension
- shakiness, weakness, falls
- drowsiness, sedation

Ask questions to determine
- onset
- duration
- compliance with prescribed regimen
- relationship to drug or meal administration

Determine health history, drug allergies, and drug hypersensitivities. Obtain a complete list of medications, both prescribed and over-the-counter drugs. Match each medication to a diagnosis or a target symptom.

B. Assess patient by review of systems:
- general appearance—extrapyramidal movements
- vital signs—elevated or decreased blood pressure, orthostatic hypotension, tachycardia or bradycardia, tachypnea, fever
- oral—gum or tongue irritation or lesions (see Mouth Lesions/Ulcers, p. 174, and Gum Irritation/Gingivitis, p. 172)
- cardiac status—history of arrhythmias
- skin—rashes, lesions, discoloration, bruises, induration or inflammation
- GI—stool for occult blood
- neurologic
  - cognition or behavior
    - confusion
    - delirium
    - agitation
    - altered level of consciousness
  - gait
  - bradykinesis
  - tremor
  - rigidity
  - motor strength
  - peripheral neuropathy

Useful laboratory determinations include
- electrolytes (especially Na and K)
- complete blood count, hemoglobin and hematocrit
- lipid profile
- prothrombin time/partial thromboplastin time (PT/PTT)
- glucose
- serum creatinine, blood urea nitrogen
- liver function tests

C. FDA form 1639 is used only to report (1) serious events that are not included in the official drug labeling, (2) a *cluster* of serious labeled events, and (3) all serious events associated with newly marketed drugs. Serious events include those that result in or prolong hospitalization, are life-threatening, or contribute to significant disability or death. If a serious ADR occurs, the prescriber or a clinical pharmacist should assist in the reporting process. The patient's medical record must be accurately updated to avoid future drug misadventures with the same or similar agents. The patient and caregiver should be appropriately informed. In the hospital setting, *all* ADRs should be reported via the hospital-wide ADR monitoring program.

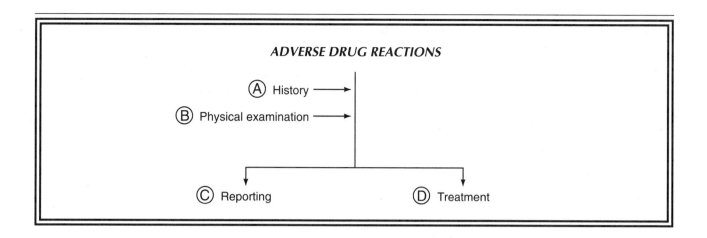

ADVERSE DRUG REACTIONS

A. History

B. Physical examination

C. Reporting

D. Treatment

D. Allergic drug reactions (usually type B) often resolve promptly once the offending medication is discontinued. Treatment includes
- discontinuation of the suspected drug or *all* drugs not absolutely necessary
- supportive care, which may include antihistamines, epinephrine
- if not contraindicated, fluids, which may enhance elimination
- steroids, which may be required for persistent or severe ADR

Common adverse reactions (type A) are usually managed by

- modifying (usually reducing) the dose
- changing to a different medication
- altering the dosage schedule
- adding another medication

References

Brocklehurst JC, ed. Geriatric pharmacology and therapeutics. Boston: Blackwell Scientific Publications, 1984.

Lamy PP. Adverse drug effects. Clin Geriatr Med 1990; 6:293.

Pagliaro LA, Pagliaro AM. Pharmacologic aspects of aging. St. Louis: CV Mosby, 1983.

DRUG INTERACTIONS

Linda Tarkowski

It is estimated that patients aged 65 years and older consume >25% of all prescription and nonprescription drugs dispensed. Approximately 30% of all geriatric hospital admissions are due to drug-related problems. Drug interactions play a key role. Drug interactions may exist between drugs or between foods and drugs. Interactions may affect drug absorption, distribution, metabolism, or elimination, causing enhanced or reduced effect, prolonged or shortened activity, or increased or decreased drug clearance.

A. Obtain a complete and accurate list of all medications the patient is currently taking:
   - Use the "brown bag" method. Ask patients to bring along all their medications for review. It is important to ask patients how they are currently taking each medication.
   - Prompt the patient about over-the-counter drugs, e.g., pain relievers, antacids, cough and cold preparations, laxatives.
   - Give specific examples: "Do you take nonprescription pain relievers such as Tylenol, Bayer, Anacin?"
   - Clarify and quantify directions such as "as needed" or "as directed."

Obtain a nutrition history, including use of caffeine and alcohol and the relationship of meals to medications, and ask about food choices with potential for food and drug interactions.

TABLE 1 Significant Medication Interactions

Class	Drug	Interacts with	Food Precautions
Anticonvulsant	Carbamazepine (Tegretol)	Erythromycin Isoniazid	None
Antimanic	Lithium	Thiazides	Avoid large fluctuations in daily salt intake.
Monoamine oxidase (MAO) inhibitors	Phenelzine (Nardil) Tranylcypromine (Parnate) Isocarboxazid (Marplan)	Fluoxetine Meperidine Decongestants	Avoid tyramine-containing foods (see the tool *Food and Drug Interaction*, p. 78)
H_2 blocker	Cimetidine (Tagamet)	Theophylline Warfarin Benzodiazepines Antiarrhythmics	None
Cardiac	Digoxin (Lanoxin)	Quinidine	None
Electrolyte replacement	Potassium	Amiloride Spironolactone Triamterene	None (see the tools *Food and Drug Interaction*, pp. 78, 79)
Antituberculosis	Isoniazid (INH)	Phenytoin Carbamazepine	Avoid alcohol
Bronchodilator	Theophylline	Cimetidine Erythromycin Ciprofloxacin Tobacco	Take with food
Anticoagulant	Warfarin	Amiodarone Antithyroid drugs Barbiturates Cimetidine Metronidazole Nonsteroidal anti-inflammatory drugs Rifampin Salicylates Sulfonamides Thyroid hormones	None

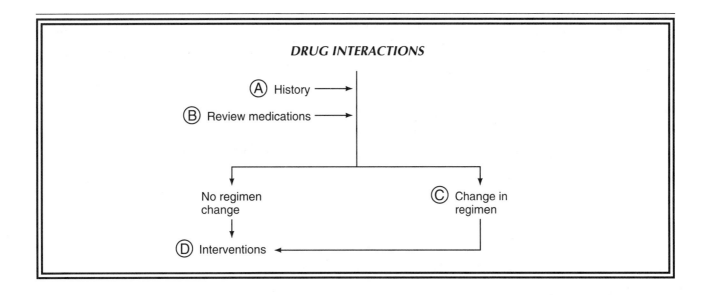

DRUG INTERACTIONS

(A) History

(B) Review medications

No regimen change

(C) Change in regimen

(D) Interventions

B. Match each medication to a specific condition or diagnosis described in the medical history. Identify medications that have no clear indication for use. Look for therapeutic duplication (e.g., ibuprofen and indomethacin). Scan the medication regimen for agents well documented in the drug-interaction literature (Table 1). If you suspect a drug interaction, consult your clinical pharmacist for additional information. Patients receiving multiple drug therapy with anticholinergic, antihistaminic, sedative, and/or alpha-blocking properties are at increased risk for dramatic side effects. This type of interaction is termed synergistic.

C. Any time a medication is added or deleted or a dose is changed, the symptom or condition that prompted the change should be reassessed. Laboratory determinations may include therapeutic drug levels, creatinine, blood urea nitrogen, and electrolytes.

D. Teach patient and caregiver about medications ordered:
- dosage regimen
- schedule
- food precautions
- purpose of medication
- potential side effects (warnings)
- stress compliance

Use a nonthreatening, nonjudgmental approach to detect noncompliance with medication regimen (see

---

Ways to Improve Compliance

Provide simple, clear instructions.
Ask patients to repeat instructions in their own words.
Periodically repeat instructions to patient.
Provide written instructions.
Assess hearing, vision, and memory loss. If necessary
- provide special instructions for the hearing impaired
- use large type to facilitate reading of written instructions
- involve family member or other caregiver in management of medication
Use established daily routines for taking medications (e.g., mealtimes).
Develop new daily routines for taking medications (use calendars, charts).
Simplify regimen where possible.
Monitor for side effects.
Invite questions.
Encourage patients to participate in their own health care.
Encourage practitioners to write the purpose of the medication on the prescription in simple terms, e.g., "for heart," "for diabetes."

---

boxes). Techniques include
- oblique questioning, e.g., "Most people have trouble remembering to take all of their medications. Do you have trouble remembering yours?"
- pill counts
- blood levels or urine assays
- prescription refill records

Reasons for Poor Compliance

Many medications prescribed
Complexity of medication regimen
Cognitive decline, poor recall
Physical limitations (failing eyesight, hearing loss)
Expense of medications
Safety-closure containers
Actual or perceived adverse drug reactions
Psychiatric diagnosis
Social isolation
Inadequate medication instructions

References

Carty MA, Everitt DE. Basic principles of prescribing for geriatric outpatients. Geriatrics 1989; 44:85.

Cooper JW. Reviewing geriatric concerns with commonly used drugs. Geriatrics 1989; 44:79.

Gainsborough N, Powell-Jackson P. Prescribing for the elderly. Practitioner 1990; 234:246.

Stewart RB, Caranasos GJ. Medication compliance in the elderly. Med Clin North Am 1989; 73:1551.

Yuen GJ. Altered pharmacokinetics in the elderly. Clin Geriatr Med 1990; 6:257.

POLYPHARMACY

Sue Miller

Polypharmacy is the use of two or more medications
- for no apparent clinical reason
- for the same purpose
- that interact
- to treat adverse reactions from another medication

The result is a combination that may interfere with or potentiate the effects of one or both drugs. Most elderly people take three to five prescribed medications a day. The risk of polypharmacy increases in proportion to the number of medications taken. Nearly one third of the elderly have adverse drug reactions because of
- multiple disease states
- use of multiple physicians
- the potential for interaction between prescription drugs and over-the-counter medications
- physiologic changes associated with aging that increase the half-life of medications taken
  - decreased body fluid
  - decreased hepatic blood flow
  - increased total body fat
  - decreased glomerular filtration rate

Cardiovascular drugs and diuretics account for the largest percentage of prescribed medications. Common over-the-counter drugs are vitamins, analgesics, antacids, and laxatives. Most of these affect body fluid distribution, stomach pH, and blood chemistry, which can alter the absorption, distribution, and elimination of other drugs taken.

A. Review all drugs.
- prescriptions
- over the counter
- alcohol intake
- caffeine use
- illicit drug use
- use of tobacco products

Ask questions to assess the patient or caregiver's ability to understand, speak, and read English and label instructions. Many medication errors may occur because of illiteracy and small print. Try to actually see all bottles. Determine whether the patient or caregiver knows about the medications currently being used with regard to

- purpose and action
- dosage and administration schedule
- adverse reactions
- precautions
- food and drug interactions
- storage

Was the medication prescribed for an acute problem that has now resolved? Was it prescribed to treat an adverse reaction to another drug? Is there a clinical indication for the medication? Obtain a health history. Ask about physiologic changes
- in bowel function
- in appetite
- in taste (see Taste Changes, p. 136)
- in smell (see Decreased Sense of Smell, p. 126)
- in hearing (see Hearing Loss, p. 122)
- rash (see Eczema/Rashes/Dermatitis p. 104)
- in vision
- in sexuality

Explore psychosocial issues with regard to
- previous coping methods
- past and present social activities
- recent changes
  - losses
  - isolationism

B. Look for symptoms of adverse drug effects (Table 1). These are easiest to determine if baseline data are available.

C. Pharmacist drug review provides information on
- identification of potential drug-drug interactions
- indications for use of a drug or dose
- length of appropriate therapy
- ways to avoid duplication
- ways to cut costs for medications by substituting generics

Concurrent review of medications as they are ordered can prevent adverse drug reactions. This process is much easier in the hospital or nursing home than in the community because of the decreased availability of other sources.

Text continued on page 74.

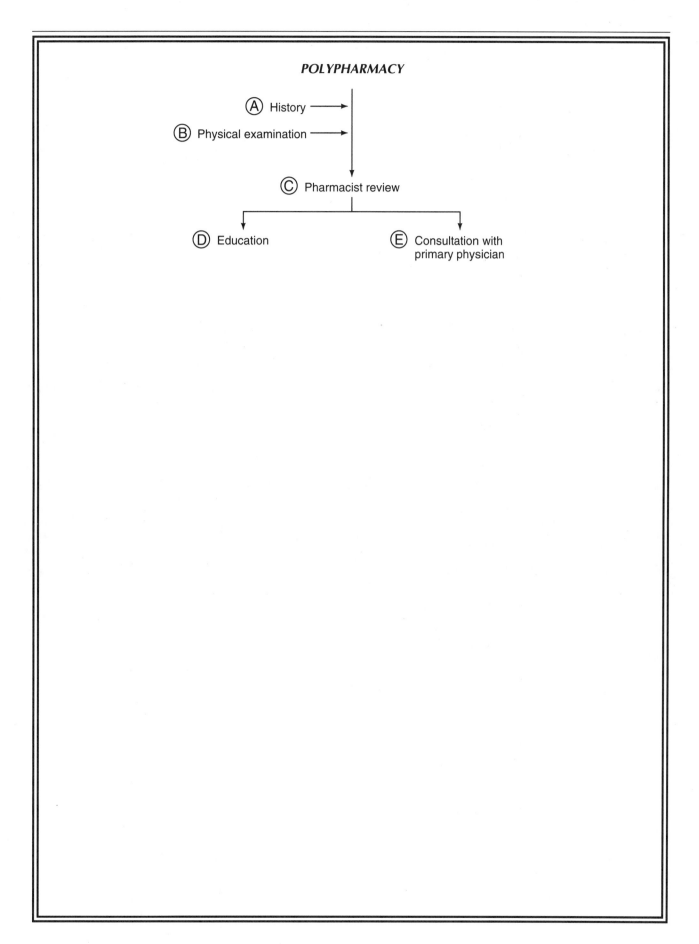

POLYPHARMACY

Ⓐ History

Ⓑ Physical examination

Ⓒ Pharmacist review

Ⓓ Education

Ⓔ Consultation with primary physician

TABLE 1 Symptoms of Adverse Drug Effect

System	Symptom	Examination Tips
Cardiovascular	Tachycardia Bradycardia ECG changes Arrhythmias Orthostatic hypotension Edema (see p. 10)	• Do not rely on radial pulse, check apical heart rate for 60 sec • Check orthostatic blood pressure, allowing patient to remain in each position at least 2 min
CNS	Lethargy Sedation Fatigue (see p. 14) Headache Confusion (see Confusion/Cognitive Changes/ Dementia, p. 254) Behavioral changes Ataxia Dizziness (see p. 140) Hyperactive reflexes Hypoactive reflexes	• Evaluate gait, balance, and coordination with heel to toe walking, observing patient getting out of a chair • Test mental status using tools available in Cognition/Perception section, pp. 268–273
Gastrointestinal	Dry mouth Constipation (see p. 184) Diarrhea (see p. 186) Changes in appetite	• Observe oral mucosa

Senses
  Ears
  Eyes
 	
  Nose
 	
  Mouth
 	
  Skin
	
	Ototoxicity
	Dry, irritated
	Dilated pupils
	Pinpoint pupils
	Blurred vision
	Loss or decreased sense of smell (see p. 126)
	Nasal congestion
	Decreased sense of taste (see Taste Changes,
	   p. 136)
	Slurred speech
	Garbled speech
	Fixed rash
	Diffuse rash
		• Have patient wear dentures, eye glasses, and hearing aid during examination
		
		• Pay particular attention to areas that receive sun exposure

Laboratory Tests	Abnormal finding	
Hematology	Anemia Decreased platelet count Elevated or decreased WBC High or low sedimentation rate	
Chemistry	Electrolyte imbalance Elevated or decreased BUN Elevated blood glucose Elevated creatinine High or low calcium High or low phosphorus High or low bilirubin (total, direct or indirect)	
Hormonal	High or low TSH Positive ANA	
Urine	High or low urine pH Elevated creatinine clearance	
Stool	Positive for occult blood	
Therapeutic drug levels	Not in therapeutic range	

TABLE 2 Patient Teaching to Prevent/Reduce Polypharmacy

Subject	Content	Rationale
Specific medication	Name Purpose Dose Schedule	Adult learning principle that knowledge will enhance compliance
Drug interactions	Physiology of absorption and excretion Side effects of prescribed drugs Effects that foods and fluids have on absorption	Provide information for informed decision making
Safety	Storage Child-proofing	Prevent degradation of medications and accidental injury to others
Alternatives to medication use	Exercise program Nutrition Use of heat and/or cold Relaxation exercises	Reduce need for multiple medication use

D. Teaching should focus on ways to prevent misuse of or noncompliance with medication regimens and to optimize drug effects (Table 2). All information should be geared to the ability of the patient or caregiver to learn and read instructions. Written information, when given, is not useful unless it is at the appropriate reading level and in a simple, direct form. Patients with little or no formal education, for whom English is not a primary or native language, or who have no dependable support system may have special educational needs. Pill containers may be helpful to remind patients to take medications as prescribed. Manufactured pill containers are available at pharmacies, grocery stores, discount stores, and through the mail. Containers can also be made at home with an empty egg carton or cups. Reminder systems may include
- calendar check-off systems
- printed medication charts (see p. 77)
- calls from members of the support system

Monitoring can be done by
- preparing medications in advance and placing in a container
- counting the number of pills left in the bottle
- reviewing any check-off system

Color coding medication bottles, with colored dots matched to a medication chart, may assist the illiterate or those with poor vision. Encouraging the patient or caregiver to have all prescriptions filled at the same pharmacy can enhance the pharmacist connection. The pharmacist can then
- remind the patient of medication schedules
- watch for potential drug interactions
- give advice on appropriate over-the-counter agents

E. Consultation with the primary physician is necessary when
- symptoms of drug interaction exist
- drug dosages need to be adjusted
  - drug toxicity
  - enhanced effect
  - decreased effect
- new symptoms occur requiring intervention

References

Hussey L, Gilliland K. Compliance, low literacy, and locus of control. Nurs Clin North Am 1989; 24:605.

Williams P, Rush DR. Geriatric polypharmacy. Hosp Pharm 1986; February:109.

Commonly Used Drugs and Their Potential Side Effects

Drugs	Side Effects
Anticonvulsants (in general)	Sedation
Antidepressants	Sedation
Antihypertensives (in general)	Sexual dysfunction
Antisecretories (oxybutynin, belladonna)	Urinary retention, constipation, increased delirium or dementia
Antipsychotics	
Chlorpromazine, thioridazine	Sedation, hypotension, anticholinergic effect
Haloperidol	Extrapyramidal symptoms
Benzodiazepines	CNS depression, worsened dementia, sleep disorders, increased falls or fractures, sedation
Beta-blockers	Lethargy, depression, heart block, decreased hypoglycemic response
Codeine and derivatives	Delirium, sedation, constipation
Digoxin	Anorexia, weight loss, electrocardiographic changes
Ethanol (alcohol)	Sedation, diuretic effect, depression, decreased appetite
Iron supplements	Constipation
K-sparing diuretics	Hyperkalemia
+K supplement	Hyperkalemia
Meperidine	Excitation or confusion, anticholinergic effect
Methyldopa	Depression
Metoclopramide	Dystonias
Mineral oil laxative	Possible aspiration, decreased absorption of fat-soluble vitamins (A,D,E)
Misoprostol	Diarrhea
Nifedipine	Peripheral edema
Nitroglycerin	Orthostatic hypotension, headache
NSAIDs (e.g., ibuprofen, naproxen)	GI bleeding, anemia, fluid retention, impaired kidney function, constipation, increased bleeding tendency
Quinidine	Tinnitus, GI upset, light-headedness
Steroids (long-term, p.o.)	GI bleeding, loss of diabetic control, infection, osteoporosis, psychiatric disturbances, fluid retention
Tetracycline	Photosensitivity
Trazodone	Sedation, priapism
Tricyclics (especially amitriptyline)	Dry mouth, urinary retention, constipation, sedation
Verapamil	Constipation
Warfarin	Bruising, bleeding
Caffeine	Diuretic effect, CNS stimulant, cardiostimulant, sleeplessness, exacerbation of incontinence
Tobacco	Worsened pulmonary function

Medication Teaching Sheet

Reason for Taking	Example of Pill	Name of Pill	No. of Pills	Times		Patient's Name:						Date:		

Food and Drug Interaction Information for Tranylcypromine (Parnate) Phenelzine (Nardil)

Your doctor has ordered a monamine-oxidase (MAO) inhibitor for you.

To prevent headaches, flushing, confusion, vision problems, and high blood pressure, you should avoid foods containing tyramine, such as:
  Cheese
  Smoked or pickled fish
  Processed meats
  Liver
  Broad beans
  Italian green beans
  Meat extracts
  Yeast extracts
  Brewers' yeast
  Fermented sausage
    Bologna
    Pastrami
    Salami
  Meat tenderizers
  Soy sauce
  Yogurt
  Sour cream
  Broth
  Bouillon
  Alcoholic beverages
    Ale
    Beer
    Chianti
    Sherry
    Sauterne
    Reisling wine

Please ask your doctor, nurse, or pharmacist if you have questions.

Food and Drug Interaction Information for Hydrochlorothiazide

Your doctor has ordered a diuretic (water pill) for you.

Please take this medicine with food.

Follow what your doctor says about using salt substitute or taking potassium supplements while on this medicine.

If your doctor asks you to eat foods high in potassium, use:
Potatoes
Fresh fruits
Fruit juices
Green vegetables
Dried beans
Dried peas
Milk

Please ask your doctor, nurse, or pharmacist if you have questions.

SLEEP/REST

SEDATION

Paula Tosch

Sedation may reflect dysfunction of one or many systems. It may refer to a variety of conditions, including fatigue, lethargy, and malaise. It may also signal a change in neurologic status.

A. History taking for sedation should include a review of
   • medications
   • environment
   • medical conditions and chronic diseases
   • sleep habits
   • nutrition, including 24-hour recall
   • impact on functioning and determination of changes in any of these factors

   Elicit information concerning onset, pattern of occurrence, and duration of sedation as well as patient/caregiver perception of the problem.

B. Physical examination should include weight, vital signs, and temperature. The neurologic examination evaluates
   • level of consciousness
   • focal findings
   • mental status (see Confusion/Cognitive Changes/Dementia, p. 254)

   Diagnostic testing is used to pinpoint or rule out systemic disease. Laboratory tests ordered usually include CBC with differential, urinalysis, serum electrolytes with BUN and creatinine, blood glucose, thyroid profile, toxicology or therapeutic drug screen, and arterial blood gases. An ECG may be warranted if there is bradycardia or a positive cardiac history. If the physical examination reveals pulmonary findings, obtain an order for a chest film.

C. If the patient is found to be unstable at the time of examination, emergency treatment is warranted. Take care to maintain an open airway and monitor vital signs until medical treatment is started.

D. Medical evaluation may be indicated if there are physiologic findings. If the history demonstrates a sleep pattern disturbance, electrophysiologic testing, including an electroencephalography and sleep studies, may be indicated.

E. Health maintenance includes continuing positive health behaviors, preventing new problems, and decreasing the risk of injury. Promoting a safe environment, meaningful activity, medication knowledge, and adherence are aspects of health maintenance. Collaboration with social service and community agency representatives may be indicated to facilitate patient well-being. In case a medical or emotional crisis occurs, emergency telephone numbers or procedures should be pre-established with the patient or caregiver and be immediately accessible.

References

Matteson MA, McConnell ES. Gerontological nursing, concepts and practice. Philadelphia: WB Saunders, 1988.

Watson CA, Wyatt NN. Altered levels of awareness. In: Concepts common to acute illness: Identification and management. St. Louis: CV Mosby, 1981:151.

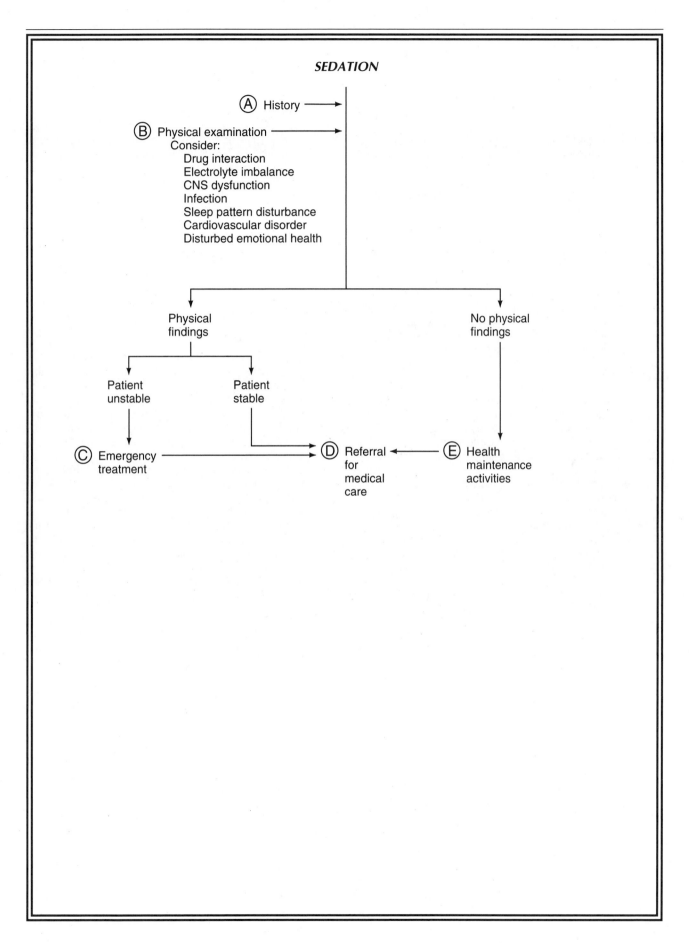

SEDATION

(A) History

(B) Physical examination
Consider:
    Drug interaction
    Electrolyte imbalance
    CNS dysfunction
    Infection
    Sleep pattern disturbance
    Cardiovascular disorder
    Disturbed emotional health

Physical findings

No physical findings

Patient unstable

Patient stable

(C) Emergency treatment

(D) Referral for medical care

(E) Health maintenance activities

SLEEP PATTERN DISTURBANCE

Paula Tosch

Sleep is divided into rapid eye movement (REM) and non–REM (NREM) sleep. NREM sleep is further divided into four stages (Table 1). In the elderly there is an increase of stages 1 and 2 and a decrease of stages 3 and 4. By age 50 years, stage 4 sleep is reduced by half. Generally, older persons take more time to fall asleep and have more frequent awakenings. Total sleep time may decrease slightly, but more time may be spent in bed either awake or napping. Sleep pattern disturbance is a disruption in a patient's typical pattern of sleep and wakefulness that causes discomfort and interferes with functioning. The sleep complaint may be too much or too little sleep. Symptoms include complaints of excessive daytime sleepiness or sleep attacks, leg movements during sleep, morning headaches, awakening earlier or later than desired, and a feeling of not being well rested.

A. History should elicit
   • normal sleep pattern
   • frequency of occurrence of disturbance
   • changes in behavior or function
   • onset and duration of disturbance
   • exacerbating and palliative measures
   • chronic diseases and related symptoms that may interfere with sleep
   • whether the patient feels rested or tired
   • whether injury has occurred
   • type of deviation from normal
   • severity of disturbance
   • medications
   Gather information from sleep partner or caregiver about behavior during sleep.

B. Clinical signs to be assessed include
   • dark circles under eyes
   • thickened speech
   • level of consciousness
   • dysarthria
   • yawning
   • tremor
   • nystagmus
   • obesity
   Evaluate mental status (see the tools in the section Cognition/Perception, pp. 268–273) to look for agitation, anxiety, irritability, or confusion. Laboratory evaluation may not be indicated until the sleep disorder is classified.

C. A sleep diary is helpful in differentiating the type of sleep disturbance. Both the patient and sleep partner are asked to record information about physical and mental activities, meals, and sleep and rest activities.

D. Disorders of the sleep-wake schedule occur when the patient's circadian rhythm does not match society's timetable for sleep. It may occur transiently in persons experiencing long-distance travel or long-term shift work. The latter is not common in the elderly.

E. Disorders of Initiating and Maintaining Sleep (DIMS) denote insomnia or poor sleep at night. Disorders of Excessive Somnolence (DOES) reflect conditions of pathologic daytime sleeping (Table 2). DOES, which are usually chronic and unlikely to cause injury or lifestyle changes, are hypersomnia and nocturnal myoclonus. Hypersomnia is chronic, uncontrollable drowsiness that occurs regardless of the sleep experienced. Spontaneous, uninterrupted sleep may last 12 to 20 hours. Patients are often confused and disoriented after awakening. Hypersomnolence may be the precursor of decreased consciousness and coma in certain medical crises, such as congestive heart failure, hypertension, increased intracranial pressure, polycythemia, uremia, drug intoxication, hypothyroidism, or diabetic acidosis, and emergent treatment is indicated. Nocturnal myoclonus is unilateral or bilateral jerks consisting of extension of the big toe and partial flexion of the ankle, knee, and sometimes the hip during sleep. It is followed by a partial awakening. Nocturnal myoclonus is associated with complaints of insomnia or daytime fatigue. Patients do not complain of sore legs, but bed partners report kicking.

F. Certain sleep pattern disturbances can cause changes in lifestyle or potential for injury. They include parasomnias such as sleep walking, sleep apnea, and narcolepsy. Lifestyle changes brought about by these disorders may be social isolation due to chronic fatigue and/or fear of injury or embarrassment, change in sleeping arrangements, and inability to participate in activities.

G. Patients should be taught that sleep behavior changes with age. Awakenings are often normal and do not impair the effectiveness of the whole sleep cycle.

Text continued on page 84.

SLEEP PATTERN DISTURBANCE

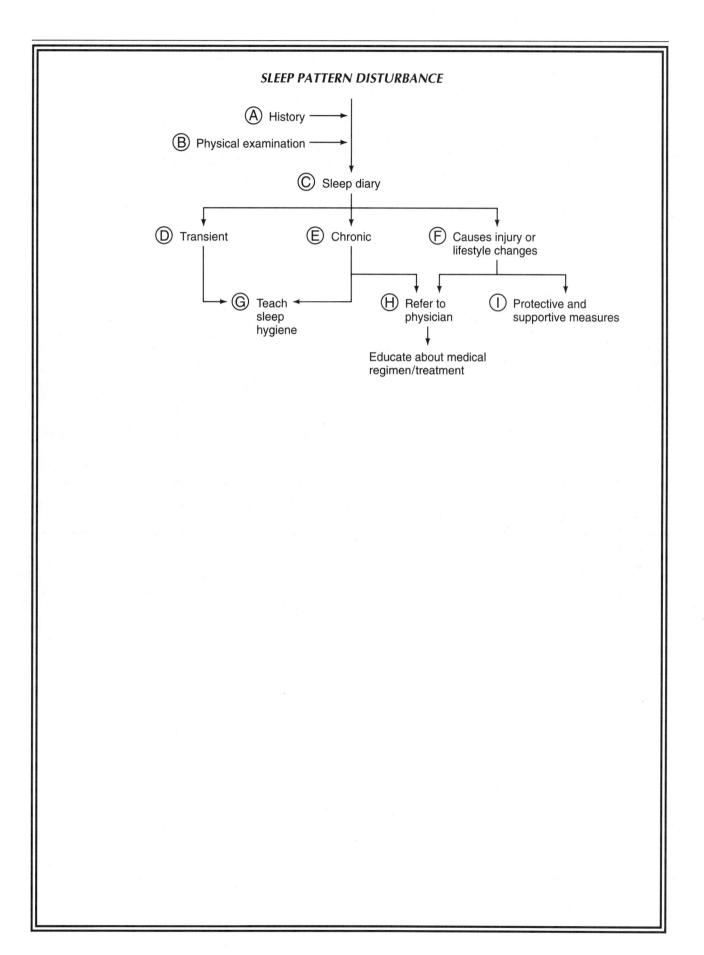

TABLE 1   Stages of Sleep and Changes in the Elderly

Stage	Definition	Characteristics	Changes in Elderly
NREM			
1	Light sleep	Drifting, easy awakening	Increased duration
2	Light sleep	Greater relaxation; short thoughts	More frequent awakenings in this stage
3	Slow wave or deep sleep	First phase of deep sleep; decreased pulse, temperature; muscle relaxation	No change
4	Deep sleep	Decreased pulse, blood pressure, respiration, metabolism; associated with restoration	Reduced by 50% by 50 years of age; almost absent in old age
REM	Deepest level of relaxation	Rapid Eye Movement sleep; muscle relaxation; increased oxygen consumption, pulse, blood pressure	Decreased proportion; distribution more uniform

TABLE 2   Sleep Disturbances

Classification	Disorder	Definition	Treatment
Disorders of Initiating and Maintaining Sleep (DIMS)	Insomnia	Recurring shortfall of sleep manifested by problems falling asleep, frequent awakenings, and waking early	Sleep hygiene
Disorders of Excessive Somnolence (DOES)	Narcolepsy	Uncontrollable recurrent attacks of deep sleep occurring during the day	Methylphenidate Amphetamines
	Sleep apnea	Apnea occuring soon after falling asleep with breathing resuming when the patient wakes up	Sleep position
	Hypersomnia	Chronic uncontrollable drowsiness despite amount of sleep obtained	Methysergide
	Nocturnal myoclonus	Unilateral or bilateral lower extremity jerking during sleep, followed by partial awakening	Clonazepam
Dysfunctions associated with sleep, sleep stages, or partial arousals (parasomnias)	Somnambulism	Sleep walking or performing complex acts while asleep with no recollection of event	Protection
	Disorders of sleep-wake schedule	Transient mismatch metween patient's circadian rhythm and society's timetable	

Individual sleep habits vary. If a patient is not adversely affected or disturbing family or caretakers by adhering to a reversal of day and night activities, a change in regimen is not indicated. Sleep hygiene education may be helpful (see the tool *Helpful Hints for a Good Night's Sleep,* p. 86).

H. Referral to a physician is necessary to make a differential diagnosis and to institute medication when appropriate. Care must be taken that a prescription for sedatives or sleeping medications is not viewed as a panacea. Medical work-up may include
   - arterial blood gases
   - complete blood count
   - toxicology screen
   - electrocardiogram
   - pulmonary function tests
   - electrolytes, glucose, blood urea nitrogen
   - computed tomography
   - ear, nose, and throat studies

   Polysomnography, the monitoring during sleep of several biologic variables and their relationships, may be ordered. Standard monitoring includes the electroencephalogram, electrooculogram, electromyogram, and electrocardiogram. Respiration, oxygen saturation, and body temperature can also be monitored. Sleep apnea may require surgical intervention to remove mechanical obstruction such as swollen adenoids or to reposition the mouth and tongue. If the situation dictates, a permanent tracheostomy is performed.

I. Measures must be taken to protect patients from injury or harm. Consideration should be given to the sleep environment, nutritional status, and partner or caregiver education. Changes in sleep environment may include removing hazardous furniture, locking doors and windows to confine a sleepwalker, and positioning a patient with sleep apnea in an upright position. Patients with sleep apnea can often benefit from diet counseling. Weight loss may decrease the potential for airway occlusion.

References

Bahr RT. Sleep-wake patterns in the aged. J Gerontol Nurs 1983; 9:534.

Guilleminault C. The polysomnographic evaluation of sleep disorders in humans. In: Aminnoff MJ, ed. Electrodiagnosis in clinical neurology. 2nd ed. New York: Churchill Livingstone, 1986:645.

Kartmann JL. Sleep and the elderly critical care patient. Crit Care Nurse 1985; 5:52.

Helpful Hints for a Good Night's Sleep

To Do:

Exercise regularly during the day

Keep a consistent schedule of when you go to bed and when you get up

Make the bedroom conducive to sleep
Adjust the light, temperature, bed firmness, bed clothes, and noise level to be comfortable for you

Use relaxation techniques such as a warm shower, music, reading, imagery, meditation, or praying

Relieve your physical pain or discomfort by taking pain medicines 30 minutes prior to sleep

Use warm or cool compresses to affected areas as needed

Eat a small snack or drink milk just before sleep if it is helpful

Report sleep problems to your doctor

To Avoid:

Caffeine or alcoholic beverages prior to sleep

Lying in bed for long periods of time worrying
If you cannot fall asleep after awhile, get out of bed and do something to try to relax; then try to go to sleep again

Drinking plenty of liquids just before sleep

Tobacco products

Watching television, reading, and eating in bed; maintain the association of the bed and sleep by not using the bed for reading, eating, or watching television.

EMERGENCY SITUATIONS

BURNS

Sue Miller

Accidents resulting in burns occur most often in the home of the older adult, particularly in the kitchen. The most frequent cause of burns is flame; next is scalding, followed by flammable liquids and electrical wiring or appliances. Burns may be more severe than they initially appear because of thinning of aging skin.

A. Ask patient or caregiver specific questions about the burn:
    • When did the accident occur?
    • What was the cause or suspected cause?

Postburn Education	
Topic	Content
Wound care	• clean wounds with a mild soap such as Dove or Caress, not a deodorant soap or Ivory • remove all the old ointment before reapplying • use only the ointment ordered by the physician • change dressings once or twice a day • apply splints made to maintain function
Exercise	• cautiously stretch the burned area only until it begins to turn white or hurt a little • hold position until pain eases and color returns • stretch a little further • massage areas as they are stretched
Nutrition/ hydration	• eat a well-balanced diet adequate in calories and protein to promote wound healing • drink at least 8 glasses of water a day
Lifestyle modification	• stay out of the sun unless using a sunscreen with SPF 15 or above • wear a hat and clothing that covers burned areas • avoid overheating; grafted skin does not sweat • drink lots of fluids • find cool places to rest • sit with burned extremities on pillows or footstool • do not stand for long periods
Safety	• check bath temperatures carefully • do not smoke in bed • evaluate kitchen safety • remove area rugs that may cause falls

• Did the injury occur in a closed space?
• Could the accident have caused other trauma?
• What first aid was used?
Determine health history affecting burn treatment or recovery.
• allergies (some burn agents contain sulfa or iodine)
• current medications (prescription and over-the-counter)
• chronic illness/problems
    • diabetes
    • cardiovascular disease
    • degenerative joint disease
    • seizures
    • drug or alcohol abuse
    • pulmonary disease
• experience with and tolerance of pain
• physical impairments (hearing loss, diminished vision, etc.)
• status of tetanus immunization
• emotional problems (to rule out self-inflicted injury)
• possibility of abuse

B. Immediately evaluate airway, breathing, and circulation. Measure and record, when possible, vital signs, height, and weight. Determine depth of burn (see Pressure Sore, p. 106) and percentage of body surface burned. If height and weight are accurate, calculate total body surface area (TBSA) using a nomogram. Estimate extent of burns using the Rule of Nines. For small or scattered burns, use the patient's palm, which represents approximately 1% of body surface, as a ruler.

C. First aid for burns is very basic.
    • Flood the area with cool water to remove chemicals or debris.
    • Do NOT use ice, cold water, butter, or ointments initially.
    • Pat burns dry with a clean towel or sheet; do NOT rub.
    • Remove clothing to assess entire body.
    • Wrap burns with a clean, lint-free cloth before patient transport.
    Burns should be evaluated in an Emergency Room or Burn Center if
    • more than 20% TBSA is burned
    • third- or fourth-degree burns on more than 5% of TBSA
    • second-, third-, or fourth-degree burns of the face, hands, feet, perineum, or genitalia
    • chemical or electrical burns
    • associated with inhalation injury

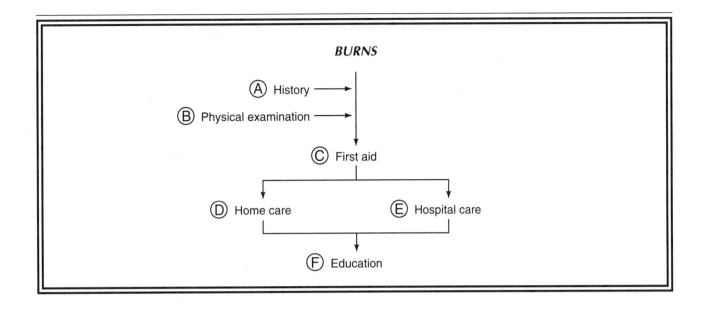

BURNS

Ⓐ History ⟶

Ⓑ Physical examination ⟶

Ⓒ First aid

Ⓓ Home care   Ⓔ Hospital care

Ⓕ Education

• burns with associated trauma
• circumferential burns

D. Home care goals are to provide appropriate wound care, prevent infection, and promote wound healing.
  • Clean burn sites once or twice daily with soap and water.
  • Apply prescribed burn ointment.
  • Cover burns and/or ointment with bulky, absorbent dressings.
  • Do NOT break blisters; they provide a sterile cover.
  • When blisters break, remove loose skin.
  • Watch for signs of infection.
  • See a physician if signs of infection appear.
  • Observe for emotional problems, self-neglect, or injury.
  • Plan well-balanced meals with adequate protein.
  • Encourage oral fluid intake to 2000 ml/day.
  • Increase oral fluids if urine appears concentrated.

E. Standard hospital care of burns in the elderly includes
  • maintenance of an adequate airway and gas exchange
  • hydration therapy
  • monitoring of vital signs and circulation
  • gastric decompression
  • monitoring appropriate lab values (e.g., carboxyhemoglobin, urine osmolarity, electrolytes, serum albumin, and CBC)
  • pain management
  • maintenance of adequate body temperature
  Special care for older burn patients may include
  • monitoring for atypical signs of secondary infection

  • confusion
  • no temperature elevation
  • observing for secondary infections
    • urinary tract infection from Foley catheter
    • donor site or trach site infections
  • watching for pneumonia from immobility
  • watching for exacerbation of preexisting conditions caused by immobility or stress
    • degenerative joint disease
    • osteoporosis
    • peripheral vascular disease
  • assessing response to stress
    • decreased cognition
    • regression
    • increased pain

F. Education provides both patient and caregiver with information about wound care, nutrition, lifestyle modifications, and safety. See the box "Postburn Education."

References

Foyt MM. Does aging magnify the danger of burn injury? Part I. J Gerontol Nurs 1985; 1:22.

Foyt MM. Does aging magnify the danger of burn injury? Part II. J Gerontol Nurs, 1985; 11:17.

Hussey L, et al. Going home/burn discharge booklet, 1989. Revised 1992. Parkland Regional Burn Center Orientation Manual. Parkland Memorial Hospital, Dallas, TX.

FALLS

Paula A. Loftis

Falls are not inevitable with aging and are often preventable. Their causes are multifactorial and can be divided into
- intrinsic risk factors (see box "Intrinsic Factors Contributing to Falls")
- extrinsic risk factors (see the box "Extrinsic Risk Factors Contributing to Falls")

Many age-related factors contribute to instability and the potential for falls. Falls occur more often in women than in men. Falls are a major cause of death, morbidity, and disability. Their consequences include fractures, severe soft tissue injury, head injury, loss of independence and mobility, and fear of falling. This fear can result in loss of self-confidence, isolation, and immobility, which in turn can lead to a vicious cycle that increases the risk of falls and of institutionalization.

A. Ascertain the risk factors (see boxes) and pertinent history, such as
   - pain, dizziness, syncope, sedation, or sensation of a rapid heart rate
   - chronic medical conditions
   - medications, prescribed and over the counter
   - patient perception of what may have caused the fall
   - account of the fall by a witness, when possible
   - detailed description of the fall
     - location
     - time of day
     - association with meal ingestion
     - activity being performed at the time of fall (e.g., exercise, shaving, dressing, toileting, using stairs)
   - loss of consciousness, including the length of time unconscious
   - loss of bowel or bladder control
   - pain or injury from the fall
   - previous falls
   - frequency of falls
   - circumstances of previous falls
   - nutritional and fluid intake recall or changes
   - association with a change in position

B. Assess
   - vital signs
     - blood pressure: supine, sitting, and standing for orthostatic hypotension with a concomitant change in pulse
     - heart rate, for tachycardia
     - respiratory rate, for tachypnea
     - temperature, for fever
   - any area with visible evidence of trauma
   - the skin for bruises, significant turgor changes
   - visual acuity
   - the neck for suppleness, range of motion, and symptoms with movement
   - the cardiovascular status for arrhythmia, murmur, signs or symptoms of congestive heart failure, carotid bruit
   - the musculoskeletal system
     - deformities including feet (see Foot Deformities, p. 54)
     - trauma
     - restricted range of motion
     - joints
       - pain
       - inflammation
       - induration (see Joint Pain and Inflammation, p. 36)
   - footwear (see the tool *Foot Care*, p. 60)
   - extremities
     - range of motion (see Limited Range of Motion, p. 8)
     - signs and symptoms of inflammation, erythema, induration
     - pain
   - neurologic status
     - mental status (see Confusion/Cognitive Changes/Dementia, p. 254, and the tools *Mini-Mental State Examination*, p. 269 and *Short Portable Mental Status Questionnaire*, p. 271)
     - focal neurologic signs
     - muscle weakness, rigidity, spasticity
     - tremor (see Tremor, p. 48)
     - peripheral neuropathy
     - ataxia, finger to nose and heel to shin ability (see Gait Disturbances, p. 42)
     - cerebellar function, including Romberg test, p. 63
   - posture and balance
     - sitting balance
     - standing balance with eyes closed (see tool *Romberg Test*, p. 63)
   - gait (Fig. 1) (see Gait Disturbances, p. 42, and the tool *Balance and Gait*, p. 61)
     - nudge test (see the tool *Balance and Gait*, p. 61)
     - get-up-and-go test (see p. 62)
     - use of assistive devices (see Gait Disturbances, p. 42)

Laboratory assessment should consist of CBC with differential, serum electrolytes, and BUN. Radiograph injured areas if asymmetry/gross deformity or restricted/painful range of motion is found. A chest film and ECG may be indicated if the history and examination suggest a pulmonary or cardiovascular cause. Noninvasive studies (e.g., a carotid Doppler) may be performed if a transient ischemic attack is suspected.

C. The value of an assessment for environmental hazards cannot be underestimated. Awareness and ameliora

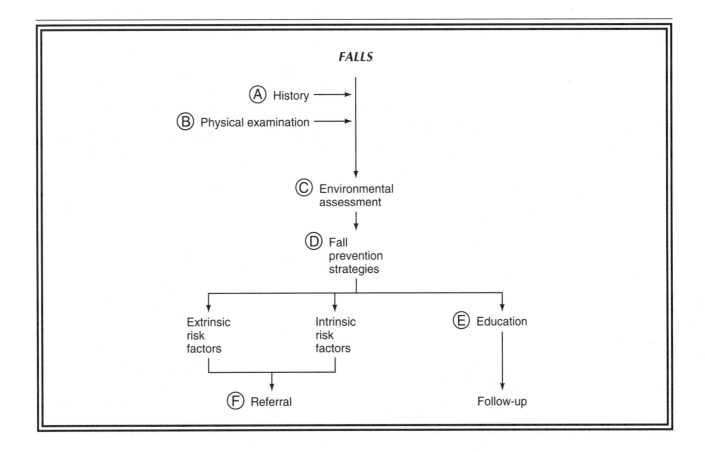

FALLS

A History
B Physical examination
C Environmental assessment
D Fall prevention strategies
Extrinsic risk factors
Intrinsic risk factors
E Education
F Referral
Follow-up

tion of extrinsic factors contributing to falls is essential (see the box "Extrinsic Risk Factors Contributing to Falls."). There are resources to obtain a home assessment in many communities through either home health care, local city and county health departments, hospital outreach services, or specialized senior citizens organizations. The home assessment should focus on

- observation of patient activities in the home
- performance of activities of daily living (ADL) and instrumental ADL (see Inability to Perform Activities of Daily Living, p. 6)
- potential hazards (see box "Extrinsic Risk Factors Contributing to Falls")

In patients who are institutionalized, consider also environmental risks such as

- recent admission
- inadequate patient-to-staff ratio
- poorly supervised patient activities, including toileting and getting out of bed
- oversedation, use of psychotropic drugs

D. The prevention of falls requires a broad approach because of the interrelation of intrinsic and extrinsic risk factors. The overall goals are to increase patient stability, decrease risk factors, and reduce environmental hazards. The following are target areas:

- critical evaluation and correction of environmental hazards
  - lighting
  - flooring
  - furniture

- temperature regulation
- stairways
- bathroom
- shelving
- appliances
- review of medications with conservative use of psychotropics
- sensory adaptation, regular testing of vision and hearing with proper correction, cerumen removal if indicated
- use of appropriate assistive devices, footwear, and clothing
- restriction of alcohol consumption

E. Education of patients, families, and health care providers is the primary method for preventing and reducing falls. Patients need to understand

- what constitutes adequate nutrition and fluid intake
- the need for caution in getting up too quickly after eating, lying down, or resting
- the need to maintain a regular program of exercise to improve strength and muscle tone
- the use of proper assistive devices (see box "Extrinsic Risk Factors Contributing to Fall", and Gait Disturbances, p. 42)

Efforts to raise the consciousness of health care providers concerning fall risk factors and hazards include attending to

- modification of the environment
- supervision of patients at risk for falls
- use of fall-monitoring devices
- selective use of restraints

Intrinsic Factors Contributing to Falls	
Category	*Discriminator*
Health related	Endocrine disorder/diabetes/neuropathy
	Postural hypotension (20 mm Hg drop in mean blood pressure when position is changed)
	Gait/balance problems (post–cerebrovascular accident, Parkinson's disease)
	Hemianopsia
	Psychiatric illnesses
	Degenerative joint disease
	Neurologic disease
	Cognitive impairment
	Foot deformities or diseases
	Sensory impairments
	Cardiovascular disease
	Cerumen impaction
	Generalized weakness
	Pain
Behavioral	Poor nutrition
	Carrying vision-blocking loads
Activity related	Sedentary lifestyle
	History of falling
	Restraints
	Immobility
	Nightime trips to bathroom
	Deconditioning
	Gait instability, paresis, orthopedic devices
Physiologic changes with aging	Decreased hearing
	Impaired vision
	Advanced age
	Faulty vestibular mechanism
	Decreased functional status or ability to perform ADL (requires assistance with two or more ADL)
	Increased incidence of pathologic conditions
	Changes in posture and gait
	Men (see Fig. 1):
	Wide-based
	Short-step
	Decreased arm swing
	Forward flexion of upper trunk
	Flexion of arms and knees
	Women:
	Narrow-based
	Short-step
	Waddling
	Inadequate height of step
	Diminished proprioception
	Slowed reflexes
	Decreased muscle mass and strength
Pharmacologic	Medications: polypharmacy, sedatives, psychotropics
	Substance abuse, alcohol

Extrinsic Risk Factors Contributing to Falls	
Category	*Discriminator*
Clothing	Improper footwear, especially slippers
	Loose, long, or flowing clothing
Furnishings	Inappropriate furniture: too low, soft cushions, with wheels, sharp corners, and susceptible to tipping if grabbed
	Low bed height
	Use of high shelving
	Low-lying objects: footstools, pets, small children
	Trailing electric cords
Structural	Unadapted bathroom: no handrails, elevated toilet seat, or safety mats
	Uneven, slippery, waxed, patterned, or glaring floor surfaces; worn carpeting, loose rugs, or throw rugs
	Deteriorated stairs and treads without rails or with insecure handrails; poorly identified and anchored stairway edges
Safety	Clutter and poor storage of items (shoes, clothing)
	Unfamiliar surroundings
	Inadequate lighting, especially of stairs and bathroom
	Worn, broken, or improperly used equipment or adaptive devices

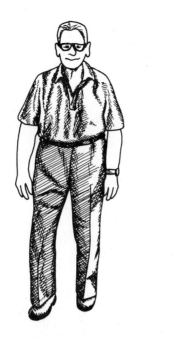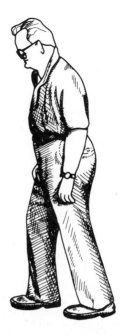

Figure 1 Gait and body alignment of elderly male. (Illustration courtesy of JoAnn Clemons Elliott, 1992.)

F. Referral to the primary care physician to rule out or treat pathologic findings is warranted. Physical medicine and rehabilitation consultation for physical and/or occupational therapy can address functional and exercise concerns. Environmental assessment is always appropriate to modify extrinsic risk factors.

References

Hernandez M, Miller J. How to reduce falls. Geriatr Nurs 1986; 7:97.

Hindmarsh JJ, Estes EH. Falls in older persons: Causes and interventions. Arch Intern Med 1989; 149:2217.

Janken JK, Reynolds BA, Swiech K. Patient falls in the acute care setting: Identifying risk factors. Nurs 1986; 35:215.

Rubenstein LZ, Robbins AS, Josephson KR, et al. The value of assessing falls in an elderly population: A randomized clinical trial. Ann Intern Med 1990; 113:308.

Tinetti ME, Williams TF, Mayewski R. Fall risk index for elderly patients based on number of chronic disabilities. Am J Med 1986; 80:429.

Whedon MB, Shedd P. Prediction and prevention of patient falls. Image: J Nurs Scholarship 1989; 21:108.

SEIZURES

Paula Tosch

Causes of new-onset seizure disorder in elderly individuals include brain tumor, stroke, hypertensive encephalopathy, and heart disease that produces cerebral emboli or ischemia. Seizures are categorized as partial (focal) or generalized. Partial seizures begin in one area of the brain, and generalized seizures involve both hemispheres, do not have a focal onset, and cause at least a brief loss of consciousness. Most seizures in elderly persons are partial (Table 1). Status epilepticus may be defined as a tonic clonic seizure lasting more than 8 minutes *or* three tonic clonic seizures in succession without full recovery between seizures. Causes include abrupt withdrawal of medicine, sepsis, or a brain lesion. Status epilepticus is a medical emergency and requires prompt recognition and treatment. Prolonged seizure activity may cause physical injury, brain damage, and death.

TABLE 1 Seizure Classification

Category	Type	Definition
Partial	Simple	Consciousness is not impaired
		May have sensory and psychic autonomic or motor symptoms
		An aura is a simple partial seizure
	Complex	Consciousness is impaired
		May begin as simple partial seizure
		Often involves staring with amnesia and/or automatisms, which are repetitive, purposeless movements
		Lasts for 30 to 90 seconds; followed by a postictal period, which may involve confusion and aphasia
	Evolving to generalized	May progress to loss of consciousness with tonic and/or clonic activity
Generalized	Absence	Altered awareness for 5 to 30 seconds (petit mal)
	Myoclonic	Abrupt muscle contractions of arms
	Clonic	Bilateral flexion and extension of extremities
	Tonic	Extension of arms and legs; back arched
	Tonic clonic	May begin with a shrill cry; lasts 2 to 5 minutes (grand mal)
	Atonic	Abrupt loss of muscle tone, resulting in a fall (drop attack)

A. The history gathers data about seizure activity from both patient and caregivers, including
   • onset
   • precipitating factors
   • presence of aura
   • duration
   • tongue or lip biting
   • level of consciousness
   • involved body parts
   • movements observed
   • incontinence
   • behavior after seizures
   Other pertinent information to collect is
   • medical history, such as metabolic disorders, cardiac dysrhythmias, infection, cerebral circulation problems, head injury, hypertension, previous seizures, and psychological or emotional disorders
   • medication history, including prescription and over-the-counter drugs, compliance with regimen, and alcohol use or abuse.

B. Seizure assessment and documentation include recording injury or fall, eye position, pupil size and reactivity to light, changes in level of consciousness, part of body seizure activity first observed, progression of seizure activity, duration, incontinence, and cyanosis or apnea. After the seizure, assess for
   • transient one-sided weakness
   • behavior changes
   • headache
   • change in blood pressure, pulse, and respiration
   • aphasia
   • mouth injury
   • level of consciousness
   For prolonged or unusual seizure activity, obtain laboratory results to evaluate the patient and rule out possible causes. Laboratory tests include complete blood count, electrolytes (glucose, sodium), and therapeutic drug levels.

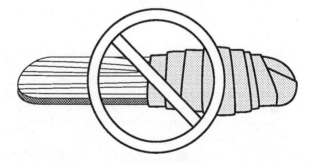

Figure 1 A padded tongue blade. A padded tongue blade or airway should not be forced into the mouth. Forcing objects into the mouth risks damaging teeth and gums. Swallowing the tongue is physically impossible, and a bitten tongue heals relatively quickly. (Illustration courtesy of JoAnn Clemons Elliott, 1992.)

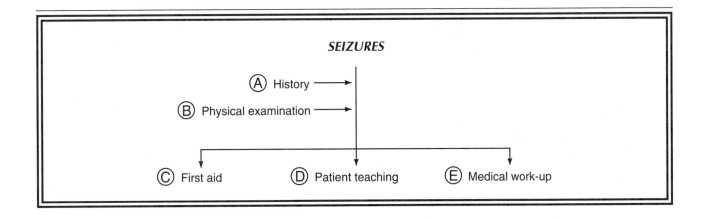

SEIZURES

(A) History →

(B) Physical examination →

(C) First aid   (D) Patient teaching   (E) Medical work-up

C. During and after a seizure, the patient is at risk for airway obstruction, aspiration, injury, and embarrassment. Emergency care during seizures includes
   • maintaining a patent airway (Fig. 1)
   • turning the patient on one side to allow drainage of secretions, saliva, vomitus, or blood
   • suctioning as required to prevent aspiration
   • loosening restrictive clothing around the neck and chest
   • administrating oxygen if needed
   Provide a safe, protected environment by
   • removing dangerous objects
   • placing a flat pillow under the patient's head
   • NOT restraining
   • maintaining seizure precautions
     • keeping padded side rails in upright position
     • keeping bed in low and locked position
     • maintaining suction and oxygen nearby
     • taping an oral airway at the bedside
     • restricting activity as appropriate based on the patient's potential for injury
   Additional interventions in status epilepticus include
   • drawing blood for laboratory tests and establishing intravenous line for administration of
     • lorazepam or diazepam to stop seizure
     • dextrose 50% to correct hypoglycemia
     • thiamine to prevent acute encephalopathy
     • phenytoin or phenobarbital to prevent further seizures
   • treating hyperthermia
   • providing close observation

D. Patient teaching aims to
   • help patients identify and avoid factors that trigger seizure
     • missed medication
     • hypoglycemia
     • hyponatremia
     • alcohol intake
     • excessive heat
     • sleep deprivation
     • excessive stress
     • febrile illness
   • provide information about
     • first aid
     • seizure type
     • activity restrictions
     • community resources
     • medications
       • name
       • dose schedule
       • adverse or toxic effects
       • interactions
   Individuals with epilepsy may have anxiety and decreased self-esteem. Arrange appropriate referrals.

E. Patients with new-onset seizures are usually admitted to the hospital for evaluation. Diagnostic studies include
   • thorough history taking
   • neurologic examinations
   • lumbar puncture
   • computed tomography
   • magnetic resonance imaging (MRI), currently preferred over CT
   • electroencephalogram (EEG)
   • blood studies

References

Callanan M. Epilepsy: Putting the patient in control. RN 1988; 51:48

Mahler ME. Seizures: Common causes and treatment in the elderly. Geriatrics 1987; 42:73.

Santilli N, Sierzant TL. Advances in the treatment of epilepsy. J Neurosci Nurs 1987; 19:144.

Sung C-Y, Chu NS. Status epilepticus in the elderly: Etiology, seizure types and outcome. Acta Neurol Scand 1989; 80:51.

TRAUMA

Sue Miller
Margaret Pasquarello

Trauma, often multiple trauma, in the elderly is usually the result of falls (see p. 90), burns (see p. 88), motor vehicle accidents, or assault. Trauma is the fourth leading cause of death in persons over the age of 55 and the fifth leading cause of death for those over age 70. Surviving elderly have more profound long-term effects, frequently requiring nursing home placement, and are more likely to die within 48 hours after emergency treatment, probably as a result of hypoperfusion secondary to the aging process. Trauma may involve soft tissue, bone, or internal organs. Types of trauma include
- surface trauma
  - contusions
  - abrasions
  - puncture wounds
  - lacerations
  - bites or insect stings
- strains and sprains
- fractures: closed or open
- internal injury with or without external signs
  - closed head injury
  - pneumothorax or hemothorax
  - cardiac bruising or tamponade
  - vessel tears
  - abdominal organ injury
- thermal injury
  - burns (see p. 88)
  - hypothermia (see p. 24)
  - heat stroke (see p. 22)
  - heat exhaustion (see p. 20)

Factors that compound the diagnosis and treatment of the elderly who have suffered trauma include
- impaired peripheral circulation
- decreased cardiac reserve
- deconditioned muscles
- degenerated joints
- changed cognition
- concurrent chronic illnesses
- decreased motor function
- changed pain perception
- hypoperfusion

A. First aid for trauma depends on the type of injury but always includes the ABCs—airway, breathing, and circulation:
- Obtain and maintain a patent airway; reposition head cautiously.
- Stop bleeding using direct pressure.
- Clean and cover open wounds.
- Protect injured areas by immobilizing and maintaining alignment.

B. Ask patient and/or caregiver specific questions:
- When did injury occur?
- Where did injury occur?
- What happened?
  - preceding or precipitating event(s)
  - sequence of events
- Were there witnesses?
- What are current symptoms, including pain?
- Was home treatment given?

Be alert to the potential of self-inflicted injury or abuse (see Abuse, p. 290). Obtain a health history:
- current medications
- allergies
- immunization status
- chronic medical problems

Determine cognitive and functional levels before injury. Also ask about degenerative changes or deformity that may have been present. Ask questions to determine caregiver or support system capabilities.

Trauma Assessment Parameters and Abnormal Findings	
Parameter	*Abnormal Findings*
Adequate gas exchange and airway	Impaired gas exchange Shallow breathing Increased or decreased respirations Cyanosis Sucking wound
Adequate circulatory perfusion	Absent pulse Overt bleeding Hypothermia or hyperthermia Decreased blood pressure (shock) Tachycardia or bradycardia Pallor Increased blood pressure
Neurologic status	Drowsiness Disorientation Slurred speech Unequal or pinpoint pupils Lethargy Confusion Enlarged or sluggish pupils
Mobility	Inability to move limbs Discoloration Tears in skin Pain Fractures Bruising

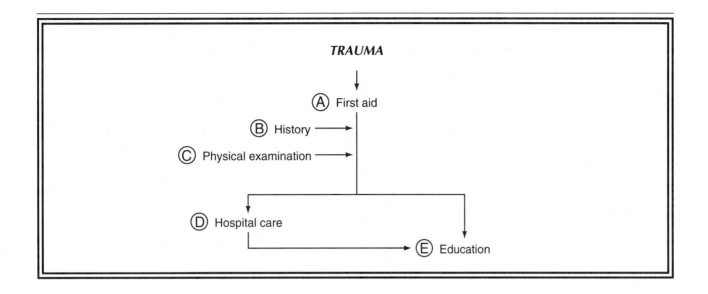

TRAUMA

A. First aid

B. History

C. Physical examination

D. Hospital care

E. Education

C. Physical examination may reveal
  - altered vital signs: hypotension, tachycardia, tachypnea
  - circulatory changes: absent pulses, skin temperature change, slow capillary refill
  - distortion of a limb
  - shallow or labored respirations
  - absent or adventitious breath sounds
  - guarding or tenderness on palpation
  - bleeding
  - open wounds
  - discoloration of skin
  - swelling

  Evaluate mental status and level of consciousness. See the box "Trauma Assessment Parameters and Abnormal Findings" for physical assessment parameters and abnormal findings.

D. Hospital care focuses on diagnosis and treatment, prevention of complications, and maintenance of function. See the box for explanation of emergency care procedures. Treatment may include casting, splinting, or traction; debridement and closure or treatment of wounds; observation; and rehabilitation. Complications can occur as a result of imposed bed rest or because of injury-induced altered function:
  - pressure areas or skin breakdown
  - pneumonia
  - infection: osteomyelitis, amputation
  - altered cognition
  - change in eating habits
  - depression

E. Patients and caregivers can be taught care procedures and safety measures to prevent recurrence of avoidable injuries:
  - wound care: dressing changes, cast care
  - use of assistive devices
  - nutrition and hydration principles
  - reevaluation of decision to continue to drive
  - safety measures based on cause of fall and functional level

Emergency Care Procedures

Procedure	Purpose
IV lines—two large-bore catheters, if possible	Replace fluid
	Monitor central venous pressure
	Replace blood, if needed
Foley catheter	Accurately measure output
	Titrate IV lines to maintain output of at least 30 ml/hour
Oxygen	Improve oxygenation
Radiographs	Determine extent of injuries
Laboratory tests	
Hemoglobin	Determine extent of blood loss
Hematocrit, blood urea nitrogen	Determine level of hydration
Arterial blood gases, oximetry	Determine oxygenation levels
Electrolytes	Determine composition of fluid replacement
Lavage	Determine presence of internal bleeding or injury
Gastric	
Peritoneal	
Monitor	
Vital signs: blood pressure, heart rate, temperature	Determine changes
	Evaluate effectiveness of emergency treatment
Neurologic status	
Vascular status	

References

Bobb JK. Trauma in the elderly. J Gerontol Nurs 1987; 13:28.

Hogue CC. Injury in late life: Part I. Epidemiology. J Am Geriatr Soc, 1982; 30:183.

Mancini ME. Decision making in emergency nursing. Philadelphia: BC Decker, 1987.

Physical

SKIN INTEGRITY

ACTINIC KERATOSIS

Sylvia Moreno

Actinic keratosis is a common precancerous skin lesion that results from chronic ultraviolet radiation exposure. Patients are usually older than 50 years of age, fair-skinned, and of Celtic ancestry. Men are affected more often than women and more often on the ears and vermilion border of the lower lip. Hyperpigmented solar lentigines, known as "liver spots," often occur in association with actinic keratosis. Malignant transformation of actinic keratosis to squamous cell carcinoma may occur after years of exposure. Metastasis is rare.

A. Ask about
  * onset of the lesion
  * the site on which the lesion first appeared
  * spread
  * itching or burning
  * exacerbating factors
  * how the lesions developed
    * color
    * appearance
    * pain
    * swelling
    * scaling
    * oozing
  * sun exposure habits
  * ability to tan
  * susceptibility to burn

B. Use the information collected to determine the skin type (Table 1). Examine the skin with particular attention to exposed areas such as
  * face: nose, ears, forehead, cheeks
  * bald scalp
  * backs of the hands
  * neckline "V" of the chest
  * forearms
  Sun-damaged skin may lose elasticity and appear
  * coarse
  * yellowish
  * weatherbeaten
  * dry
  * wrinkled

  * freckled
  * atrophic
  * hyperpigmented or depigmented
  * telangiectatic
  Is the distribution
  * linear?
  * symmetric?
  * circular?
  Is there a spread? Measure the size. Actinic keratosis is usually 1 cm in diameter or larger. Observe
  * color
  * warmth
  * swelling
  * macular versus papular lesions
  * scaling
  * oozing
  The types of actinic keratosis are listed in Table 2.

C. Education of the patient with actinic keratosis helps them prevent further skin damage. Encourage them to
  * avoid excessive sun exposure
  * use sunscreens with an SPF of 15 or greater
  * apply a sunscreen in the morning before any sun exposure
  * reapply the sunscreen as needed but at least every 3–4 hours
  * cover bald heads and ears with a hat
  After medical treatment, caution patients against self-treatment of skin problems. Ensure that medical follow-up appointments are scheduled at least yearly.

TABLE 1 Skin Type Chart

Skin	Burns	Tans
I	Always	Never
II	Usually	With difficulty
III	Mild	Average
IV	Rarely	Easily
V	Never	Tan (brown skin)
VI	Never	Tan (black skin)

TABLE 2 Types of Actinic Keratosis

Type	Characteristics
Erythematous	Begins as telangiectatic area of <0.5 cm
	Base of mature lesion has an erythematous halo
Keratotic	Adherent, yellow-brown-gray scaly surface
	Attached to skin
	Round to irregular shape
Cornu cirtaneum (cutaneous horn)	Thick, sharp-edged
	Dark yellow to dark brown
	Straight, bent, screwlike, coiled or peglike
Lichen planus	Begins as erythematous patch progresses to brownish color
	Solitary
	Indurated
	Sharply defined
	5 mm or greater
	Scaly or keratotic surface
	May appear smooth

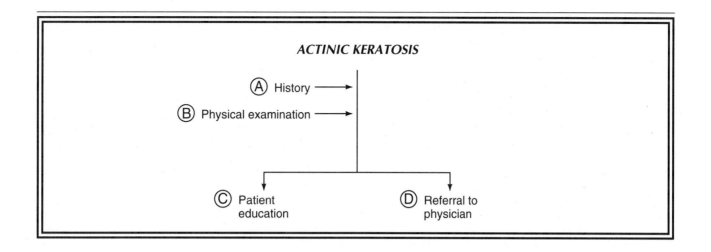

ACTINIC KERATOSIS

(A) History
(B) Physical examination

(C) Patient education
(D) Referral to physician

D. Medical intervention may take many forms:
  - excision
  - curettage/electrodesiccation
  - cryotherapy
  - chemical peel
  - dermabrasion
  - etretinate
  - topical chemotherapy

Send any lesion removed for pathologic evaluation to rule out malignancy. Topical chemotherapy is done with 5-fluorouracil (5-FU) and may last 3–8 weeks. Response to treatment is classified into four phases: phase I, early inflammatory; phase II, severe inflammatory; phase III, tumor or lesion disintegration; phase IV, healing. Local toxicities that may occur include
  - edema
  - erythema
  - superficial necrosis
  - oozing

Patients should anticipate intense discomfort and pain during phase III. Avoidance of sun exposure is strongly recommended. Cool tapwater compresses may provide relief from discomfort. The physician may prescribe bland emollients or topical corticosteroid cream.

References

Arndt KA. Manual of dermatologic therapeutics. Boston: Little, Brown, 1989.

Braun-Falco O, Plewig G, Wolff HH, Winkelmann RK. Dermatology. Berlin: Springer-Verlag, 1991.

Fry L. Skin problems in the elderly. Edinburgh: Churchill Livingstone, 1985.

Habif TP. Clinical dermatology: A color guide to diagnosis and treatment therapy. St. Louis: CV Mosby, 1985.

Marks R. Skin disease in old age. Philadelphia: JB Lippincott, 1987.

Newcomer VD, Young EM. Geriatric dermatology: Clinical diagnosis and practical therapy. New York: Igaku-Shoin, 1989.

Sauer GC. Manual of skin diseases. Philadelphia: JB Lippincott, 1991.

DRY SKIN

Ruby Taylor

The integument is the largest organ in the body. Its functions are to provide a semipermeable barrier for water, to aid in temperature regulation, and to protect the body from infection. Any change in skin integrity interrupts the body's first line of defense. Local and systemic skin changes related to aging include
• decreased elasticity
• altered water loss related to decreased sebum production
• increased fragility
The elderly can suffer from excessive dryness of the skin (xerosis), which can lead to pruritus.

A. Question patients reporting dry skin about
   • onset
   • duration
   • area affected
   • actions that relieve or exacerbate symptoms
   • nutritional intake
   • medication hypersensitivity
   • present medication regimen
   • use of over-the-counter medications or preparations
   • skin-related diseases
   • medical history of other chronic illnesses
   Hygiene-related questions include
   • bathing frequency
   • soaps and laundry products used
   • skin care products
   • purchased or home remedies for dry skin
   Ascertain environmental factors that might affect skin health, such as
   • type of heating/air conditioning
   • presence of hot and cold water
   • exposure to sun and wind
   • presence or absence of protective clothing

B. General skin inspection reveals
   • appearance
   • tone
   • elasticity
   • scars
   • chapping
   • cracks
   Compare similar or symmetric anatomic and functional areas. Skin turgor is not a valid measurement, unless asymmetric, in the elderly because of decreased overall skin elasticity.

C. The elderly often exist on a diet deficient in nutrients essential to good health (see Nutritional Deficits Requiring Supplementation, p. 154). Interventions to improve nutritional status must focus on the underlying problems discovered (see Nutritional Assessment, p. 166).

D. Patient teaching focuses on hygiene and environmental factors. Hygiene habits are often long standing and difficult to change. Tell patients that
   • frequent use of water can dry skin
   • hot water is more drying than warm or tepid water
   • harsh soaps or detergents should be avoided
   • alcohol and witch hazel are drying agents and should be avoided
   • frequent use of emollients can build up on the skin and prevent it from "breathing"
   • rejuvenating preparations should be avoided unless recommended by their physician
   • use of topical over-the-counter preparations should be discussed with their regular pharmacist to avoid drug interactions or reactions
   Environmental precautions should also be taught, as follows:
   • avoid prolonged exposure to ultraviolet rays (sun)
   • avoid extreme cold
   • humidify the air in winter, because heating tends to dry the skin
   • avoid wool clothing if the skin is dry, because it can be irritating

E. Referrals should be made on the basis of the identified problem. For nutritional problems, patients may need help from a
   • dietitian for nutrition counseling
   • home-delivered meal service
   • community pantry
   • social worker to obtain financial assistance for purchasing food
   Environmental issues may require different referrals, such as
   • social work to obtain assistance with
     • utility bills
     • housing
   • community service agencies for help with clothing
   Referral to a physician or dermatologist may be necessary if
   • skin integrity is compromised
   • an infection occurs
   • treatment is required for an underlying medical problem

References

Andress R, Bierman E, Haggard W. Principles of geriatric medicine. New York: McGraw-Hill, 1985.

Frantz RA, Kinney CK. Variables associated with skin dryness in the elderly. Nurs Res 1986; 35:98.

Marks R. Skin disease in old age: Itching and other dry skin disorders. Philadelphia: JB Lippincott, 1987.

Roe DA. Nutrition and the skin. New York: Alan R Liss, 1986.

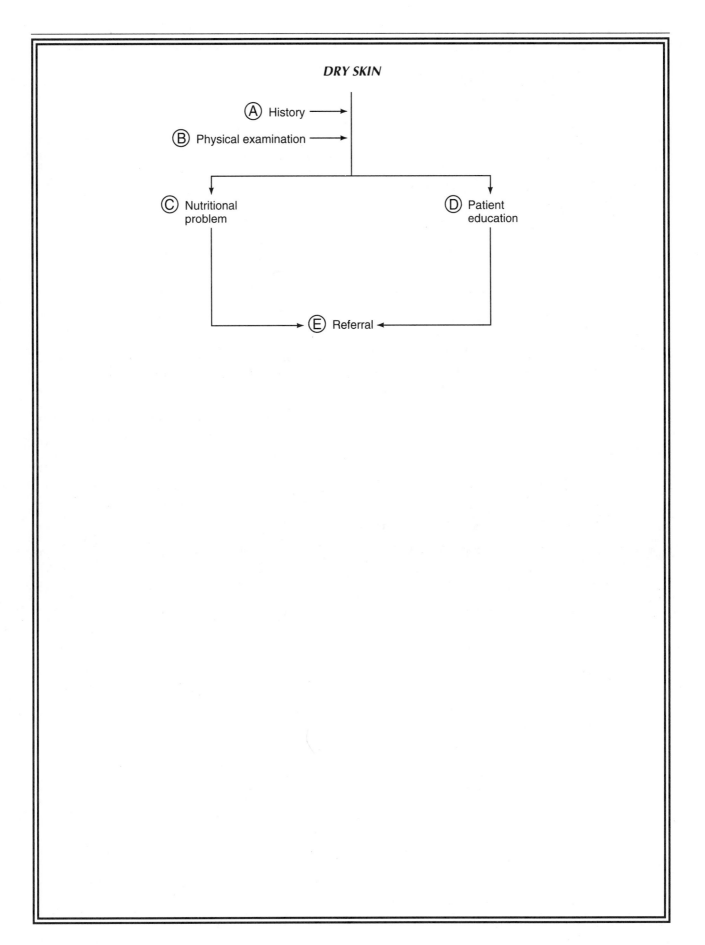

DRY SKIN

Ⓐ History

Ⓑ Physical examination

Ⓒ Nutritional problem

Ⓓ Patient education

Ⓔ Referral

ECZEMA/RASHES/DERMATITIS

Dennis M. Bellett

Characteristics of eczema, a superficial inflammatory process involving the epidermis, are exaggerated in the elderly, possibly because of changes in the skin (Table 1). The principal complication of eczematous dermatoses is infection with *Staphylococcus aureus* and herpes simplex. With advancing age, susceptibility to superficial fungal infection also increases.

TABLE 1 Eczema

Type	Cause/Origin	Appearance	Location	Incidence	Treatment/ Education	Comments
Seborrheic eczema	Unknown May be due to disturbance of microflora of skin	Reddened, scaling eruption	Scalp Facial flexures Upper trunk Major body flexures	Common in elderly Both sexes	Use antiseborrheic shampoo 2 to 3 times weekly Leave shampoo lather on scalp 5 minutes before rinsing May use cream rinse or conditioner for dryness	Can be controlled, not cured Titrate frequency of shampoo for maintenance Rotate shampoo to avoid tachyphylaxis
Asteatotic eczema (eczema craquelé)	Low humidity	Cracked "paving" of epidermis Speckled pattern	Limb extensor aspects Lateral lower legs Trunk	Debilitated patients Winter months Air-conditioning	Moisturize after bathing Avoid harsh soaps Avoid hot baths	Humidify home when possible
Gravitational eczema	Venous hypertension Obesity Past leg injury	Vessel tracking Brown discoloration of tissue Thickened skin Pitting edema Ulcers	Lower leg above medial malleolus Medial ankle aspect Dorsum of foot	Elderly Hypertension More often women	Control hypertension Maintain ideal body weight Promote venous return Avoid injury to ankles Wear thick socks and comfortable shoes Dress ulcers occlusively	Occlusive dressings can inhibit bacterial growth, absorb exudate, and debride necrotic tissue
Allergic eczema (contact dermatitis)	Reaction to agent causing specific, acquired hypersensitivity	Rash Eruption	Site of contact	Repeated exposure Specific allergy	Identify and avoid allergen Use over-the-counter creams or antihistamines Wear protective clothing Wash clothes and skin after contact	Contact with toxins or pollen causes reaction

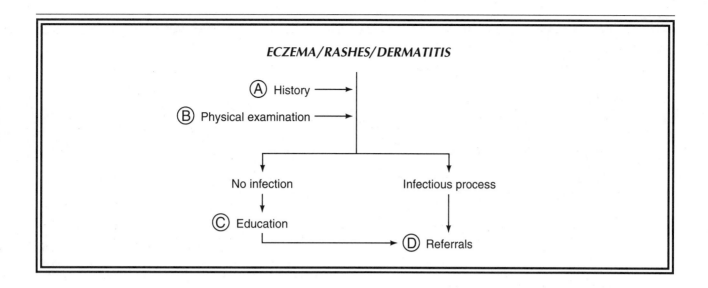

ECZEMA/RASHES/DERMATITIS

(A) History →

(B) Physical examination →

No infection

(C) Education

Infectious process

(D) Referrals

A. History includes
- onset and duration of skin changes
- nutritional intake
- medications: prescribed and over-the-counter drugs
- medical history
- other symptoms: pain, fever, rash
- prolonged exposure to dry, air-conditioned environments
- changes in hygiene activities
- changes in soaps
- changes in laundry detergent
- exposure to allergens
- exposure to caustic agents

B. Physical assessment identifies and describes skin characteristics and changes by location and appearance:
- erythema or inflammation
- dryness
- thickening
- loss of function
- greasy yellow crusting
- vascular insufficiency
- scaling
- cracking
- fissures
- exudate
- weeping or oozing
- ulcers
- signs of infection
  - purulent drainage
  - foul odor
  - fever

Complete blood count will determine the presence of leukocytosis. Viral, bacterial, and fungal cultures should be taken of suspicious vesicles with exudate.

C. Table 1 identifies patient education and therapeutic interventions.

D. Referral to a primary physician or dermatologist is indicated for
- signs of infection
- exacerbation of symptoms
- open wounds
- failure to improve on prescribed regimen

Medical treatment may include
- antihypertensives
- antibiotics
- antihistamines
- steroids
- elastic stockings to promote venous return
- occlusive dressings
- debridement of necrotic tissue

Physical therapy and home health care agencies may also be involved in treatment.

References

Lavecker R. Structural alterations in exposed and unexposed aged skin. J Invest Dermatol 1979; 75:59.

Marks R. Skin diseases and old age. Philadelphia: JB Lippincott, 1987.

Newcomer VD, Young EM. Geriatric dermatology: Clinical diagnosis and practical therapy. New York: Igaku-Shoin, 1989.

Shuster S. The etiology of dandruff and the mode of action of therapeutic agents. J Invest Dermatol 1984; 111:235.

PRESSURE SORE

Ruby Taylor

A pressure sore results when a bony prominence rests against a resistant surface, impeding the blood flow. The process of skin breakdown can be staged to determine appropriate treatment.

A. Ask questions to determine
   - general physical condition
   - mobility
   - functional level
   - bowel and bladder continence
   - nutritional intake history (see p. 148)
   - information about the pressure sore
     - onset
     - duration
     - prescribed or home remedies tried
     - pain

B. Assess
   - ability to move, transfer, and bear weight
   - position in chair or bed
   - sensation
   - skin
     - character
     - color
     - temperature
     - capillary refill
   Measure and describe all pressure sores for
   - size
   - appearance
   - location
   - stage (See Stages of Skin Ulceration, p. 167)
   - signs and symptoms of infection
   Photographs are beneficial to document progress and supply information to other health care providers. Laboratory data collected should reveal infection, anemia, and malnutrition:
   - CBC

   - albumin
   - wound culture
   X-ray films of the involved area are probably indicated when a stage IV ulcer is seen.

C. The goal of treatment of pressure sores is to clean and protect the wound as well as enhance nutritional status to promote healing (Table 1). Ongoing restaging, measurement, and photographing of pressure sores should continue at specified intervals, no less often than once a month.

D. Use pressure relief measures to prevent extension of the current pressure sore and formation of new ulcers (Table 2).

E. The patient or caregiver will need education about
   - nutrition
     - increasing protein intake
     - reporting when the patient is not able to tolerate prescribed diet
   - wound care
     - dressing changes
     - aseptic technique
     - observe for and report redness, tenderness, swelling, or changes in exudate
   - prevention of recurrence
     - avoidance of restrictive clothing
     - keeping the skin clean and dry
     - maintaining adequate nutrition
     - avoiding weight fluctuations
     - positioning to avoid pressure to one spot

F. Refer pressure sores of stage II or higher to a physician or skin care nurse for surgical debridement. A physician's order may be required for whirlpool therapy and antibiotic therapy if indicated.

TABLE 1 Treatment for Pressure Sores

Modality	Type	Purpose
Dressings	Moist saline gauze	Prevent adherence to dressings
	Transparent membrane	Protect from contamination
	Hydrophilic	Keep wound moist
	Absorptive	Absorb drainage
Cleaning	Whirlpool or wound irrigation	Remove bacteria
		Visualize wound
Nutrition	Calories	Provide energy for healing
	Protein	Enhance tissue formation

TABLE 2 Pressure Relief Measures

Measure	Purpose	Techniques
Positioning	Prevent pressure	Change position often: side, prone, supine
		Use small pillows, towels, foam to form bridge
Padding	Prevent skin contact with hard surface	Mattress overlays
		Heel and elbow pads
		Bridging/splints

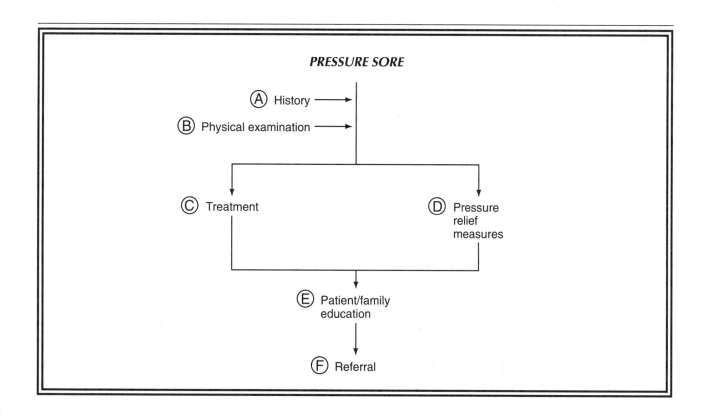

PRESSURE SORE

Ⓐ History ⟶

Ⓑ Physical examination ⟶

Ⓒ Treatment

Ⓓ Pressure relief measures

Ⓔ Patient/family education

Ⓕ Referral

References

Bergstrom N, Braden BJ, Laguzza A, Holman V. The Braden scale for predicting pressure sore risk. Nurs Res 1987; 36:205.

Bobel LM. Nutritional implications in the patient with pressure sores. Nurs Clin North Am 1987; 22:382.

Cerrato PL. How diet helps fight pressure sores. RN January 1986; 49:67.

Gosnell D. Assessment and evaluation of pressure sores. Nurs Clin North Am 1987; 22:399.

Guralnik JM, Harris TB, White LR, Cornoni-Huntley JC. Occurrence and predictors of pressure sores in the National Health and Nutrition Examination Survey follow-up. J Am Geriatr Soc 1987; 36:807.

Panel on the Prediction and Prevention of Pressure Ulcers in Adults. Pressure ulcers in adults: prediction and prevention. Quick reference guide for clinicians. AHCPR Publication No. 92-0050. Clinical Practice Guideline. AHCPR Publication No. 92-0047. Rockville, MD: Agency for Health Care Policy and Research, Public Health Service, U. S. Dept of Health and Human Services, May 1992.

Sebesn M. Home-team strategies for treating pressure sores. Nursing 87. April 1987; 17(4):50.

Sieggreen MY. Healing of physical wounds. Nurs Clin North Am 1987; 22:439.

SHINGLES/HERPES ZOSTER

Tom Emanuele

Varicella-zoster can disrupt the well-being of patients both physically and emotionally. The primary infection, chickenpox (varicella), is a viral infection of children and of young adults who have not previously been exposed to the virus. After the initial infection resolves, the virus becomes dormant in the dorsal root or cranial nerve ganglia and may become reactivated after many years in latency. Precipitating factors are thought to be physical or emotional stress and depressed immunity. Zoster is a self-limiting, localized disease that causes discomfort to severe pain for several days to a week but usually heals.

A. History taking should elicit both physiologic and psychologic information. Physiologic data include
   • when symptoms began
   • progression of symptoms
      • prodromal tingling or itching
      • initial location of rash
      • pain before or after rash occurred and duration
   • medical history
   • infectious disease history
   • medications
   • recent physical stress
   • malaise or fatigue
   Relevant psychosocial information includes
   • recent emotional stress
   • previous coping patterns
   • support systems

B. Clinical signs and symptoms to assess are
   • fever
   • infection
   • ulceration and tenderness of mucous membranes
   • satellite lesions
   • ptosis, possibly from third cranial nerve involvement
   • conjunctivitis with lid margin vesicles
   • episcleritis
   • keratitis and iritis occurring 2–3 weeks after the rash
   • rash characteristics
      • begins as erythematous and macular
      • progresses to vesicles and crusts
      • unilateral, not crossing the midline
      • follows the plane of a ganglion, dermatome

C. Respiratory isolation is required if papules and vesicles are present or weeping. The varicella virus is present in the vesicular fluid. Visitors and caregivers should be screened for a positive history of chickenpox. Herpes zoster is highly contagious at this stage, especially to an immunocompromised host. Once all lesions are dry and crusted, universal precautions are appropriate. A patient is considered noninfectious when only one skin surface is involved and when all lesions are dried and can be covered by an occlusive dressing. If the patient is at home, teach caregivers

   • the need to avoid viral transmission among contacts
   • good handwashing technique after care or before touching unaffected skin surfaces
   • that oozing areas are infectious

D. Symptomatic relief may be obtained with
   • skin care: wash lesions two or three times a day with a povidone-iodine aqueous solution
   • moist compresses
   • drying lotions containing alcohol, menthol, and phenol
   • analgesics
   • loose-fitting clothing
   • avoiding extreme temperatures, since perspiration may increase discomfort

E. Observation for complications or spread is essential. Look for signs of
   • bacterial superinfection of lesions
   • pneumonia
   • encephalitis
   • keratoconjunctivitis if the fifth cranial nerve is involved
   • postherpetic neuralgia (pain lasting >1 month), which occurs in 9–14% of patients

F. Medical evaluation and treatment may include
   • pain relief (opiates may be required)
   • a steroid regimen to reduce or prevent postherpetic neuralgia
   • treatment of infection with IV or systemic antibiotics
   • local, topical, or systemic therapy for postherpetic neuralgia (e.g., topical capsaicin cream three or four times a day)
   • antiviral agent use such as intravenous acyclovir sodium at 5 mg/kg over one hour every eight hours
   • ophthalmology evaluation is imperative for differentiation of herpes zoster keratoconjunctivitis and herpes simplex keratitis
   Referral to counseling or social work services is warranted for psychosocial problems.

References

Arndt KA. Manual of dermatologic therapeutics. 4th ed. Boston: Little, Brown, 1989:82.

Balfour HH Jr. The clinical significance of viral infections in the immunocompromised patient: Varicella-zoster virus infections. New York Burroughs-Wellcome, 1988:1.

Klaus BJ. Protocols handbook for nurse practitioners. New York: John Wiley, 1979:193.

Krause PR, Straus SE. Zoster and its complications. Hosp Pract 1990; 25:61.

Marks R. Skin diseases in old age. Philadelphia: JB Lippincott, 1987:144.

SHINGLES/HERPES ZOSTER

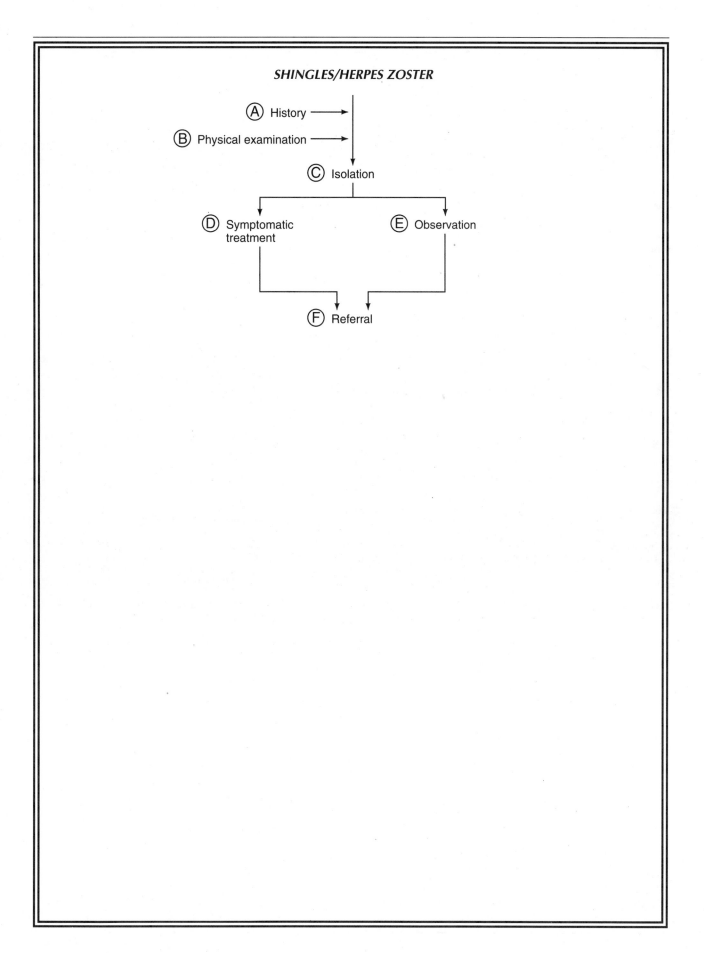

(A) History ⟶

(B) Physical examination ⟶

(C) Isolation

(D) Symptomatic treatment

(E) Observation

(F) Referral

SKIN CANCERS AND TUMORS

Sylvia Moreno
Etta Hall

Development of skin cancer may be preceded by benign keratosis or precancerous lesions. Both carcinoma and benign tumors of the skin develop after middle age. Basal cell carcinoma and squamous cell carcinoma arise from the inner, active cells of the epidermis. Melanoma develops from premalignant lesions or preexisting melanocytic nevi caused by cumulative exposure to solar radiation. Table 1 provides information about the four most common skin lesions.

TABLE 1   Differentiation of Skin Cancers and Tumors

	Basal Cell Carcinoma	*Squamous Cell Carcinoma*	*Melanoma*	*Seborrheic Keratosis/ Basal Cell Papilloma*
Incidence	Most common type	More common in men Increases after age 60 Variable with latitude	<0.25% per diagnosis of actinic keratosis	Most common cutaneous tumor
Growth	Slow	Rapid More rapid on lip, tongue, intraoral mucosa, vulva, and glans penis	Extremely variable	May fall off and recur
Metastasis	Rare	To regional lymph nodes	Lymphatic system Blood-borne	Not applicable
Surrounding Tissue	Erosion or ulceration Local tissue destruction	Minimal change Rare pain or itching Usually asymptomatic	Itch, tender or painful Erythematous, inflamed, and/or altered pigmentation	Secondary infection may produce malodorous discharge
Appearance	Nodular Edge: pearly, shiny, raised Surface: unbroken or ulcerated Bleeds easily if crust removed	Nodular Surface: warty, flat, scaly, indurated Ulceration if >1–2 cm Papillomatous Metastatic nodes Malodorous exudate	Size: 5 mm or greater Border: asymmetric, irregular, scalloped, notched, angular Color: mixture of tan, brown, pink, white, or dark black Surface: scaling, oozing Bleeding in later stages	Papules, single to multiple Edge: sharply circumscribed Color: brown to black Surface: cryptlike depressions Greasy, latex to firm "Stuck on" Secondary infection
Location	Exposed areas: face, especially temples; scalp; forearms; trunk	Exposed areas: face, tongue, lower lip, neck, back of hands, lower legs	Exposed areas: face, bald scalp, ears, dorsa of forearms, hands	Covered areas Trunk Arms, neck, and face less often
Treatment	Surgical excision Radiotherapy Cryosurgery Electrodesiccation and curettage Mohs' surgery Cytotoxic agent	Surgical excision Radiotherapy Cryosurgery Electrodesiccation and curettage Mohs' surgery	Surgical excision Cytotoxic agent	Surgical excision Cryosurgery Electrodesiccation and curettage
Purpose of Treatment	Remove malignancy	Remove malignancy Prevent metastasis	Remove malignancy Prevent metastasis Prolong life	Cosmetic Eliminate source of irritation

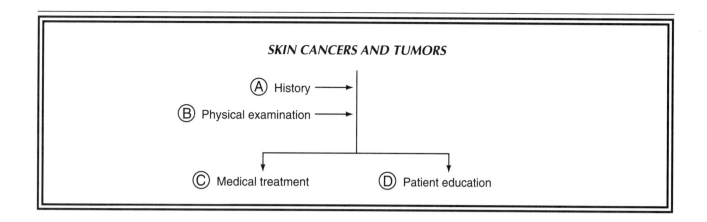

SKIN CANCERS AND TUMORS

(A) History →

(B) Physical examination →

(C) Medical treatment

(D) Patient education

A. Ask the patient about
- exposure to sunlight, heat, wind
- exposure to radiologic procedures
- exposure to heavy metals
- exposure to chronic irritants
- history of precancerous lesions
- susceptibility to burning
- tobacco use
- oral hygiene habits
- genetic disorders
- immunosuppression
- ability to tan

Identify risk factors for melanoma
- diagnosis of keratosis
- age over 40
- sun-damaged skin
- fair skin
- female

B. Assess appearance and location of lesion (see Table 1). Wound culture may be warranted if infected ulcerations are seen.

C. Treatment of choice depends on tumor size, location, cell type, presence of metastatic nodes, and previous treatment. Diagnosis of tumor type requires biopsy and histologic evaluation since size of tumor when first treated and histologic grade determine prognosis. Prognosis of patients with melanoma is poor if tumor depth is 2.5 mm or greater. The involvement of one lymph node indicates a 53% 5-year survival rate. Prompt treatment may enhance the possibility of a cure. The physical condition of the patient and cosmetic desires are considered in the treatment plan.

D. Patient education focuses on prevention of recurrence and wound care and encourages appropriate follow-up with the physician. To prevent recurrence, teach
- avoidance of sun exposure
- use of sunscreens
- covering of bald head and ears with a hat

Teaching about wound and graft care includes
- signs and symptoms of infection
- dressing changes
- pain control

References

Fry L. Skin problems in the elderly. 1st ed. New York: Churchill Livingstone, 1985.

Steinburg FU. Care of the geriatric patient. 6th ed. St. Louis: CV Mosby, 1983:199.

SKIN LESIONS/ULCERATIONS

Ruby Taylor

Venous or arterial impairment can place an older adult at risk for skin lesions or ulcers. Vascular insufficiency causes >90% of all ulcers below the knee. Many people over age 60 years assume that pain in the legs and skin ulceration are a part of growing old, and fail to notice the development of a problem. Chemical, mechanical, thermal, and surgical factors can precipitate skin breakdown (Table 1).

A. History taking should elicit
    • onset and duration of the lesion
    • occurrence of trauma or bleeding
    • preferred body positioning
    • presence of pain or claudication
    • topical agents used
    • use of heat or cold
    • current ulcer treatment, including home remedies
    • medical history
    • food and fluid intake
    • current level of activity
    • incidence of swelling

B. Assess the lesion for
    • location
    • size: length, width, depth
    • undermining
    • drainage
    • odor
    • inflammatory halo
    • stage
    • appearance of wound bed
    • surrounding tissue
    Evaluate circulation to the area by
    • skin temperature
    • capillary refill
    • edema
    • blood pressure ankle/arm indices
    • Doppler (see p. 236)

Check the neurologic status of affected area in relation to
    • differentiation of heat and cold
    • pain sensation
    • awareness of pressure or position
Culture of drainage may be helpful. A biopsy is sometimes performed to diagnose a chronic bacterial or fungal skin infection.

C. Educational efforts include
    • proper hygiene and skin care
    • local wound care using a nonirritating cleanser (*note:* never put anything in a lesion that could not be placed in an eye)
    • elevation of the involved extremity (see p. 237)
    • avoidance of prolonged periods with the involved extremity in a dependent position
    • proper use of antiembolic stockings
    • daily inspection of extremities
    • observation for signs and symptoms of infection
    • medication regimen
    • injury precautions
    • adequate nutrition and fluids
    • pain relief measures (Table 2)
    Since skin lesions are often slow to heal, reassure and offer ongoing support to the patient and caregiver.

D. Goals of treatment are
    • appropriate wound care
    • promotion of wound healing
    Appropriate wound care requires that a clean, warm, moist wound environment be maintained. Ways to accomplish this include
    • debridement of devitalized tissue
    • scheduling of dressing changes
    • management of incontinence
    • placement of occlusive dressings

TABLE 1 Precipitating Factors for Skin Lesions and Ulcers

Type	Definition	Manifestation
Chemical	Interaction of elements applied to skin	Blisters, rash, secondary infection
Mechanical	Injury to skin due to pressure, loss of circulation, or external object	Scratch, laceration, puncture, pressure ulcer (see Pressure Sore, p. 106)
Thermal	Heat or cold applied to skin with impaired circulation	Blisters, ischemia
Surgical	Operative procedure that opens skin	Incision, wound dehiscence

TABLE 2 Pain Management Methods

Method	Purpose
Analgesics	Pain relief Reduction of inflammation
Compression devices	Reduction of swelling Enhancement of circulation
Cordotomy	Surgical interruption of anterolateral quadrant of spinal cord; used for intractable pain in lower extremities
Psychological Music Biofeedback Relaxation	Alteration of pain response
Neuromodulation	Pain suppression by electrical stimulation

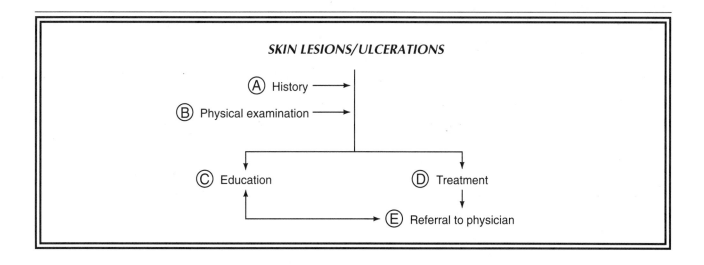

SKIN LESIONS/ULCERATIONS

Ⓐ History

Ⓑ Physical examination

Ⓒ Education

Ⓓ Treatment

Ⓔ Referral to physician

Wound healing is promoted by
- providing optimal nutrition
- improving circulation
- reducing pressure on the lesion

E. Medical evaluation and management is indicated for
- signs and symptoms of infection
- pain management (Table 2)
- deep debridement
- whirlpool
- use of occlusive dressings or Dome paste bandages

References

Bok L. Chronic ulcers of the skin. New York: McGraw-Hill, 1985:93.
Brunner LS, Suddarth DS. The Lippincott manual of nursing practice. Philadelphia: JB Lippincott, 1982:333.
Stanford L. Dermatology in primary care. Philadelphia: WB Saunders, 1986:358.

SKIN TAGS (ACROCHORDONS)

Sylvia Moreno
Etta Hall

Skin tags are benign proliferations of dermis and overlying epidermis. They consist of loose fibrous tissue connected to the skin by a narrow pedicle and with thin epidermis. They are flesh colored or slightly darker and are frequently found with typical sessile seborrheic warts. Skin tags appear pedunculated and often constricted at the base. They are round, soft, elastic, and frequently pigmented. The surface may be smooth or irregular and may vary in size from 1 to 10 mm in diameter. They are generally asymptomatic unless the pedicle twists and infarction occurs. Skin tags are common in menopausal and postmenopausal women. Recent research indicates that men with diabetes may be predisposed to skin tags.

A. Ask the patient about
   • onset
   • medical and menopausal history
   • pain
   • location
   • changes in skin color
   • irritation from clothing

B. Examine closely areas where skin tags are commonly found, such as the
   • lateral neck
   • eyelids
   • axillae
   • upper trunk
   • groin
   In obese patients, also check
   • areas of flexion
   • the front of the neck

Laboratory screening may include glucose level testing.

C. Patient education should focus on care of the skin tag areas. Tell patients to
   • avoid clothing that irritates
   • keep the area clean and dry
   • report any changes in color or development of pain

D. Common medical treatment for skin tags is excision by snipping with scissors or cauterization. Other forms of treatment include electrodesiccation, cryosurgery, and chemical cauterization. Pain during these procedures is minimal. Local anesthesia is optional. Skin tags removed are sent for histologic examination to rule out cutaneous papillomas. After medical treatment the patient should be taught signs and symptoms of infection to report.

References

Balin AK, Kligman AM. Aging and the skin. New York: Raven Press, 1989.

Fry L. Skin problems in the elderly. London: Butler & Tanner, 1985.

Marks R. Skin disease in old age. Philadelphia: JB Lippincott, 1987.

Newcomer VD, Young EM Jr. Geriatric dermatology/clinical diagnosis and practical therapy. New York/Tokyo: Igaku-Shoin, 1989.

SKIN TAGS (ACROCHORDONS)

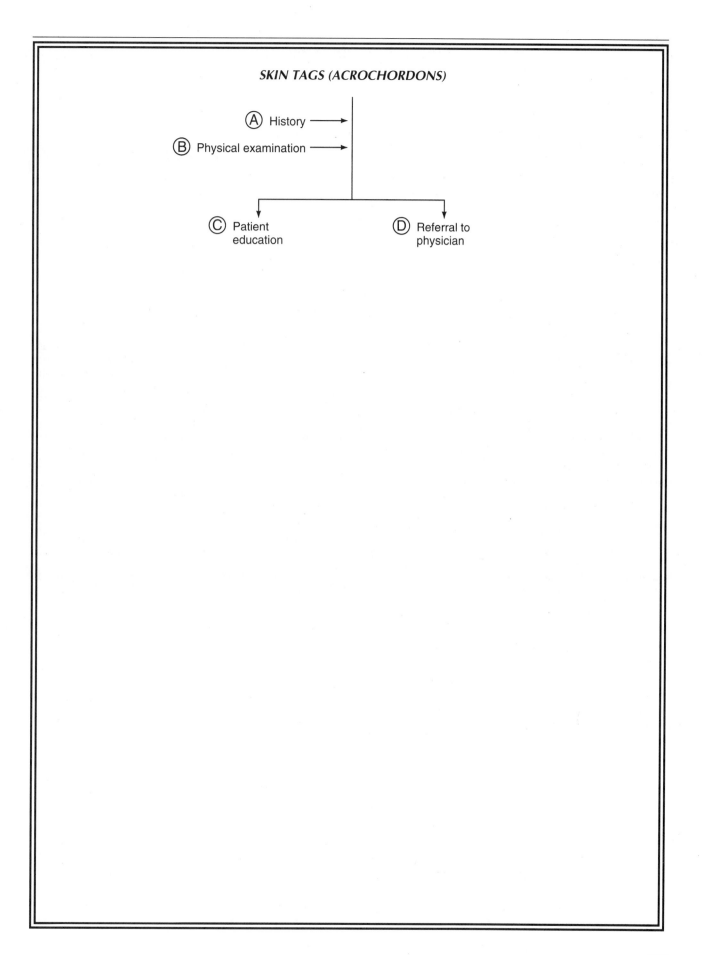

(A) History ⟶

(B) Physical examination ⟶

(C) Patient education

(D) Referral to physician

WARTS

Tom Emanuele

Warts are a common problem. They are caused by viruses and transmitted by direct contact during viral shedding. Elderly patients who have large numbers of warts may be immunosuppressed.

A. History taking focuses on
- current skin problems
  - onset
  - duration
  - precipitating factors
  - treatments tried
- past skin problems: warts, plantar warts
- sun exposure
- medical history
  - communicable diseases
  - presence of a pacemaker
  - autoimmune disorders
    - rheumatoid arthritis
    - lupus erythematosus
    - diabetes mellitus
    - malignancy/cancer
    - sexual history
    - medications
      - steroids
      - chemotherapy

B. Physical examination evaluates the warts' location, distribution, and appearance (Table 1). Determine if the lesions cause functional disability.

C. Refer the patient to a physician when warts are discovered. A podiatrist may be an appropriate referral for plantar warts. Treatment will be determined by the type of warts and location (Table 1).

TABLE 1 Warts: Differentiation, Treatment, and Nursing Care

Type	Appearance	Location/Distribution	Treatment	Comments	Nursing Care
Common warts	Primary—pinhead size, flesh-colored, translucent papules Secondary—larger, raised surface; hyperkeratotic; flesh-colored or darker	Common on hands and fingers May appear on skin and mucous membranes	Cantharidin Salicylic acid (SAL) Podophyllin resin 10% Curettage Cryotherapy Electrodesiccation	Change size over weeks to months	Leave Podophyllin resin on overnight Cover lesions with adhesive tape to increase effectiveness of chemicals
Seborrheic warts (basal cell papilloma)	Well defined, irregular, nodular thickened, roughened surface Usually light brown, but may be fawn to jet black	Hair-bearing skin Sun-exposed skin	Curettage Electrodesiccation Cryotherapy	Increase in size over time May appear suddenly	Encourage sunscreen
Giant condyloma of Buschke (virus-induced papilloma)	Exuberant warty nodule	External genitalia and perineal region	Surgical excision Cryotherapy	Specific to elderly Requires cytology to differentiate from squamous cell carcinoma	Provide support
Plantar warts	Hyperkeratotic, firm elevated or flat lesions with central nodule Interrupts natural skin lines	Weight-bearing soles of feet	Dichloroacetic acid 50% to 80% 10% SAL plaster	Unusual as new lesion in elderly Surgical excision is not recommended	Pare lesion before acid Remove crusts Treat every 1–2 weeks Keep area covered
Venereal warts (condyloma acuminata)	Small papillomas develop into soft, friable, vegetating clusters	Foreskin, penis, vaginal walls, labial folds, urethral meatus	Podophyllin 20%–25% Electrodesiccation Interferon into lesion	May get large if untreated Grow in warm, moist areas	Maintain patient confidentiality
Molluscum contagiosum (caused by pox virus)	Small cratered or umbilicated pearly nodules Central core contains white, cheesy, waxy material	Alone or clustered Face, neck, trunk, lower abdomen, pubis, inner thighs, genitalia	Cryotherapy Electrodesiccation Surgical excision/ curettage Manual expression of core Podophyllin 20%–25%	May arise in elderly alone or multiple Lesions near eyes may cause keratosis and conjunctivitis	Encourage cryotherapy which leaves no scar

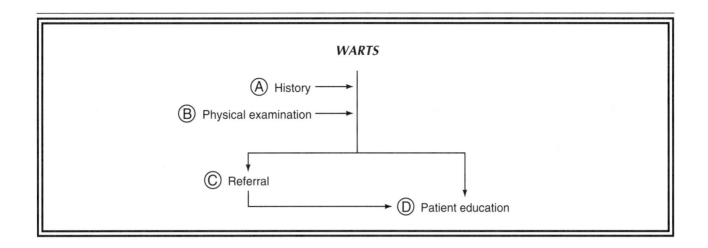

WARTS

Ⓐ History

Ⓑ Physical examination

Ⓒ Referral

Ⓓ Patient education

Instructions Based on Type of Treatment
Chemical treatment • expect a stinging or burning sensation • do not get chemicals on healthy skin • may apply petroleum jelly to healthy skin for protection Electrodesiccation • high-frequency cautery may deactivate a pacemaker Interferon • flulike symptoms may develop • be sure to drink plenty of fluids, especially if fever is present

D. Specific instruction (see box) depends on the treatment prescribed. General instructions relate to
   • Shaving and direct contact with lesions, which can transmit or inoculate other areas.
   • Care of surgical areas
   • Comfort measures (administration of analgesics and warm packs or sitz baths)

References

Arndt K. Manual of dermatologic therapeutics. Boston: Little, Brown and Company, 1989.

Marks R. Skin disease and old age. Philadelphia: JB Lippincott, Co., 1987.

SENSORY/COMMUNICATION

DECREASED VISION

Sue Miller

Decreased vision is a symptom resulting from systemic disease or physical changes that alter the light path, prevent light from passing through the eye, or distort image formation.

A. History includes
- onset: sudden or gradual
- chronic medical problems
- unilateral or bilateral
- date of last visual test
- ability to read newspaper print
- current medication use, over-the-counter and pre-scription drugs
- occurrence of motor vehicle accidents or citations
- duration
- changes in lifestyle
- use of corrective lens
- previous eye surgery
- allergies

B. Examination includes external eye assessment, eye function tests, and ophthalmic examination. Common external eye findings are
- arcus senilis
- dry eyes due to impaired tear production
- cataracts
- senile ptosis

TABLE 1   Conditions and Diseases Affecting Vision

Disease	Visual Symptoms	Clinical Findings
Cataract	Complaints of intolerance to glare Progressive dimming of vision not corrected with prescription change Colors faded or muted Loss of detail No complaints of pain	Reduction of visual acuity to 20/30 or less Ophthalmoscope shows lens opacity as dark areas with pupil dilated.
Macular degeneration	Loss of central vision Peripheral vision remains unchanged Visual acuity may decrease within days	Straight line appears crooked, bent, or missing a central segment Ophthalmoscope shows small yellow-white spots around the macula as disease progresses, dark pigmentary areas clump and scar
Glaucoma, open-angle (chronic)	Asymptomatic Halos around lights Intolerance to glare Blurred vision not corrected with glasses Slow, progressive loss of peripheral vision	Narrowed visual fields High intraocular pressure (>21 mmHg) Degeneration and cupping of optic disc Atrophy of optic nerve head
Glaucoma, acute-angle (closed)	Symptoms occur more rapidly than with open-angle glaucoma Colored halos around lights May have severe headache, nausea or vomiting, pain in eyes, blurring of vision Usually occurs in one eye	Pupil fixed in mid-dilation Eye is tender Eye feels firm as compared to unaffected eye Visual fields narrow
Diabetes	Blurred vision may occur as blood sugars fluctuate	Elevated or unstable blood sugars Increased incidence of cataracts
Hypertension	Blurred vision Headache	Elevated blood pressure Ophthalmoscope reveals ocular vessel constriction, hemorrhages, exudate, and papilledema
Chronic hypocalcemia	Symptoms associated with cataract formation	Decreased serum calcium Increased incidence of cataracts

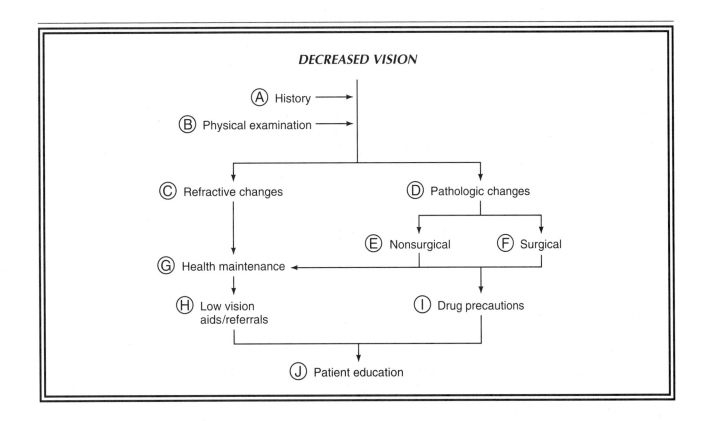

DECREASED VISION

A. History
B. Physical examination

C. Refractive changes   D. Pathologic changes

E. Nonsurgical   F. Surgical

G. Health maintenance

H. Low vision aids/referrals   I. Drug precautions

J. Patient education

Medications Contraindicated or Used with Caution in Glaucoma

- antianxiety agent
- anticholinergic
- anticonvulsant
- antidepressant
- antihistamine
- antiparkinsonian
- antipsychotic
- antispasmodic
- bronchodilator
- central nervous system stimulant
- decongestant: systemic and local
- mydriatic
- psychotropic drugs
- sedative or hypnotic
- skeletal muscle relaxer
- vasodilator
- vasopressor

Eye function testing consists of
- visual acuity
- extraocular movements
- responsiveness to light
- accommodation
- peripheral vision

The Snellen's test (Fig. 1) may be used for testing distance vision. Test each eye individually, with and without glasses. The Rosenbaum Pocket Vision Screener (Fig. 2) may be used to test reading vision. All causes of decreased vision require investigation when a change of glasses does not improve vision. A quick evaluation can include determining if the patient can see facial expressions at 2 and 10 feet. Lens opacity will impair the examiner's ability to visualize the inner eye. Table 1 lists diseases that contribute to visual changes or loss.

C. Age changes in the lens cause the loss of accommodation. Items held closer than 1 or 2 feet may appear fuzzy because of the lens' inability to thicken and focus light from the object to the retina. Refractory changes are usually corrected by prescribed reading glasses or bifocals.

D. Visual acuity can be maintained with treatment. An immediate ophthalmology examination is indicated for acute vision changes.

E. Nonsurgical treatment needs an understanding of the disease disorder and treatment plan. Laser treatment and drugs usually control vision loss if the patient adheres to a strict routine.

F. Judicious surgical intervention can improve or maintain vision. Cataract surgery may provide sight restoration. Lens implants can improve vision to 20/30 in many cases. Surgical procedures for acute-angle glaucoma (iridotomy) and retinal detachment are usually performed as an emergency. Retinal detachment occurs quickly, sometimes as a result of trauma to the eye or as a complication of cataract surgery. Symptoms of retinal detachment are flashes of light, floaters, distortion of images, and loss of vision.

G. A complete eye evaluation of visual acuity, visual fields, tonometry, and dilation of the pupil at least 6 mm in diameter is recommended every 2 to 3 years or as recommended for a known ophthalmic disease. Use of over-the-counter eye drops should be discussed. The eye drops may mask eye problems or precipitate an exacerbation of visual disorders. Safety goggles should be encouraged for individuals engaged

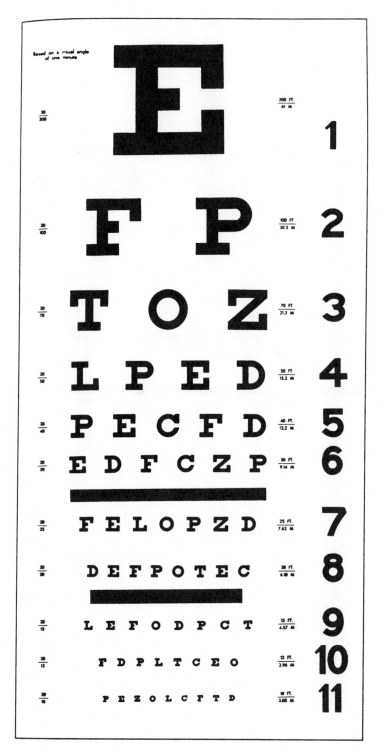

Figure 1 Snellen eye chart.

in activities with flying debris, such as welding, machinery, carpentry, and yard work.

H. Patients with visual losses can benefit from low-vision aids such as
- glasses with reading prism, high-power bifocals or reading lens, microscope, reading telescope
- magnifiers: handheld and with adjustable stand
- telescopes for distance vision
- large-print books

Referrals to community agencies such as the State Commission for the Blind, American Foundation for the Blind, Lighthouse for the Blind, and the Lions Club may increase life satisfaction and enjoyment. Specialized services for the visually impaired can offer training for activities of daily living and adaptation to changes presented by a loss of sight.

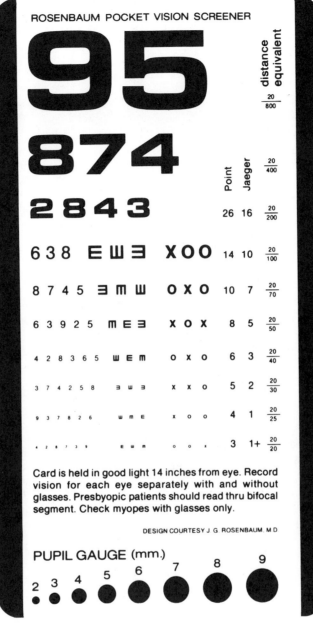

Figure 2 Rosenbaum Pocket Vision Screener. Card is held in good light 14 inches from eye. Record vision for each eye separately with and without eyeglasses. Presbyopic patients should read through bifocal segment. Check myopic with glasses only. (Design courtesy of JG Rosenbaum, M.D.)

I. Any drug that increases intraocular pressure should be avoided by patients with glaucoma. See the box on the preceding page for classes of medications contraindicated or used with caution. Consult a pharmacist for specific drugs in each classification. Patients taking systemic corticosteroids have an increased incidence of cataract formation.

J. Patient education focuses on
   • use of medications, including technique for instilling eye drops
   • use of visual aids
   • smoking cessation
   • adherence to follow-up care

   • signs and symptoms requiring emergency care: rapid, complete, or partial vision loss.

References

Ebersole P, Hess P. Toward healthy aging: Human needs and nursing response. 3rd ed. Baltimore: CV Mosby, 1990:286.

Eliopoulas C. Caring for the elderly in diverse care settings. Philadelphia: JB Lippincott, 1990:210.

Reichel W. Clinical aspects of aging. 3rd ed. Baltimore: Williams & Wilkins, 1989:445.

HEARING LOSS

Carolyn Cole

Hearing loss is not necessarily due to aging alone. Many causes of hearing loss are treatable. Consonants with high frequency, such as *t, f, z, g, th,* and *sh* are generally not heard by older persons. Determining conductive versus sensorineural hearing loss is crucial to the nursing assessment and subsequent management of this common problem.

A. Ask about
- current and previous ear infections
- medications, particularly ototoxic drugs
  - loop diuretics
  - aminoglycosides
  - salicylates
- childhood illnesses
- family health history
- symptoms of eighth cranial nerve disease
  - sudden or unilateral hearing loss
  - accompanied by
    - vertigo
    - tinnitus
    - aural fullness
- prolonged noise exposure

B. Hearing screening includes the spoken voice or an audioscope, Weber's test, Rinne's test, and an otoscopic examination (Table 1). Have the patient repeat words presented in a soft whisper, a normal spoken voice, or a shout, preferably in a quiet room. Test each ear separately by having the patient occlude the opposite ear with a finger.

A 40-db audioscope can be used to test frequencies of 500, 1000, 2000, and 4000 Hz. High frequencies, particularly 4000 Hz, may not be heard.

Otoscopic examination includes inspection of the external canal and middle ear. Observe for
- redness
- bulging of the membrane
- discharge
- foreign bodies
- cerumen
- extreme tenderness during examination
- perforated tympanic membrane
- scarring

Test cranial nerves.

C. Patients who can hear only a shout or have difficulty hearing pure tones at more than one frequency on an audioscopic examination should be referred to an otolaryngologist or audiologist. Patients with conductive hearing loss may benefit from a variety of listening devices. A referral should be made to an appropriate center specializing in communication disorders to obtain the most useful device for the individual. Financially disadvantaged senior citizens may benefit from referral to social service agencies to obtain hearing aids or other amplification devices at reduced cost.

Patient Teaching for Hearing Loss	
Topic	Content
Pathophysiology	• cilia in the external ear become coarse and stiff with aging • cerumen buildup and impaction occur more frequently as the self-cleaning properties of the ears diminish with age • any medication or solution put into the ear should be warmed to body temperature to prevent dizziness, nausea, or fainting
Hygiene	• cleanse ears gently with a washcloth over the finger • hairpins, swabs, and other instruments may cause injury, secondary infection, or further cerumen impaction if used for cleaning • moderate amounts of cerumen can be treated with over-the-counter cerumenolytics or mineral oil before gentle irrigation with tap water at body temperature
Communication facilitation	• restate words not heard in conversation rather than repeating the same word several times • face the patient on the same level • be aware that eating, chewing, or smoking while talking will make speech more difficult to understand • reduce background noises by turning off the radio or television • keep hands away from face while talking • never talk from another room • get the patient's attention before starting to speak • speak in a normal fashion, without shouting • check that light is not shining in the eyes of the patient during conversation • recognize that patients with hearing loss who are tired or ill understand and hear less

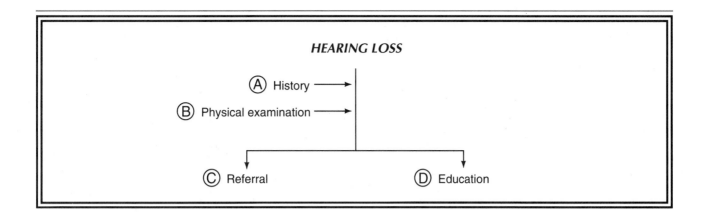

HEARING LOSS

Ⓐ History

Ⓑ Physical examination

Ⓒ Referral

Ⓓ Education

TABLE 1 Specialized Hearing Tests

Test	Equipment	Technique	Analysis
Weber's	512-Hz tuning fork	Tap tuning fork lightly. Place vibrating tuning fork gently on patient's forehead.	In unilateral conductive loss, sound will lateralize to the affected ear. Sound lateralizes to the good ear in sensorineural loss.
Rinne's	512-Hz tuning fork	Tap tuning fork lightly. Place vibrating tuning fork on the mastoid bone. Have patient state when the sound is no longer heard. Move tuning fork next to patient's ear. Compare length of time sound is heard in each position. Test each ear.	Air conduction is greater than bone conduction in normal hearing or in sensorineural loss. Bone conduction is greater than air conduction in conductive loss.

Cases of cerumen obstruction in the presence of chronic otitis media, perforated drum, or other middle ear anatomic anomalies should be referred to an otolaryngologist for safe removal after 1 week's treatment with mineral oil to soften the impaction. If the nurse cannot treat infections or if the patient has chronic, resistant otitis media, the patient should be referred to a physician for treatment.

D. Patient teaching includes pathophysiology, hygiene, and ways to facilitate communication (see box on facing page).

References

Mahoney DG. One simple solution to hearing impairment. Geriatr Nurs (New York) 1987; 8:242.

Scura KW. Audiological assessment program. J Gerontol Nurs 1988; 14:19.

TINNITUS

Carolyn Cole

Tinnitus is often associated with presbycusis (decreased hearing due to old age), but it can be due to illness. Physiologically, tinnitus can arise from the outer ear, middle ear, or cochlea and neural pathways. Previous noise exposure, ear infections, and medication can cause tinnitus, but frequently the underlying cause is undetermined.

The effects of tinnitus on an individual's life-style can be far-reaching and may include
- sleep disturbances (see p. 82)
- hearing interference
- difficulty understanding telephone conversations
- tiredness
- irritability
- loss of concentration
- depression (see p. 282)
- psychological illness

A. Ask questions about
- current or previous occupational noise exposure
- trauma
- infections
- allergies
- medical history
  - hypertension
  - diabetes
  - hypoglycemia
  - hypothyroidism
  - syphilis
- medications: prescription and over-the-counter drugs (see box "Drugs That May Cause or Aggravate Tinnitus")
- depression (see p. 282)

Obtain information about specific symptoms:
- pulsatile tinnitus may be associated with vascular anomalies
- aural fullness, deafness, vertigo, and other neurologic symptoms can be indicators of eighth cranial nerve disorders
- auditory hallucinations

B. Physical examination consists of
- vital signs to detect uncontrolled hypertension
- otoscopic examination
- common reversible causes of tinnitus
  - otitis media
  - trauma
  - occluding cerumen
- foul-smelling discharge
- blood
- foreign body
- perforated tympanic membrane
- Weber's test (see Table 1 in Hearing Loss, p. 122 or 123)
- Rinne's test (see Table 1 in Hearing Loss, p. 122 or 123)
- hearing screening
- neurologic testing, particularly of cranial nerves, looking for
  - ataxia
  - nystagmus
  - papilledema
  - other signs of increased cerebral pressure

Laboratory tests that may prove helpful are
- therapeutic drug levels
- blood chemistries

C. Education focuses on reducing further damage or aggravation of symptoms. Tinnitus may not always be resolved, but increasing a patient's resourcefulness and ability to care for oneself can decrease the impact of tinnitus on the patient's life (see the box "Education for Patients with Tinnitus").

D. Referrals may be made on the basis of findings from both physical examination and history (see the box "Potential Referrals for Tinnitus").

Drugs That May Cause or Aggravate Tinnitus

Aminoglycosides
Loop diuretics
Salicylates
Quinine
Tricyclic antidepressants
Quinidine
Antineoplastic drugs
Beta-blockers
Nonsteroidal anti-inflammatory drugs
Immunosuppression drugs

Education for Patients with Tinnitus

Topic	Content
Noise exposure	Noise-induced tinnitus can arise from prolonged or a single episode of noise exposure
	Use protective ear devices to reduce occupational and recreational noise exposure
Diet	Stimulants that may aggravate tinnitus include
	• caffeine
	• chocolate
	• foods that cause allergic reactions
Life-style	Soft external noise from a radio or stereo can mask tinnitus especially at night when that symptom is most severe
	Habits that decrease overall health can aggravate tinnitus
	• smoking
	• excessive alcohol
	Regular exercise and stress reduction can improve overall health and promote a sense of well being

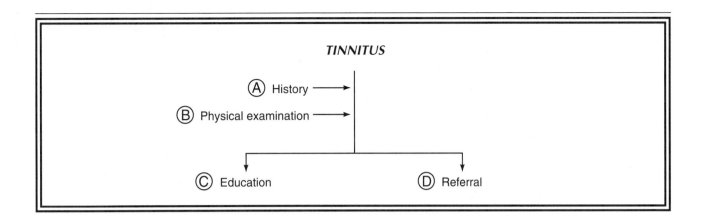

TINNITUS

Ⓐ History ⟶

Ⓑ Physical examination ⟶

Ⓒ Education   Ⓓ Referral

Potential Referrals for Tinnitus	
Refer to	*Purpose*
Primary physician	Review or change of medication regimen
Otolaryngologist	Treatment of hearing loss
	Treatment of significant ear findings
	• infection
	• cerumen impaction
Neurologist	Evaluation of cranial nerve function
Psychosocial counseling	Treatment of depression
	Evaluation of psychological disorders
Community resources	Decrease social isolation
	Stop-smoking clinics
	Alcohol addiction recovery (i.e., Alcoholics Anonymous)
Audiologist	Hearing screening
	Audiogram
	Assistive device

References

Cole RE, Hallam RS. Tinnitus and its management. Br Med Bull 1987; 43:983.

Gulya AJ. Ear disorders: hearing loss. In: Abrams WB, Berkow R, eds. Merck manual of geriatrics. Rahway, NJ: Merck and Co., 1990:1083.

Klotch DW. Otolaryngology in the geriatric patient. Primary Care 1982; 9:167.

LaMarte FP, Tyler RS. Noise-induced tinnitus. Ann Am Occup Health Nurs 1987; 35:403.

Stephens DG. Tinnitus. Practitioner 1987; 231:1115.

DECREASED SENSE OF SMELL

Cynthia Sommer

Changes in sense of smell can affect quality of life, safety, and adequacy of nutrition. Ability to distinguish pleasant as well as unpleasant odors affects emotional response, appetite, and social responses and forewarns of danger. Patients who have impaired ability to smell often become unsure of themselves socially. Sense of smell affects:
- ability to determine presence of odors
  - objectional body odor
  - smoke
  - spoiled foods
  - escaping gas
- dietary habits and ability to appreciate food flavors
  - eating more to compensate for lack of flavor
  - using excessive salt or sugar to offset losses
  - avoiding food, resulting in weight loss (see Weight Change, p. 158)

After the age of 70 years there is an accelerated decline in smell sensitivity partly because of a decrease in olfactory receptors. Forty percent of persons over age 80 have difficulty identifying common substances by smell. Decrements in smell occur more often in men, in late old age, and with illness. Conditions and medications associated with impaired sense of smell are listed in the box "Conditions and Medications Associated with Decreased Sense of Smell."

A. History should seek to determine past or present
- nasal obstruction
- epistaxis
- occupational exposures
- snoring
- neurologic disorders
- lesions
- rhinorrhea, rhinitis, or coryza
- trauma to nose or head
- chronic upper respiratory infections
- liver disease
- change in or difficulty with sense of smell
- diagnosed or suspected allergy manifested in the nose
  - onset
  - cause
  - frequency
  - measures taken
- medication use, particularly type and frequency of nose drops and sprays

B. Physical examination is meant to look at the nose and identify abnormalities. Gloves should be worn during examination. Inspect and palpate externally for
- nasal symmetry
- lesions or drainage
- nasal septal deviation
- nasal bone and cartilage tenderness

Inspect internally with a nasal speculum or penlight and blade-type speculum for

TABLE 1 Differential Findings in Nasal Examination

Condition/Cause	Color	Appearance
Normal mucosa	Pink	Free of swelling, lesions, drainage
Allergy	Pale, gray	Swollen
Rhinitis (upper respiratory infection)	Red	Swollen

Conditions and Medications Associated with Decreased Sense of Smell

Condition	Medication
Congenital/genetic	Opiate analgesics
Infectious: upper respiratory infection*	Antithyroid drugs
Acute viral hepatitis	Methimazole
Cirrhosis	Propylthiouracil
Alzheimer's disease	Cardiovascular drugs
Seizure disorders	Dipyridamole
Multiple sclerosis	Beta-blockers
Meningiomas	Nifedipine
Parkinson's disease	Diltiazem
Korsakoff's disease	Dextroamphetamine
Head trauma*	Tetracycline
Occupational exposure	Acetylcholine HCl
Nasal/sinus disease*	Menthol
Allergies*	Strychnine

*Most common causes

Patient and Caregiver Instructions

Topic	Content
Maximize function	• sniff foods before eating • call up memory of smells before eating • stimulate appetite with aesthetic food preparation • use pleasant smells: cologne, flowers, sachet • follow a daily hygiene regimen that will eliminate body odor
Use other senses	• date spoilable foods and discard appropriately • check pilot lights visually
Environmental precautions	• check gas appliances for leaks frequently • contact gas company for leak detector • maintain smoke detectors in working order • use electric heat and cooking if possible

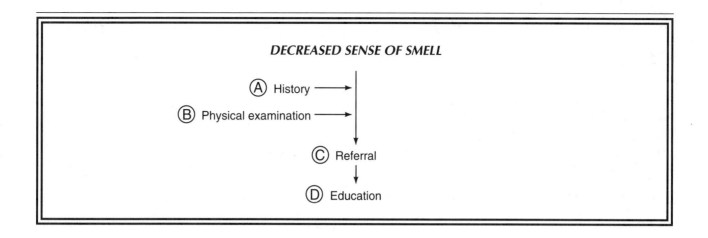

DECREASED SENSE OF SMELL

Ⓐ History

Ⓑ Physical examination

Ⓒ Referral

Ⓓ Education

• lesions or drainage
• appearance of septal wall and turbinates
• presence of polyps, usually protruding from middle turbinate

Differential findings are shown in Table 1. Assess patency of the nares; one may be slightly larger than the other.

• Have patient hold one naris shut and breathe through the other.
• Observe circles of condensation on a small mirror beneath naris.
• Look for differences in size of condensation to indicate blockage.

Assess olfaction (cranial nerve I) through neurologic testing.

• Have patient hold one naris shut to test each one separately.
• Place a substance with a familiar odor under the open naris, such as
  • cinnamon
  • lemon or orange
  • cloves
  • garlic
  • cocoa
  • peanut butter
  • coffee
  • vanilla

• Ask patient to identify the substance.
• Use different substances for each naris.

C. Refer pathologic findings to primary care or ear, nose, and throat physician. Dietary consultation may be warranted if decreased appetite puts the patient at risk for malnutrition.

D. Education of the patient and caregiver focuses on maximizing remaining function, using other senses, and modifying the environment (see the box "Patient and Caregiver Instructions").

References

Doty RL, Perl DP, Steele JC, et al. Olfactory dysfunction in three neurodegenerative diseases. Geriatrics 1991; 46(Suppl 1):47.

Kee CC. Sensory impairment: Factor X in providing nursing care to the older adult. J Community Health Nurs 1990; 7:45.

Kopac CA. Sensory loss in the aged: The role of the nurse and family. Nurs Clin North Am 1983; 18:373.

Malkiewicz J. Examining the nose. RN 1982; 45:55.

Scott AE. Clinical characteristics of taste and smell disorders. Ear Nose Throat J 1989; 68:297.

Zegeer LJ. The effects of sensory changes in older persons. J Neurosci Nurs 1986; 18:325.

HOARSENESS

Kathy B. Wright

Changes in stiffness or tension of the vocal folds in the larynx affect traveling wave motion, causing hoarseness. Hoarseness can result from inflammatory responses, tumors, traumatic injury, neurologic disease, or other underlying causes such as functional aphonia. Hoarseness is the prime, and often, sole symptom of laryngeal disease (Table 1).

A. History should include
    • onset of hoarseness
    • cough
    • snoring or earaches
    • dysphagia, dyspnea
    • cancer, any type
    • exposure to tuberculosis or syphilis and treatment
    • history of sore throats, frequency including duration, and cause, such as mild pharyngitis versus streptococcal infection
    • presence of contributing factors such as
      • cigarette smoking
      • vocal straining
      • chronic laryngitis
      • alcohol consumption
      • chemical fumes or dust exposure
      • family predisposition
    • reports of pain or discomfort: radiating to the ear, on swallowing, or associated with drinking hot liquids
    • medication and drug history, particularly antihistamines, decongestants, birth control pills, steroid sprays, marijuana, or cocaine
    • chronic illnesses
    • presence and amount of sputum
    • history of hoarseness or aphonia
    • habitual clearing of throat
    • weight loss or debilitation
    • heartburn or gastric reflux

Antireflux Regimen

Lifestyle Modification
  • reduce or stop smoking
  • do NOT use more pillows
  • do NOT bend from waist
  • elevate head of bed on 6-inch blocks or use large foam rubber wedge under shoulders and back
  • restrict alcohol
  • avoid slouching while sitting
  • avoid tight garments or belts

Nutrition Alterations
  • eliminate or decrease foods causing symptoms:
    • fats
    • citrus juices
    • tomato products
    • chocolate
    • coffee or tea
    • carminatives—peppermint, garlic, onion
  • eat small or lighter, more frequent low-fat meals
  • lose weight, if indicated; even 5 to 10 pounds can help
  • do not lie down until 2 to 3 hours after a meal
  • follow a bowel management regimen to avoid constipation

Pharmacologic Measures
  • use antacids regularly, 1 to 2 tablespoons or 1 to 2 tablets, well chewed, 30 to 60 minutes after each meal and at bedtime
  • discuss with physician decreasing or discontinuing drugs such as theophylline, diazepam, calcium channel blockers, nitrates, and anticholinergics

Measures If No Relief Occurs from Dietary or Lifestyle Changes
  • pharmacologic agents
    • histamine H_2—receptor-blocking agents (cimetidine, ranitidine, famotidine, nizatidine, omeprazole)
    • promotility or prokinetic agents (bethanechol, metoclopramide, domperidone, cisapride)
    • enhance mucosal resistance (sucralfate)
  • surgery—construction of new sphincter for an effective antireflux barrier

HOARSENESS

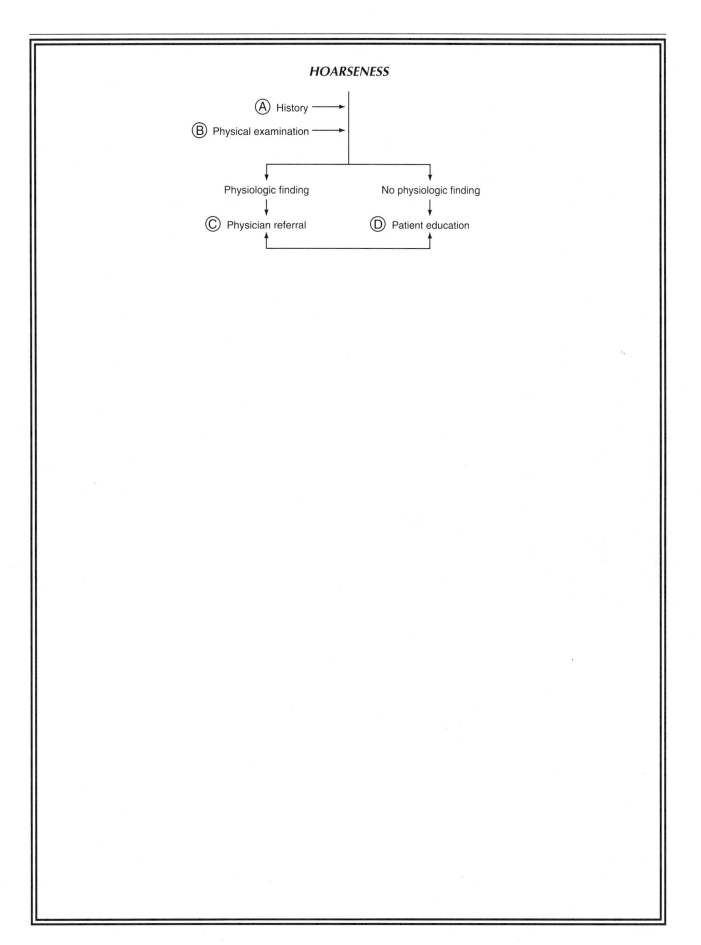

TABLE 1 Potential Causes of Hoarseness

Cause	Recent Onset	Chronic Problem
Overuse	Shouting, cheering	Occupational: singer, teacher
Infection, inflammation	Laryngitis Upper respiratory infection Epiglottitis Diphtheria Smallpox Measles	Nonspecific chronic laryngitis Alcoholism Gout Tobacco use, smoking Singer's nodes Sarcoidosis
Edema	Insect bite Potassium iodide	Myxedema Chronic nephritis Allergy
Dryness, lack of mucus	Atropine-like drugs Antihistamines Decongestants	Sjögren's disease
Surface ulcers, lesions, burns	Aspirin aspiration Inhalation of irritant gases Swallowing hot or caustic liquids	Keratosis Pachyderma Herpes Leukoplakia Tuberculosis Syphilis Leprosy Lupus erythematosus Typhoid fever
Trauma	Intubation damage Foreign body	Foreign body X-ray radiation of neck region
Neoplasm of cords		Benign or malignant tumors: papilloma, fibroma, angioma, lipoma, epithelioma, and carcinoma
Innervation of cords	Severed nerve during thyroidectomy	Compression of nerve by aortic aneurysm, large left atrium, mediastinal neoplasm, lymphadenopathy or retrosternal goiter
Weakness of cords		Severe anemia
Weakness of muscles		Myasthenia gravis Myxedema
Compression of larynx		Thyrotoxicosis Retropharyngeal abscess Neoplasm of pharynx Goiter Actinomycosis of neck

B. Physical examination focuses on the head and neck
- inspect for signs of infection, previous surgery, or injury
- observe breath odor
- palpate the neck for swelling, tenderness, or changes in thyroid cartilage
- examine the oropharynx (see the tool *Oral Examination*, p. 183)
- perform indirect laryngoscopic examination

Laboratory evaluation may include a complete blood count and serum analysis for syphilis. Tuberculin skin test may be indicated by history.

C. Referral to a primary care physician or otolaryngologist is indicated for treated hoarseness lasting longer than 2 weeks. In the presence of pathologic findings, immediate referral to a physician is indicated to rule out neoplastic or infectious disease. Viewing of the vocal cords is highly recommended unless hoarseness is attributed to a cold or voice misuse. The larynx can be inspected directly using rigid or flexible laryngoscopy. A biopsy may be performed if indicated. Diagnostic examinations may include barium swallow; chest radiograph if hoarseness is accompanied by cough; CT scan or MRI for suspected tumor; and pH monitoring for suspicion of reflux. Objective measurements of hoarseness permit evaluation of laryngeal function for documentation and quantification purposes and include imaging, and aerodynamic or acoustic measurements.

D. Patient education addresses
- smoking cessation
- steam inhalation
- voice rest for several days
- constant environmental heat and humidity
- increased fluids
- throat lozenges
- avoidance of antihistamines and decongestants because of drying effect
- use of antibiotics as prescribed
- antireflux regimen, if needed (see box on p. 128)

Speech pathology may be indicated for voice abuse, dysphagia evaluation, or cineesophagram.

References

Chasin WD, Feder RJ, Koufman JA. What a problem voice tells you. Patient Care 1987; 21:60.

Curtis LG. Common ear, nose, and throat problems, part II: Disorders of the nose and throat. Physician Assistant 1990; 14:11.

Meyerhoff WL, Rice DL. Otolaryngology—head and neck surgery. Philadelphia: WB Saunders, 1992.

SPEECH AND LANGUAGE IMPAIRMENT

Cynthia Sommer

Speech or language impairment includes disorders that interfere with the production, comprehension, or expression of words. *Speech* is the mechanics of producing words; *language* is the comprehension and expression of ideas. Hearing and vision loss as well as certain neurologic and degenerative neuromuscular diseases, advanced pulmonary disease, dementia, and psychiatric disorders may produce serious deficits in communication ability when imposed on age-related changes. People can have speech problems, language problems, or a combination of the two (Table 1). The goals of treatment are to establish a reliable communication system, readily understood by as many people as possible, promote normality, and assist the individual to cope.

A. History should include inquiry about
   • changes in vision or hearing
   • education and reading ability
   • communication pattern concerns
   • changes in cognitive abilities
   • illness, treatment, residual effects
   • difficulties with articulating words or expressing ideas
   • cultural background
   • primary language spoken
   • language barriers
   • medications
   • recent traumatic losses

B. Determine limitations and capabilities. Losses in acuity of *vision and hearing* are assessed first (see Decreased Vision, p. 118, and Hearing Loss, p. 122). *Speech and language abilities* are determined next. Note distortions, slurring, and symmetry of function throughout testing. *Speech assessment* includes
   • lip motor control: Have patient repeat "ma, ma, ma"
   • pharynx: Use "ga, ga, ga."
   • tongue motion: Have patient say "la, la, la"
   • voice strength and quality
   • gag reflex, swallowing
   • respiration: Assess adequacy
   • Articulation (general): Note speed and quality
   Language assessment should be kept appropriate to educational level and cultural framework. It includes

   • comprehension of the spoken word: Ask the patient to follow simple commands ("Touch your nose, raise your right hand")
   • comprehension of written language: Read aloud, follow a written command
   • ability to name: Ask patient to name objects in the room
   • ability to write: Ask patient to "write what you had for lunch" or to write a dictated sentence
   A useful and efficient assessment tool for determination of speech and language disorders and need for a speech pathology consultation is the Nursing Communication Assessment tool (see p. 146).

C. Consequences of untreated impaired verbal communication include social isolation, misdiagnosis as cognitively impaired, excess dependency, lowered self-esteem, coping problems, powerlessness, and altered family processes. The person may be seen as uncooperative, noncompliant, stubborn, or withdrawn. Early rehabilitative measures can decrease psychological trauma and promote normal function and independence. Questions to ask include
   • Is the patient able to express basic needs?
   • Is the patient able to express a full range of messages in a widely understood manner?
   • Are remedial techniques employed before turning to compensatory techniques?
   • Are patient and caregiver taught techniques to facilitate verbal communication? Do they understand and comply with these measures?
   • Is counseling provided to facilitate coping with the remaining disability? Have effective coping mechanisms been attained?

D. Environmental control includes
   • describing the impairment to the patient, family, and caregivers
   • maintaining a quiet, relaxed atmosphere
   • providing a routine schedule of activities
   • instituting anxiety-reduction measures
   • stimulating communication during routine care periods
   Modify the preceding approaches when a comprehension deficit exists.

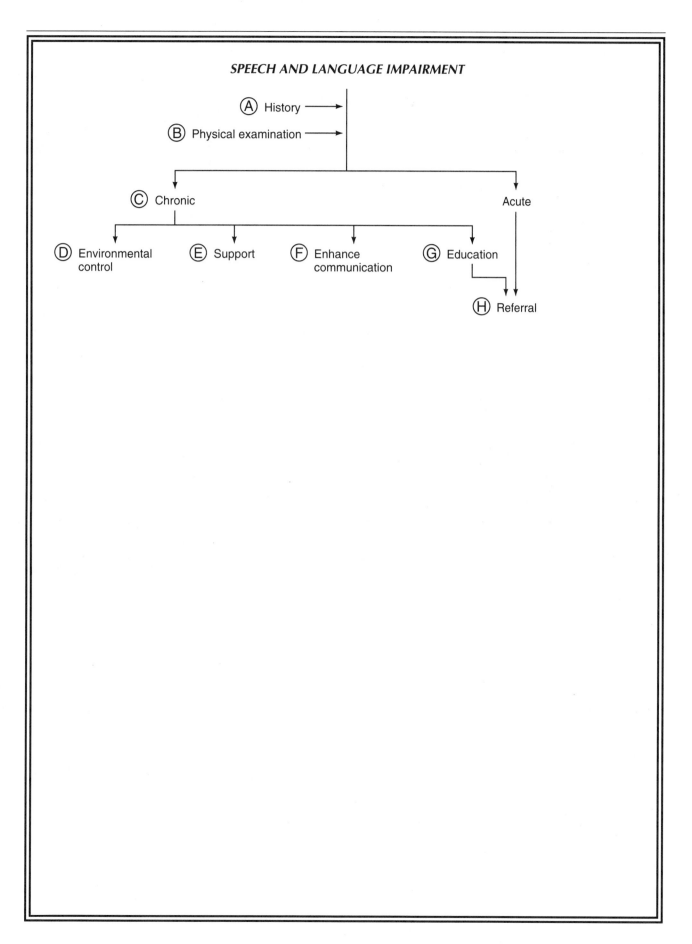

SPEECH AND LANGUAGE IMPAIRMENT

Ⓐ History

Ⓑ Physical examination

Ⓒ Chronic

Acute

Ⓓ Environmental control

Ⓔ Support

Ⓕ Enhance communication

Ⓖ Education

Ⓗ Referral

E. Support includes
- exhibiting genuine concern
- encouraging visitations
- emphasizing capabilities
- performing nursing activities in an unhurried manner
- treating patient as an adult, even when behavior is regressed
- encouraging all efforts and praising all successes, however small
- promoting socialization and diversion, as indicated
- being honest regarding prognosis and difficulties
- recognizing frustrations
- avoiding being solicitous
- being patient and accepting

F. Enhancement of communication includes
- keeping glasses clean, hearing aid battery functioning, ear mold clean
- keeping questions and instructions simple and direct
- using an interpreter when needed
- keeping the patient oriented
- encouraging attempts at communication
- providing appropriate feedback to patient

- allowing the person ample time to process words, speak, and respond
- allowing the person to talk for himself or herself
- serving as a good speech model—speak slowly, avoid using slang or medical jargon, and face the patient when talking
- not speaking louder if misunderstood; rewording what was said
- using nonverbal forms of expression, such as gestures, pantomime, or pointing if language comprehension is extremely limited
- using written communication if no reading deficit exists—paper and pencil, typewriter, or communication board
- using pictures if written and verbal language comprehension is severely impaired

Special circumstances require the following:

Apraxia: If a phrase is partially unintelligible, let the patient know what part you understood and ask the patient to try again.

Dysarthria: Let the patient know if you are having difficulty understanding; he or she may be able to increase the precision of speech.

TABLE 1 Speech and Language Disorders

Problem	Characteristics	Pathology	Causes
Speech Disorders			
Dysarthria	Slurred speech Unintelligible speech Impaired swallowing Receptive language rarely impaired	Weakness or paralysis of speech muscle	Stroke Degenerative muscle disease
Dyspraxia (apraxia)	Hesitant speech Reduced rate of speech Problems with fluency Clusters of speech sounds affected Possible existence of islands of clear speech Self-correction by patient	Failure to carry out motor movements required for speech	Dementia Cerebral infarction Brain tumor
Aphonia	Loss of voice	Malignancy Trauma	Laryngectomy
Language Disorders			
Dysphasia	Slow or halting speech that contains only nouns Speech with good rhythm or intonation that makes no sense	Damage to central speech or language center	Stroke Cerebral infarction Dementia Brain tumor
Expressive aphasia	Inability to use speech or writing to communicate	Damage to central speech or language center	Stroke Cerebral infarction Dementia Brain tumor
Receptive aphasia	Inability to understand what is heard or read	Damage to central speech or language center	Stroke Cerebral infarction Dementia Brain tumor

Aphasia: Determine which sensory modality is easier for the patient (auditory or visual), and use that modality preferentially. Aphasic patients learn to be very perceptive to gestures, tone of voice, and facial expressions. These should be emphasized in all attempts to communicate except during initial testing.

G. Education includes
- teaching patients about the communication deficit, how to help themselves, and how to help others learn to assist them
- teaching environmental management
- providing caregivers with extensive explanation and reassurance
- instructing family and caregivers in useful communication techniques

H. Referral to a primary physician is made when acute pathology or severe speech or language impairments exist. Psychiatric or psychosocial consultation is obtained for behavioral, social, or coping distress. When the sole communication impairment results from hearing or visual deficits, referral is made for examination and prescription of prosthetic aids. Referral to a speech and language pathologist is indicated when the individual cannot make basic needs known or express other messages. In advanced dementing disorders, the speech pathologist's primary focus is on caregiver education and support. Patients able to express themselves may still benefit from speech therapy and should be referred for comprehensive evaluation. Need for home care services for continued speech therapy or nursing follow-up should be assessed and timely referral initiated.

References

Boss BJ. Managing communication disorders in stroke. Nurs Clin North Am 1991; 26:985.

Matteson MA, McConnell ES. Gerontological nursing: Concepts and practice. Philadelphia: WB Saunders, 1988:320.

Reichel MD. Clinical aspects of aging. Baltimore: Williams & Wilkins, 1989:461.

TASTE CHANGES

Ellen Zignego-Smith

The four primary taste sensations are sweet, sour, bitter, and salty. The most common taste change is the reduced ability to taste sweet, sour, bitter, and salty substances. Some patients are unable to detect any taste at all or perceive tastes differently. The aroma, appearance, temperature, consistency, and texture of food also affect perception of taste. Four common causes of taste changes are poor dental health, medications, injury, and illness.

A. To help identify a taste disorder, ask questions about
   - taste preferences
   - reactions to tastes
   - medication intake
   - denture use and fit
   - condition of the teeth and mouth
   - food preparation facilities
   - food storage areas

   Ask patients about their current medication regimen and any unusual taste sensations with drug therapy (burning, salty tastes, dry mouth) when trying to determine if medications are the underlying etiology. Symptoms that may be described include
   - oral pain
   - gingival or tongue swelling
   - mobile teeth
   - halitosis
   - metallic or other taste in the mouth
   - decreased saliva
   - nasal drainage
   - fever
   - difficulty breathing

   Smell plays a large role in taste perception and can alter appetite.

B. Examine and document the appearance of the tongue, palate, and gingiva. Note tooth movement, which may indicate destruction of periodontal tissue, decreased saliva, and resultant halitosis. To determine taste changes, touch the patient's tongue in different places with a cotton-tipped applicator dipped in assorted flavors and liquids. The tongue should be brushed before beginning the taste testing and the mouth should be rinsed between tastes with distilled water (the patient should hold the solution for 15–30 seconds and expectorate). Sugar is used to assess sweetness, lemon juice for sourness, quinine for bitterness, and salt for saltiness.

C. Poor dental health can affect taste sensation significantly. Disease processes such as periodontal disease can destroy teeth and impair supportive structures. Microorganisms residing in the mouth can change food particles into virulent, fetid substances. Adequate oral hygiene, plaque removal, and fluoride treatment are important preventive dental techniques.

D. Drug use is the largest single reason for decreased salivary flow. As a result, soft tissues can crack and become dry, making the patient more prone to infection and decay. Antidepressants, anticholinergics, antispasmodics, antihypertensives, antipsychotics, and bronchodilators are among the 250 types of medications that have dry mouth, or xerostomia, as possible side effects. Chemotherapy can cause a decrease in salivary flow. Certain medications alter taste sensation. Anticonvulsants and diuretics can interfere with taste perception. Insulin can create a bitter or metallic taste. If a medication is the possible cause, discuss stopping or changing it with the patient's primary physician.

E. Injury or illness can alter taste sensation. Polyps in the nasal or sinus cavities, upper respiratory infections, hormonal disturbances, and head injuries can all lead to taste disorders. A patient may be told to let the illness run its course, if possible, after which taste sensation may return spontaneously. Hormonal disturbances such as diabetes, thyroid disease, adrenal cortex disease, and acromegaly can affect salivary flow and composition. These medical conditions should be evaluated by an endocrinologist or primary physician. Polyps in the nasal or oral cavities should be referred to an ENT specialist.

F. Patients with reduced salivary flow or taste dysfunction should be evaluated by their primary physician. It should be determined whether gland pathology, endocrine changes, therapeutic interventions, or drug use are causing the problem.

G. Oral hygiene is an important part of patient education. Encourage patients to brush their teeth and tongue at least once a day, and instruct them to rinse their mouth thoroughly after eating. Meals should be well balanced, properly prepared, and attractively served in a pleasant environment. Foods should be chewable to avoid injury to teeth or gingiva. Sugar-free gum and candy can be offered to increase salivation and avoid dental caries. Commercial products are also available for oral moistening, to supplement natural saliva. A nutritionist or dietitian can be consulted if there is concern that the patient is not receiving adequate nourishment.

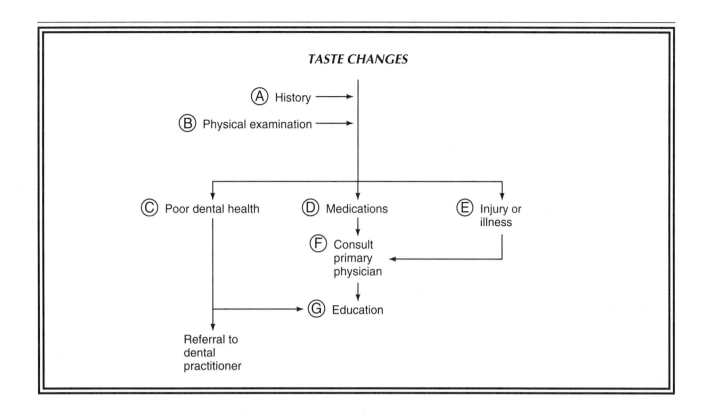

TASTE CHANGES

- (A) History
- (B) Physical examination
- (C) Poor dental health
- (D) Medications
- (E) Injury or illness
- (F) Consult primary physician
- (G) Education

Referral to dental practitioner

References

Burggraf V, Stanley M. Nursing the elderly: A care plan approach. Philadelphia: JB Lippincott, 1989.

Crow M. Pharmacology for the elderly: The nurse's guide to quality care. New York: Teachers College Press, 1984.

Esberger K, Hughes S. Nursing care of the aged. Norwalk, CT: Appleton & Lange, 1989.

Focus: Smell and taste disorders. Am Assoc Occup Health Nurs 1987; 35:463.

Longman A, Dewalt E. A guide for oral assessment. Geriatr Nurs 1986; 7:252.

Ofstehage J, Magilvy K. Oral health and aging. Geriatr Nurs 1986; 7:238.

Yurick A, Spier B, Robb S, Ebert N. The aged person and the nursing process. Norwalk, CT: Appleton & Lange, 1989.

DECREASED SENSATION

Ellen Zignego-Smith

An individual's sense of touch relies on sensory input from the inner ear, the eye, and receptors in muscles and joints. Changes in tactile sensitivity result in difficulty in discriminating temperature, decreased pain sensation, and loss of fine motor discrimination and vibratory sensitivity. Older people have slower reaction time, slower response to stimuli, and inability to localize stimuli. Stronger stimuli are needed by the elderly to produce the same response as in the younger population. These changes place the elderly at risk for potential injury due to trauma, delayed responses to noxious agents, and temperature extremes. Elderly patients may have decreased sensitivity to pain due to degenerative changes in the pain receptors and peripheral nervous system. Warnings indicating pathology may be ignored. The inability to cope with extreme environmental temperatures, especially low temperatures, is a result of the degeneration of capillaries and a loss of subcutaneous tissue. Capillaries close to the body's surface are responsible for skin nourishment and heat dissipation. The combined loss of capillaries and of subcutaneous tissue can predispose the elderly to feel cold. The loss of sensitivity to vibration begins around 50 years of age. Vibratory loss is more severe in the lower than in the upper extremities because of changes in the microcirculation of the legs or lower spinal cord.

A. History taking should include
   - reactions to extreme temperatures (especially cold)
   - experiences with pain
   - previous methods for coping with pain
   - personal perceptions of sensitivity, especially of the hands and feet
   - touches the individual enjoys (e.g., smoothness of silk, coarseness of wool)
   - present medications
   - trauma and falls (see Falls, p. 90)
   - other chronic illness (neurologic, cardiovascular, endocrine disorders)

   Patients may need to be coaxed to answer questions because they think tactile changes are inevitable with age. Ask about past illnesses and treatments when completing the history. Diabetes, hypertension, arteriosclerosis, and stroke severely affect sensation. Abdominal and cardiac problems are not always properly diagnosed because the patient may not have the same sensitivity to pain as a younger person.

B. Physical examination should focus on tactile, painful, thermal, and vibratory sensitivity. Throughout the examination, compare right to left and lower to upper extremities (see box).

C. Safety is the primary nursing concern for patients with reduced thermal sensitivity. Instruct elderly patients to avoid hot temperatures of bath water, foods, and serving dishes. Bathwater temperatures can be tested

Examination for Decreased Sensation	
Sensitivity	*Observation/Testing*
Tactile	• changes in sensitivity of skin on palms of hands and soles of feet • sensitivity to light touch: • have patient close eyes • use a wisp of cotton to touch patient's skin • ask patient to say when and where cotton is felt • test skin rather than hair on skin
Pain	• use a safety pin or neurologic tester • have patient close eyes • touch the skin with dull and sharp edges of the pin • ask patient to state whether touch is sharp or dull
Thermal	• test differentiation of warm and cold: • have patient close eyes • vary application of warm and cold: • fill test tubes with warm and cold water and place the tubes against patient's skin • fill bowls of warm and cold water and immerse patient's hands and feet in water • touch the extremities with a warm cloth and a cool cloth
Vibratory	• use a tuning fork: • have patient close eyes • apply the fork to bony prominences such as • the elbow, knee, finger and toe • have patient state when vibration starts and stops • use ear plugs for patients who respond to sound

with the patient's elbow or by a family member or friend. Heating pads should be discouraged. Nurses can help patients develop a method to remember that burners are in use: e.g., a colorful magnet with a message (HOT) can be placed near the burner when in use. Careful daily inspection and documentation of the patient's hands and feet for skin integrity, color, and warmth is a necessity. Protective measures for patients with reduced tactile sensitivity include avoiding the use of plastic forks and spoons. Heavier metal utensils are preferred because of the weight of the instruments. Patients should also be cautioned to protect their extremities. Hands and feet should be

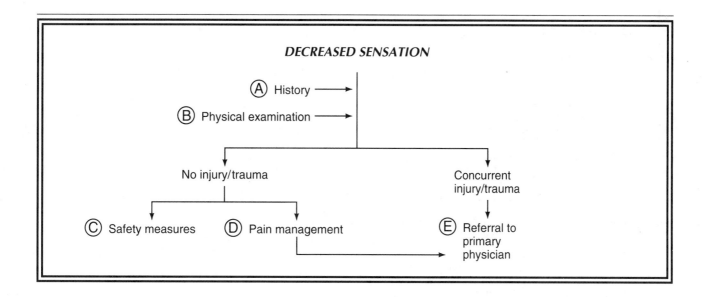

DECREASED SENSATION

Ⓐ History

Ⓑ Physical examination

No injury/trauma — Concurrent injury/trauma

Ⓒ Safety measures — Ⓓ Pain management — Ⓔ Referral to primary physician

covered during cold weather. Shoes and feet should be inspected for foreign objects; new shoes should be worn for short intervals (2 hours). Patients should note any redness, swelling, drainage, or open wounds on their feet. Use of a mirror for inspection may be helpful. Nursing interventions involving the lower extremities for patients with limited tactile sensitivity also apply to those with reduced vibratory sensitivity.

D. Pain management should focus on patients' response to pain. Be an active listener and do not assume that aches and pains are an expected part of the aging process. Encourage patients to use methods of pain relief that proved effective in the past. Remember that anxiety and fear can increase patients' pain response. General comfort measures (e.g., changing positions, a backrub) can reduce anxiety. Various relaxation techniques (imagery, progressive relaxation, cutaneous stimulation) may prove beneficial.

E. Tactile changes may vary. Consult the primary physician if losses are related to pathology, injury, or circulatory insufficiency. Patients' responses to analgesics may also vary considerably, with the possibility of toxic accumulation leading to respiratory depression and cardiac irritability. Close follow-up by a health care professional is indicated.

References

Bozian M, Clark H. Counteracting sensory changes in aging. Am J Nurs 1980; 80:473.
Burggraf V, Stanley M. Nursing the elderly: A care plan approach. Philadelphia: JB Lippincott, 1989.
Esberger K, Hughes S. Nursing care of the aged. Norwalk, CT: Appleton & Lange, 1989.
Yurick A, Spier B, Robb S, Ebert N. The aged person and the nursing process. Norwalk, CT: Appleton & Lange, 1989.

DIZZINESS

Beth Goode Moffett

Dizziness is a subjective feeling of lightheadedness or a swimming sensation. About 70% of patients complaining of dizziness have a labyrinthine or other benign cause, 12% have multiple sensory loss, 4 or 5% have cardiovascular causes, and about 12% have CNS disease. Dizziness is a frequent cause of falls in the elderly (see Falls, p. 90).

A. Ask about
- onset
- duration
- interference or occurrence with activities of daily living (ADL) (bathing, grooming, shaving)
- nausea
- vomiting
- diaphoresis
- unsteadiness of gait or falls (see Gait Disturbances, p. 90, and Falls, p. 42)
- sensation of falling or moving (see Vertigo, p. 142)
- medical history
- current medications, both prescription and over the counter
- ear problems
  - earache
  - hearing loss (see Hearing Loss, p. 122)
  - fullness
  - tinnitus (see Tinnitus, p. 124)
- allergies
- vision changes
- loss of feeling
- causative factors
  - straining at stool
  - voiding
  - change of position
  - looking up
  - moving the head
- prolonged bed rest with deconditioning
- nutrition and fluid intake
- headaches
- loss of consciousness
- psychosocial stressors
- alcohol use
- cold or flulike symptoms or exposure

B. Physical examination includes
- vital signs
  - blood pressure measurement lying, sitting, and standing for postural hypotension
  - heart rate
  - respirations for tachypnea
  - temperature for fever
- cardiopulmonary assessment
- carotid artery examination for bruits and sinus sensitivity
- peripheral pulses
- Valsalva maneuver (pinched off nostrils with forced expiration) for changes in cardiac output
- skin and mucous membranes for hydration status
- observation for anxiety or hyperventilation
- otologic inspection
- hearing evaluation (see Hearing Loss, p. 122)
- visual acuity
- proprioception testing (see Romberg test, p. 63)
- neurological examination
  - gait and balance assessment (see Gait Disturbances, p. 42)

Table 1 lists systems to be considered in assessment. Procedures may include electrocardiography for cardiac irregularity and carotid Doppler for suspected vascular etiology. Beneficial laboratory tests include CBC, glucose, thyroid function tests, and electrolytes.

C. Causes of sudden dizziness include
- labyrinthitis
- disorders of the vertebral, basilar, or internal acoustic artery
- physical or emotional stress
- vascular disorder

D. Chronic dizziness may be classified as either episodic or unremitting (see box). Fainting or syncope may be associated with unremitting dizziness.

TABLE 1 Differentiating Symptoms of Dizziness

System to Evaluate	Symptoms
Cardiovascular	Orthostasis Dizziness when neck hyperextended Arrhythmia
Hematologic	Anemia Hypoglycemia Hypothyroidism Hyperthyroidism Electrolyte imbalance
Neurologic	Loss of consciousness Paresis Seizure Decreased visual fields Rigidity Sedation
Sensory	Fullness Tinnitus Hearing loss Otitis Visual changes Proprioception

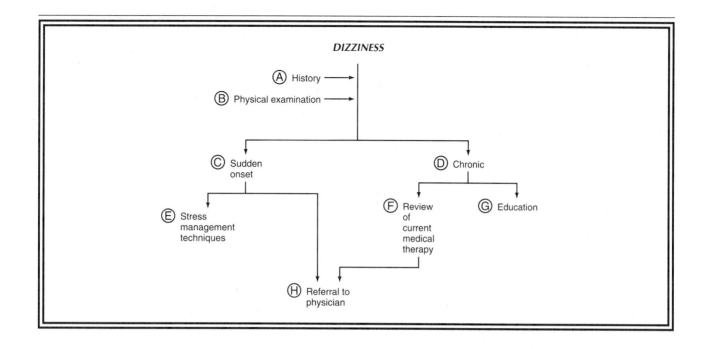

DIZZINESS

Ⓐ History →

Ⓑ Physical examination →

Ⓒ Sudden onset

Ⓓ Chronic

Ⓔ Stress management techniques

Ⓕ Review of current medical therapy

Ⓖ Education

Ⓗ Referral to physician

Possible Causes of Chronic Dizziness	
Episodic	*Unremitting*
Positional	Acoustic neuroma
Sensory deficit	Vertebrobasilar arterial
Otitis	insufficiency
Mastoiditis	Carotid arteriosclerosis
Meniere's disease	Carotid sinus sensitivity
Osteophytes of cervical	Hypertension
spine	Anemia
Acoustic neuroma	Diabetes
Hyperventilation	Seizures
Drugs	Thyrotoxicosis
Cervical trauma	Blood dyscrasias
Menopause	Psychoneuroses
Migraine	
Arrhythmias	

E. Stress management techniques may be used to decrease stress and help patients feel in control. Techniques that may be helpful include
  • biofeedback
  • relaxation tapes
  • music therapy
  • pet therapy
  • professional counseling

F. Current medical therapy to review includes
  • management of sensory losses
  • drug therapies
  • control of chronic illness
  Multiple sensory deficits that occur with aging include decreases in vision, hearing, and proprioception. Accommodation for these losses through increased sensory input may be possible with proper glasses, hearing aids, a cane, or other assistive devices. Evaluate drug therapies for interaction, side effects, and adequacy. Common drugs to consider are
  • antihypertensives
  • estrogen

  • antidiabetic agents
  • thyroid
  Patients' use of alcohol and over-the-counter drugs may require further evaluation. Chronic disorders that, when not well controlled, can result in dizziness are
  • hypertension
  • arrhythmias
  • diabetes
  • anemia
  • thyroid disorders

G. Patient education focuses on
  • avoiding sudden changes in position
  • medication use and side effects
  • nutrition and fluid intake
  • maintenance of sensory input (corrective lenses and amplification)
  • routine health maintenance
  • blood pressure monitoring and control

H. Physician referral is indicated for
  • acute onset
  • impaired ADL
  • syncopal episodes
  • falls
  • acute neurologic changes

References

Baloh R. Dizziness in older people. J Am Geriatr Soc 1992; 40:713.

Clairmont A, Turner J, Jackson R. Dizziness: A logical approach to diagnosis and treatment. Postgrad Med 1974; 56:139.

Kane R, Ouslander J, Abrass I. Essentials of clinical geriatrics. 2nd ed. New York: McGraw-Hill, 1989:191.

Kupp M, Chatton M. Current medical diagnosis and treatment. Los Altos, CA: Lange, 1984:584.

Walshe T. Manual of clinical problems in geriatric medicine. Boston: Little, Brown, 1985:49.

VERTIGO

Elizabeth Mackrella

Vertigo is sometimes incorrectly used synonymously with dizziness (see Dizziness, p. 140). Vertigo involves the feeling of rotational movement. It may be objective, the world is revolving around the patient, or subjective, the patient is revolving in space. Vertigo symptoms occur in the vestibular or equilibrium system because of physiologic or pathologic causes (Table 1).

A. History should include
- onset
- duration
- hearing loss
- allergies
- falls
- trauma
- head injury
- provoking factors (head position and movement)
- occurrence with abnormal stimuli of air, sea, and auto travel
- acute and chronic illnesses
- environmental toxin exposure
- first versus recurrent episodes
- ear infections or rhinitis
- tinnitus (see p. 124)
- nausea and vomiting
- description of sensation
- medications, including over-the-counter drugs
- alcohol and illicit drug use

B. Physiologic assessment includes
- ophthalmology examination for visual acuity, extraocular movements, and nystagmus on central and lateral gaze
- ear examination for
  - cerumen in ear canals
  - hearing screen
  - tympanic membrane integrity and appearance
  - signs of infection
  - air and bone sound conduction
- vital signs—blood pressure while lying down, sitting, and standing; assess for orthostatic changes and heart rate
- cardiovascular—insufficiency, congestive heart failure
- respiratory compromise—infection
- abdomen and neck—bruits, masses

TABLE 1 Causes of Vertigo

Type	Physiology	Condition(s)
Physiologic	Induced by irregular or rhythmic motion	Motion sickness Alcohol intoxication
Pathologic	Affecting the labyrinth of the inner ear	Benign positional vertigo (BPV) Vestibular disorders Ménière's disease Drug toxicity
	Affecting the central nervous system	Stroke Transient ischemia Vascular insufficiency Herpes zoster Migraine Drug toxicity Cervical spondylosis Cervical arthritis

- extremities—peripheral neuropathy
- neurologic examination—cerebellar function tests (Romberg's, past-pointing, and test of rapid alternation of movements) and cranial nerve evaluation

See Table 2 for description and examination criteria for common vertigo conditions. Laboratory tests to rule out systemic causes include complete blood count with differential, serum glucose, thyroid profile, and serologic tests for syphilis.

C. Promote patient safety by providing instructions for changes in activities, clothing, and the environment (see the box "Instructions for Dealing with Vertigo").

D. Referral should always be made to a primary care physician or neurologist if activities of daily living are affected. Further evaluation of underlying pathology may be necessary. Therapeutic drug levels may indicate a need to titrate or change drug therapies. Meclizine (Antivert) may be prescribed, although it is not always successful. Physical and occupational therapy consultations may be helpful for body mechanics, assistive devices, and positional treatment protocols.

Text continued on p. 144.

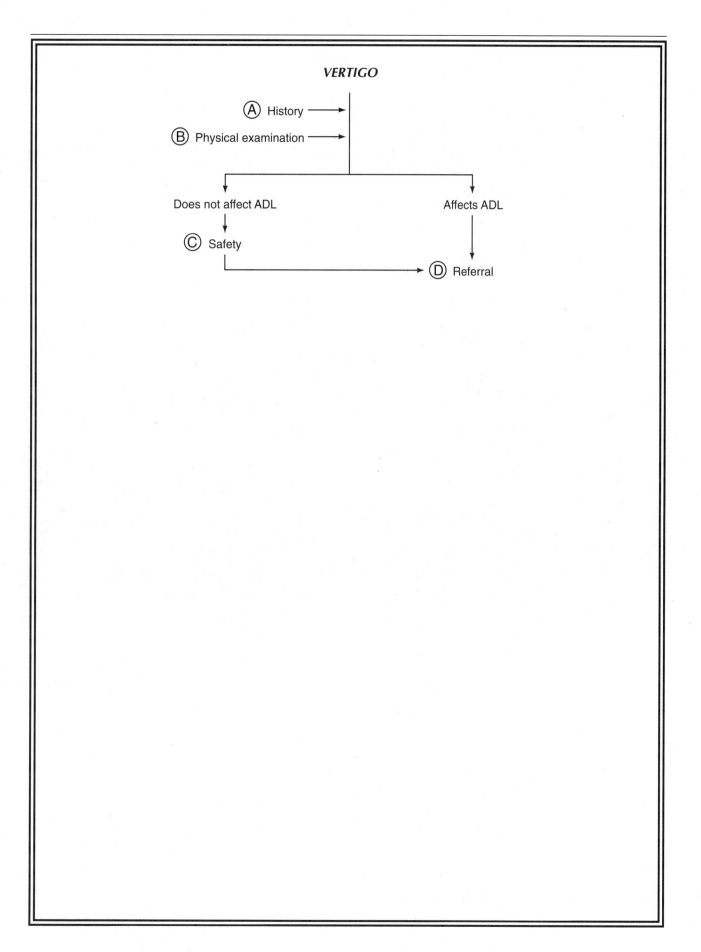

VERTIGO

Ⓐ History →

Ⓑ Physical examination →

Does not affect ADL   Affects ADL

Ⓒ Safety

Ⓓ Referral

TABLE 2   Differentiation of Vertigo

Condition	Description	Testing Procedures
Ménière's disease	Inner ear disturbance with auditory and vestibular symptoms Progressive, recurrent Usually unilateral hearing loss Episodic intense vertigo lasting 30 minutes to several hours or months, with nausea and with or without vomiting Periodic tinnitus	Otologic examination Blood screening
Labyrinthine damage due to drug toxicity Herpes zoster infection	Auditory and vestibular symptoms Vertigo and hearing loss Presence of herpetic vesicles in external canal	Onset of symptoms in relation to administration of medication
Acute labyrinthitis	Inflammation of internal ear due to infection, otitis media, influenza, or meningitis	Otologic examination
Benign paroxysmal positional vertigo	Most common inner ear syndrome Vertigo episodes lasting a few seconds May be caused and prolonged by viral infections	Hallpike-Dix maneuver (see box) Repeat any activity reported to cause vertigo

---

Instructions for Dealing with Vertigo

Topic	Instructions

Daily activities	• slow down
	  • sit up slowly
	  • turn over in bed gradually
	  • stand still when you stand up, before you start to walk
	• use support when standing, such as a heavy chair, chest, or sink edge
	• turn your head slowly side to side
	• do NOT tilt head backward or look up quickly
	• ask someone else to drive

Clothing	• wear sturdy, supportive shoes with little or no heel • do NOT wear scuffs, backless shoes, or sandals • avoid long, flowing clothing with full sleeves that may catch on furniture or footwear

Safe environment	• put kitchen supplies and equipment most used at eye level
	• if getting something lower than eye level
	  • keep your head and back straight
	  • bend at your knees
	  • hold onto a sturdy chair or cabinet
	• do NOT reach above shoulder height (it will make you tilt your head back to see what you are reaching for)

Hallpike-Dix Maneuver

Purpose: To detect head-positional vertigo

Steps:
1. Explain procedure to patient
2. Grasp patient's head on each side
3. Seat patient on bed or examination table
4. Instruct patient to look upward with eyes open
5. Tilt head backward
6. Instruct patient to lie down quickly and turn head to the right
7. Return to sitting position
8. Repeat steps 6 and 7 but turning head to left
9. Repeat steps 6 and 7 with head hyperextended over edge of table, return to sitting position
10. Rest patient, awaiting resolution of vertigo

Observations:
Observe for nystagmus

Rating:
• Nystagmus and vertigo that resolves after the maneuver in 10–60 seconds indicate the patient has benign paroxysmal positional vertigo. Average resolution is 40 seconds.
• Maneuver does not cause vertigo and nystagmus in healthy patient.

References

Atkins H, ed. When the world turns. Emerg Med 1989; 21:113, 116.

Herdman S. Treatment of benign paroxysmal positional vertigo. Phys Ther 1990; 70:56–63.

Olsky M, Murray J. Dizziness and fainting in the elderly. Emerg Med Clin North Am 1990; 8:295–306.

Ross V, Robinson B. Dizziness: Cause, prevention and management. Geriatr Nurs (New York) 1984; 5:290–304.

Nursing Communication Assessment

Alertness for Communication:

1. Does patient look at the speaker when spoken to?   Yes___   No___

2. Does patient make any social response to speaker, such as head nod, smile, outstretched hand, vocalization, or attempt gestures?   Yes___   No___

3. Does patient make any attempt to send messages?   Yes___   No___

4. Does patient say any intelligible, appropriate words?   Yes___   No___

Sensory Check for Communication:

5. Does patient seem to see well?   Yes___   No___
6. Does patient seem to hear well?   Yes___   No___

Understanding for Communication:

7. Does patient answer five or more yes/no questions correctly? (Must be better than 50%)
   - a. Are you in a hospital?   Yes___   No___
   - b. Are you at home?   Yes___   No___
   - c. Is it dark outside?   Yes___   No___
   - d. Is your name_____?   Yes___   No___
   - e. Have you eaten supper?   Yes___   No___
   - f. Do dogs bark?   Yes___   No___
   - g. Is grass green?   Yes___   No___
   - h. Do birds swim?   Yes___   No___
   - i. Do cars have wheels?   Yes___   No___
   - j. Do boats fly?   Yes___   No___

   Correct total: ___   ___

8. Does patient follow five simple commands?   Yes___   No___
   - a. Point to your nose.   Yes___   No___
   - b. Where is your window?   Yes___   No___
   - c. Point to your ear.   Yes___   No___
   - d. Point to the ceiling and then the floor.   Yes___   No___
   - e. Close your eyes and nod your head.   Yes___   No___

   Correct total: ___   ___

9. Does patient seem to recognize his own speech errors?   Yes___   No___

10. Does patient follow a written command, such as: "Make a fist," "Close your eyes"?   Yes___   No___

Expressive Communication:

11. Does patient name five objects he can see?   Yes___   No___
12. Does patient say his name?   Yes___   No___
13. Does patient give his address?   Yes___   No___
14. Does patient tell the current day of the:
    - Week?   Yes___   No___
    - Month?   Yes___   No___
    - Year?   Yes___   No___
15. Does patient express ideas in at least three-word sentences?   Yes___   No___
16. Is patient's speech clear?   Yes___   No___
17. Does patient write his name legibly?   Yes___   No___

Swallowing:

18. Does patient swallow without choking at least nine of ten times?   Yes___   No___

Assessment:

1. Communication problem?   Yes___   No___
2. Swallowing problem?   Yes___   No___
3. Hearing problem suspected?   Yes___   No___

Plan:

1. Speech pathology consult?   Yes___   No___
2. Audiology consult?   Yes___   No___
3. Other?   Yes___   No___

From Bashor PH. A nursing communication assessment guide. Reprinted from *Rehabilitation Nursing*, Volume 8, Issue 1, with permission of the Association of Rehabilitation Nurses, 5700 Old Orchard Road, First Floor, Skokie, IL 60077-1057. Copyright 1983 Association of Rehabilitation.

NUTRITION

CHANGE OF APPETITE AND EATING HABITS

Sheral Cade

A change in eating patterns or habits may be a sign of a physical or psychosocial change. A decrease in taste sensitivity (attributed to loss of taste buds, salivary secretion, and teeth) and a decrease in smell sensitivity have been correlated with a decreased enjoyment of food. The resultant decrease in appetite can have serious consequences: malnutrition (see Nutritional Deficits Requiring Supplementation, p. 154).

A. Elicit any history of changes in
    • weight
    • medications
    • mental status
    • social/environmental factors
        • death of spouse, pet, or friends
        • relocation
    • ability to perform instrumental activities of daily living (see the tool *Scale for Instrumental Activities of Daily Living*, p. 30)
    • economic status
    Try to determine the onset and duration of changes as well as recent health problems or surgery. Investigate problems affecting the ability to eat, such as
    • ability to chew
    • nausea/vomiting
    • diarrhea/constipation
    • food intolerance, real or perceived
    • decrease in smell or taste (see Taste Changes, p. 136, and Decreased Sense of Smell, p. 126)
    • fatigue (see Fatigue, p. 14)

B. Accurate height/weight measurement is essential to determine ideal body weight and whether weight changes (see Weight Change, p. 158) have resulted from changed eating habits. Physical examination focuses on abilities and disabilities. Assess
    • dentition
    • bowel sounds
    • abdominal distention/bloating
    • mental status: cognition, mood/affect
    • manual dexterity
    Laboratory data for review include
    • hemoglobin/hematocrit
    • serum albumin or thyroxine-binding prealbumin or retinol-binding protein
    • transferrin
    • total lymphocyte count

C. Nutritional assessment is most easily done by a dietitian. See the tool *Nutritional Assessment*, p. 166 for parameters to consider. The important thing to determine is whether the patient's nutritional needs are still being met despite a change in overall intake. As people age their metabolic rate decreases and their caloric needs therefore decrease. Nutrient needs do not differ greatly from those of other age groups, so selection of high nutrient density foods is important. The social and physical changes that occur in aging often lead to a limited variety of foods and thus a poor nutritional intake.

D. If a nutritional problem is evident or a more thorough nutritional assessment is indicated, referral to a dietitian is recommended. Liquid nutritional supplements are indicated for patients at risk or with malnutrition (see Nutritional Deficits Requiring Supplementation, p. 154).

E. Refer patients with continued inadequate nutrient intake to a primary physician. Explore causes of appetite and eating habit change (both physiologic and psychological). Dietary supplements may be indicated for patients with deficiencies due to decreased nutritional intake. Tube feeding to restore or maintain nutritional health may be warranted. Consultation with a dietitian concerning a recommended tube feeding formula is helpful.

F. Follow-up has a variety of purposes:
    • assessment of the intake changes the patient has made
    • ongoing evaluation of nutritional status
    • continuing education

References

Natow A, Heslin J. Nutritional care of the older adult. New York: Macmillan, 1986.

Roe D. Geriatric nutrition. Englewood Cliffs, NJ: Prentice-Hall, 1987.

CHANGE OF APPETITE AND EATING HABITS

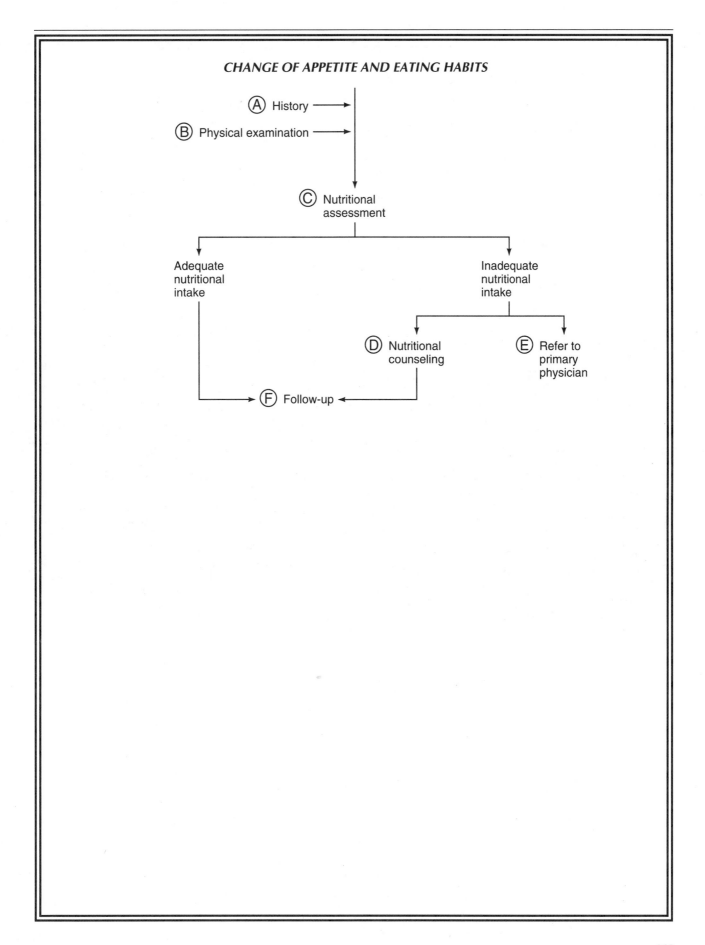

(A) History

(B) Physical examination

(C) Nutritional assessment

Adequate nutritional intake

Inadequate nutritional intake

(D) Nutritional counseling

(E) Refer to primary physician

(F) Follow-up

DEHYDRATION/VOLUME DEPLETION

Coni Francis

Water is the body's most essential nutrient. It is lost daily in the urine and stool as well as by evaporation from the skin and respiratory tract. Water is replaced by the foods and beverages consumed, and a small amount is produced by the oxidation of food.

A. Information collected in the history should include
   - medical history
   - recent illness or infections
   - current medications
   - nutrition/fluid intake history
   - weight history
   - intake/output history
   - GI problems such as nausea, vomiting, diarrhea, and constipation

B. Perform physical examination to distinguish between acute and chronic dehydration. Symptoms of dehydration may go unrecognized or be attributed to other causes in the elderly. Some clinical signs of dehydration are not useful in diagnosing dehydration in the elderly. Sunken eyes and decreased skin turgor may be present in a well-hydrated elderly person. In addition, hypovolemia may coexist with subcutaneous edema. The most useful clinical signs for dehydration in elderly people include
   - low urinary output
   - weak and rapid pulse
   - orthostatic hypotension
   - decreased state of consciousness
   Use laboratory evaluation to determine electrolyte imbalance associated with dehydration. Baseline determination of hematocrit and specific gravity is helpful when rehydration begins. Signs of improvement with rehydration in acute dehydration include urinary volume of 50 ml/hr with falling specific gravity and osmolality.

C. Sudden onset of dehydration can be caused by lack of intake or abnormal losses. Intake may not meet needs when the following are present
   - vomiting
   - diarrhea
   - fever
   - excessive sweating
   - fistula losses
   - hemorrhage
   - hypertonic IV or enteral infusions
   Rapid weight loss in acute dehydration is mainly extracellular fluid (ECF). An acute episode of dehydra-

tion can be life threatening, compromising renal function and blood pressure.

D. Chronic dehydration is usually due to inadequate intake. Water may not be easily obtained by patients who are arthritic, paralyzed, or confused. Those with incontinence may deliberately limit fluid intake. Increased losses from diuretic therapy, laxative abuse, and deficiency of or resistance to antidiuretic hormone may cause chronic dehydration. Weight loss in chronic dehydration is evenly distributed between extracellular and intracellular fluids. The effects of slow fluid depletion are less severe.

E. Intervention for acute dehydration is best accomplished by infusing water containing ECF electrolytes. Isotonic sodium chloride without glucose is the best solution to replace fluid loss due to vomiting. Ringer's lactate without glucose is preferred for diarrhea, fistula, or hemorrhage. Urinary volume of 50 ml/hr and a falling hematocrit in the absence of blood loss or falling specific gravity are useful indications of improvement in acute-onset dehydration. If the patient is alert, diminishing thirst is a useful sign of improvement. Potassium may need to be replaced once rehydration is under way. Rehydration in chronically dehydrated patients requires fluid replacement to raise urinary output to 25–50 ml/hr and return hematocrit to normal. Repletion should occur over several days rather than hours. Once rehydration is well under way, potassium will need replacing. Change in diuretic dose and reduction in laxative use will help prevent recurrence. When hypertonic IV solutions or enteral feedings cause dehydration, provide at least 1 ml fluid per calorie of formula or at least 30 ml of fluid per kilogram of body weight. Patients losing fluids by fistula also require replacement of these fluid losses.

F. Referrals should be made to the appropriate resource: physician, pharmacist, or registered dietitian. The dietitian can recommend feeding changes; the pharmacist can recommend medication changes. A physician's order may be necessary to change the feeding regimen or medication.

Reference

Shils ME, Vernon RY. Modern nutrition in health and disease. 7th ed. Philadelphia: Lea & Febiger, 1988.

DEHYDRATION/VOLUME DEPLETION

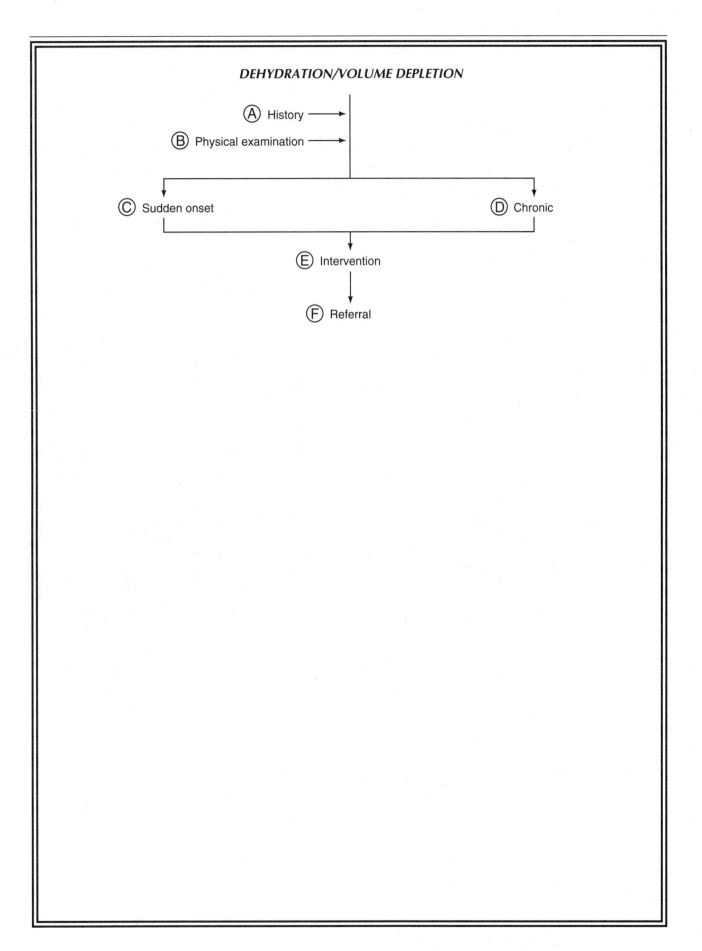

HUNGER

Coni Francis

Hunger has been described as a craving or sensation that arises from a need for food. Hunger is most commonly associated with the physiologic need for food, but many individuals have learned that food can also be used to subdue psychological "hunger."

A. Information collected in the history should include
   - onset
   - precipitating factors
   - eating habits
     - 24-hour food recall/food diary (see p. 165)
     - how many meals and snacks
     - meal spacing
   - fluid intake
   - weight history
   - food preparation and storage methods
   - current medications
   - alcohol consumption
   - psychological/emotional crisis
   - recent change in socioeconomic status
   - medical history
   - bowel movements
   - GI changes

   Careful evaluation of energy intake is important. Deficiency can cause protein calorie malnutrition (PCM), which is common in the elderly and often goes unnoticed.

B. General physical observations should include
   - appearance
   - muscle wasting
   - weakness
   - edema
   - psychological affect/mood (see Depression, p. 282)
   - abdominal tenderness/bloating

Perform a laboratory evaluation to rule out disease states that may cause hunger.

C. Physiologic causes of hunger may be increased metabolism or decreased absorption due to a variety of disease states such as
   - malnutrition
   - overgrowth of bacteria in the bowel
   - parasitic disease
   - liver disease
   - kidney disease
   - sprue
   - diabetes
   - bowel cancer
   - inflammatory bowel disease

   Malabsorption is usually characterized by diarrhea/steatorrhea. Little stool may be produced with in-

Nutritional Interventions for Causes of Hunger	
Problem	*Nutritional Intervention*
Sprue	Gluten-free diet
Liver disease	Omit alcohol
	Adequate diet
Kidney disease	Low-protein diet
Diabetes	Restrict sugar, saturated fat, and calories
Cancer	May require elemental, enteral products, or parenteral feedings to allow for bowel rest
Inflammatory bowel disease	May require elemental, enteral products, or parenteral feedings to allow for bowel rest

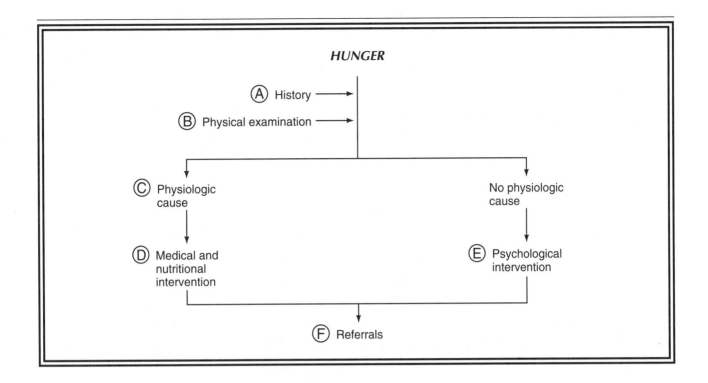

HUNGER

A. History

B. Physical examination

C. Physiologic cause

No physiologic cause

D. Medical and nutritional intervention

E. Psychological intervention

F. Referrals

creased metabolism. Weight change and poor dietary intake can contribute to feelings of hunger. Patients on enteral, elemental, or parenteral formulas may complain of feeling hungry even when they are receiving adequate calories. Some medications are known to increase appetite (Table 1).

TABLE 1   Medications that May Increase Appetite

Classification	Drug(s)
Antidepressants	Amitriptyline HCl (Elavil, Endep)
	Amoxapine (Asendin)
	Desipramine HCl (Norpramin, Petrofane)
	Doxepin HCl (Adapin, Sinequan)
	Nortriptyline HCl (Aventyl, Pamelor)
	Protriptyline HCl (Vivactil)
Antipsychotics	Thiothixene (Navane)
	Trifluoperazine HCl (Stelazine)
Antianxiety agents	Diazepam (Valium)
	Lorazapam (Ativan)
	Prazepam (Centrax)
Corticosteroids	Corticotropin (ACTH, Acthar)
	Prednisone (Deltasone, Orasone)
	Medroxyprogesterone acetate (Provera)
	Megestrol acetate (Megace, Progestin)
Anticonvulsants	Clonazepam (Klonopin)
	Valproic acid (Depakene)
Antilipemic	Clofibrate (Atromid-S)
Antihistaminic/antipruritic	Cyproheptadine (Periactin)
Antidiabetic	Insulin
	Glyburide (Diabeta, Micronase)
	Chlorpropamide (Diabinese)

D. Medical and nutritional intervention for hunger should be aimed at correcting the problem. Provide antibiotic therapy for bacterial overgrowth or parasitic disease. See the box on facing page for some of the nutritional interventions to consider. If patients are receiving enteral or parenteral nutrition, it is important to adjust calorie and nutrient levels to meet their needs with changes in weight and medical condition (see also Weight Change, p. 158). A change in medication or dosage may reduce hunger to some extent.

E. When no physiologic cause for hunger can be found, consider psychological, environmental, or social intervention. The emotional aspects of stress and mood can affect the perception of hunger. The elderly frequently eat due to boredom, loneliness, or depression or when stressed, using food to fill an emotional need. Sometimes, hunger is triggered by the environment. Food availability, climate, and habit can all affect the desire for food or what is perceived as hunger. If the patient is feeling hunger because of loneliness or boredom, increased socialization is helpful. Coping with depression or stress is usually best handled by professionals trained in psychology or psychosocial interventions.

F. Base referrals on the cause of hunger. Consider using the physician, registered dietitian, social worker, and psychiatric professional and community resources.

References

Powers DE, Moore AO. Food medication interactions. 6th ed. Phoenix, AZ: Food Medication Interactions, 1988.

Shils ME, Vernon RY. Modern nutrition in health and disease. 7th ed. Philadelphia: Lea & Febiger, 1988.

NUTRITIONAL DEFICITS REQUIRING SUPPLEMENTATION

Sheral Cade

Nutritional deficits leading to malnutrition have two basic causes:

1. A medical or physical problem that interferes with eating or assimilation
    • prolonged illness
    • effects of drugs
    • pain
    • decreased/altered sense of taste (see Taste Changes, p. 136)
    • poor dentition (see Poor Dentition/Caries, p. 170)

2. Factors interfering with the patient's willingness to eat
    • lack of socialization at meals
    • depression
    • fear/anxiety
    • stringent diet prescription

Deficits can relate to any nutrient:
• protein
• carbohydrate
• fat
• vitamins
• minerals

TABLE 1 Enteral Nutrition

Approach	Cautions	Comments
Modification of present diet with between-meal and/or bedtime snacks	Do not repel patient with too much food at one time	Preferred method
Commercial nutritional supplements	Monitor patient tolerance (taste, lactose, etc.) and acceptance	Widely available, reliable
Tube feeding/oral feeding	Monitor patient for food allergy or intolerance due to osmolarity or viscosity	Consider: nutrient requirement metabolic limitations functional capability of GI tract cost availability convenience anticipated route of delivery

A. History taking should attempt to uncover physiologic or psychological factors contributing to inadequate nutrition, such as
    • chronic illnesses
    • medications
    • nausea and vomiting
    • constipation/diarrhea
    • food intolerances
    • ability to perform activities of daily living (ADL)

B. Physical examination should assess
    • chewing/swallowing
    • skin condition (see section Skin Integrity, pp. 100 – 117)
    • bony deformity
    • health of mucous membranes
    • reflexes
    • edema (see Edema, p. 10)
    • ability to perform ADL
    • anthropometric measurements (see p. 160)
    Biochemical assessment includes
    • serum albumin
    • hemoglobin/hematocrit
    • electrolytes
    An ECG should also be performed.

C. Nutritional assessment uses information from the history and physical as well as
    • food intake history
    • food frequency recall (see the tool *Nutritional Assessment*, p. 166)
    In a malnourished patient, a dietitian or physician should always be involved in the assessment and treatment plan. Medical evaluation is particularly helpful when nutritional assessment has failed to detect a cause for low oral intake.

D. Supplementation should never be considered a substitute for a well-chosen diet and should be based on actual patient need. When calorie intake is not adequate, an initial increase of 500 calories/day is recommended; higher levels may be required in acute illnesses. A generic multivitamin-mineral supplement is convenient and inexpensive when nutritional intake is inadequate. Large supplements (more than ten times the RDA) are not recommended at any time without medical supervision.

E. The functional capability of the GI tract determines the route of nutritional support. The tract must be capable of processing and absorbing needed nutrients if the enteral route is to be used. Enteral nutritional support is preferred because it generally entails less cost and

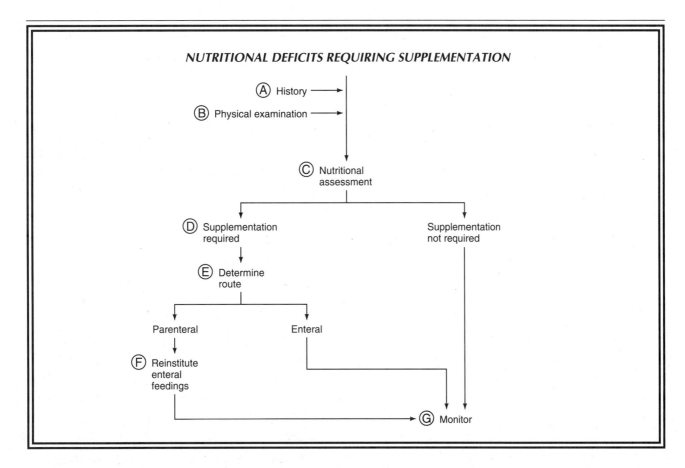

NUTRITIONAL DEFICITS REQUIRING SUPPLEMENTATION

(A) History

(B) Physical examination

(C) Nutritional assessment

(D) Supplementation required

Supplementation not required

(E) Determine route

Parenteral

Enteral

(F) Reinstitute enteral feedings

(G) Monitor

risk than parenteral nutrition. Enteral nutrition can be provided orally or by feeding tube (Table 1) using food or nutritional supplements. When using commercial supplements, monitor the patient carefully for food allergy or intolerance due to osmolarity or viscosity. Contraindications for use of the enteral route include
• uncontrolled GI hemorrhage
• an obstruction or fistula distal to the feeding site
• peritonitis
• ileus
• intractable vomiting or diarrhea
• insufficient small bowel function to absorb nutrients
Traditional IV feeding of glucose and water, even if vitamin and mineral fortified and supplemented with amino acids, is not adequate to prevent tissue breakdown and sustain body weight. Total parenteral nutrition (TPN) should be considered if after 10–14 days the patient is unable to eat adequately. Parenteral alimentation solutions are formulated to provide the correct ratio of water, electrolytes, protein, calories, essential fatty acids, vitamins, and trace elements to meet specific nutritional requirements.

F.   The transition from parenteral feeding to oral feeding should be made as quickly as possible without compromising overall nutritional status. Only when the patient is capable of eating enough protein and calories to prevent protein catabolism should parenteral nutrition be stopped. Parenteral nutrition should also be discontinued gradually; sudden cessation would put the patient at risk for recurrent malnutrition and hypoglycemia.

G.   During supplementation, maintain careful biochemical and physiological monitoring of
• weight
• intake and output
• hydration status
• blood chemistries
• vital signs
• calorie counts
The functional capability of the GI tract should be reassessed so that the patient can return to normal oral intake as quickly as possible. Monitoring should also look for complications of parenteral nutrition, such as problems with
• venous access
• indwelling catheters
• hyperosmolar feedings
Patients receiving TPN may require treatment with insulin and should have blood sugar levels monitored regularly.

References

Massachusetts General Hospital Department of Dietetics, Boston. Diet Reference Manual. Boston: Little, Brown, 1984:14.

Natow A, Heslin J. Geriatric nutrition. Boston: CBI Publishing, 1980.

Natow A, Heslin J. Nutritional care of the older adult. New York: Macmillan, 1986.

THERAPEUTIC DIET: COMPLIANCE/ADHERENCE

Sheral Cade

A modified or therapeutic diet may be indicated for certain medical diagnoses. The modification may be specific (detailed guidelines regarding types of food and amounts) or general/basic (foods to limit/foods to include). Dietary changes at any age can be difficult, but older adults can and will make changes if these are perceived as being beneficial. The reasons most often given for change are medical and social.

A. History taking may discover
   * accessibility of recommended food
   * food preparation techniques
   * food fads
   * family support for dietary restrictions
   * past experience with dietary restrictions
   * medications
   * chronic illnesses (e.g., congestive heart failure, GI disease)
   * other health problems
   * economic level
   * potential impact of change
   * level of comprehension
   * depression
   * decreased smell and taste (see Taste Changes, p. 136, and Decreased Sense of Smell, p. 126)
   * social isolation

B. Physical examination seeks to determine
   * current nutritional state (see p. 166)
   * functional level
   * mental status: cognition, mood and affect
   * dental and gingival disease
   Laboratory assessment includes
   * serum albumin
   * hemoglobin and hematocrit
   * total lymphocyte count
   * transferrin

C. A 24-hour recall allows comparison of eating patterns with those recommended or prescribed (see the tool *Food Diary*, p. 165). Food frequency recall looks at specific foods in relation to recommended usage. A 100% adherence to a therapeutic diet may be an unrealistic goal. Any change or improvement in eating patterns should be given positive reinforcement.

D. Nonadherence can be attributed to
   * poor comprehension
   * lack of food accessibility
   * patient nonacceptance
   * negative outcome to recommended diet
   The patient's acceptance of information and willingness to make changes plays an important role in dietary compliance.

E. Nutrition counseling may require a dietitian to perform a thorough nutritional assessment or give specific individualized diet instruction.

F. Follow-up should be available to reinforce positive changes, clarify questions and concerns, and provide continued education. A 24-hour recall/food frequency recall provides a mechanism for ongoing assessment of changes that have been made in eating patterns.

G. Specific barriers to dietary adherence may be ameliorated by referral to social service or community resources. Interventions aimed at improving social, environmental, and financial problems may be warranted.

References

Natow A, Heslin J. Geriatric nutrition. Boston: CBI Publishing, 1980.

Roe D. Geriatric nutrition. Englewood Cliffs, NJ: Prentice-Hall, 1987.

THERAPEUTIC DIET: COMPLIANCE/ADHERENCE

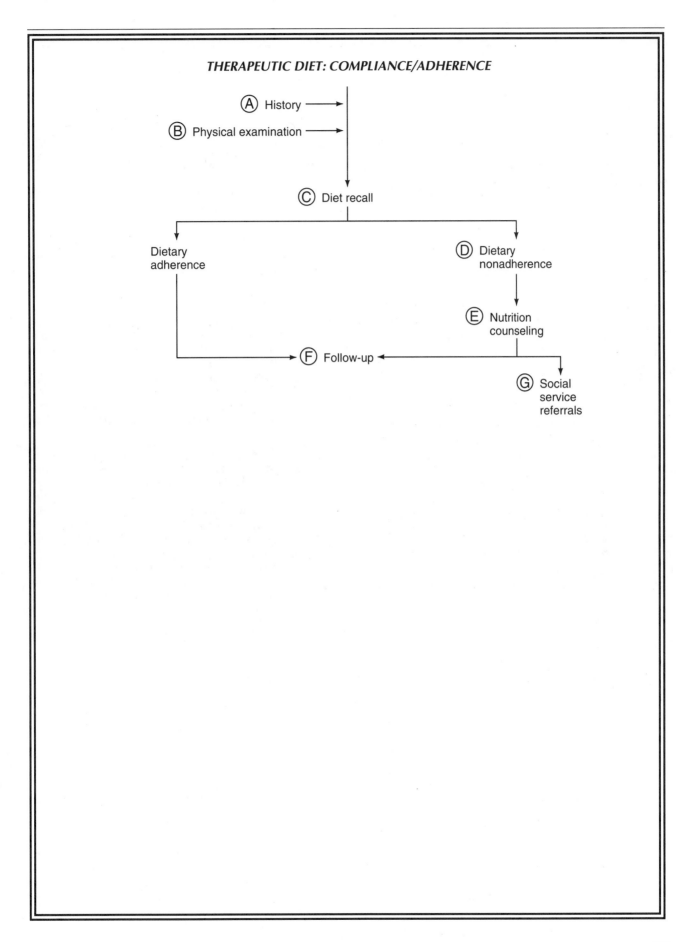

A History

B Physical examination

C Diet recall

Dietary adherence

D Dietary nonadherence

E Nutrition counseling

F Follow-up

G Social service referrals

WEIGHT CHANGE

Sheral Cade

Weight increases consistently with age for both sexes. Men reach their maximum weight around ages 34–54 years and women at ages 55–65 years. Weight stabilizes for the next 15–20 years, then progressively decreases, more slowly in women than in men. A gradual and small amount of weight loss is normal. An unplanned weight loss > 5% within 6–12 months may indicate declining nutritional status. Significant weight change can indicate a dietary change, a metabolic rate change, or the nutritional impact of a disease process. Emotional status, mental status, and physiologic changes can affect food intake or energy needs. It may not always be possible to determine the causes of weight change, but nutritional counseling is always in order.

A. Ask questions about health history and food intake.
- history of chronic disease
- appetite history
- height/weight history, including normal weight
- changes in taste (see Taste Changes, p. 136)
- changes in smell (see Decreased Sense of Smell, p. 126)
- digestive problems
- GI surgery
- laxative/purgative use
- food preparation facilities
- dentition (see Poor Dentition/Caries, p. 170)
- medications
- alcohol use
- finances
- mobility
- isolation
- proximity to family and friends
- recent losses or life crises

B. Physical examination should evaluate
- general appearance
- actual height and weight
- recent weight change
- level of hydration (see p. 150)
- skin assessment (see pp. 100–117)
- mobility
- edema (see p. 10)
- ascites

Weight change is the single most useful assessment tool. Measure actual height and weight whenever possible; a chair or bed scale may be necessary. Make estimates of height and weight using anthropometric measures (p. 160). Laboratory studies include CBC, albumin, creatinine clearance, transferrin, total lymphocyte count, and hemoglobin/hematocrit. Consider difficulties in obtaining tests and factors that may affect biochemical measurements. These include
- collecting 24-hour urine specimens
- cost
- measuring height
- obtaining weight if the patient is chair- or bed bound
- age-related decline in renal function
- over- or underhydration
- drug-drug or drug-nutrient interactions
- coexisting diseases

C. Weight loss may be a sign of a life-threatening disorder. Over time, it can be a guide for monitoring nutritional state. Consider psychiatric disorders, depression, dementia, physical deficit, systemic/pathologic disorders, or malignancy as causes.

D. Weight gain results when energy intake exceeds energy output. Factors that contribute to weight gain or obesity in the elderly are
- decrease in metabolic rate
- decreased physical activity
- altered hunger/satiety

Consider depression, isolation, decreased activity, fluid retention, and hypothyroidism as causes.

E. Nutritional assessment is most easily made by a dietitian. Interpretation of height and weight to determine ideal body weight is not a simple matter because of age-related changes that must be considered. The tool *Nutritional Assessment*, p. 166, shows parameters to consider if performing a nutritional assessment. Weight is the single most useful assessment tool. Make every attempt to obtain an accurate weight. The Body Mass Index, p. 162, contains information on how to estimate weight if measurement is not possible. See weight tables on pp. 163 and 164. The Masters and Lasser and O'Hanlon weight tables (see p. 161) are more age sensitive. Other components of a nutritional assessment are
- health history information
- food intake analysis
- anthropometric measurements (see p. 160)
- biochemical indices

Food intake analysis compares information obtained from 24-hour recall and food frequency questionnaires with established recommended daily allowances.

F. Nutrition counseling and instruction may succeed in changing the patient's eating habits. Goals are for the patient to
- make rational decisions about foods
- enjoy a wide variety of foods
- choose healthful foods
- eat in moderation

When counseling the elderly, respect lifelong food preferences. Attempts to re-educate the patient to a new style of eating will be less successful than modifying existing habits and presenting new combinations that will meet nutritional needs while satisfying established food preferences.

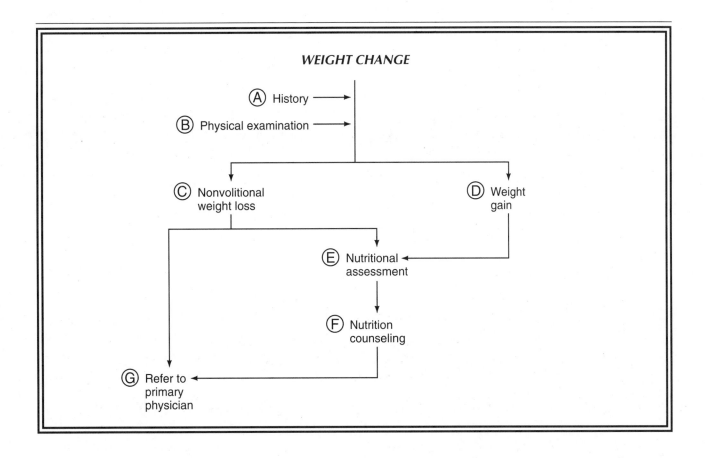

WEIGHT CHANGE

G. Medical evaluation is required when weight loss is nonvolitional or when nutrition assessment has failed to detect a cause of weight change.

References

Chernoff R, ed. Geriatric nutrition. The health professionals handbook. Gaithersburg, MD: Aspen, 1991.

Fisher J, Johnson M. Low body weight and weight loss in the aged. J Am Diet Assoc 1990; 90:1697.

Hazzard W, Andres R, Bierman E, Blass J, eds. Principles of geriatric medicine and gerontology. 2nd ed. New York: McGraw-Hill, 1990.

Morley J, Glick Z, Rubenstein L, eds. Geriatric nutrition: A comprehensive review. New York: Raven Press, 1990.

Robbins L. Evaluation of weight loss in the elderly. Geriatrics 1989; 44:31.

Anthropometric Measurements

Parameter	Measured	Calculations/Interpretation
Height	Standing upright without assistance	None
Knee height	Have patient lie supine with left ankle and left knee at right angles Measure in cm under the base of foot to knee using a sliding, broad-blade caliper	Men $(2.02 \times$ knee height$) - (0.04 \times$ age$) + 64.19$ Women $(1.83 \times$ knee height$) - (0.24 \times$ age$) + 84.88$
Weight	Upright balance scale or movable wheelchair balance beam scale or bed scale	None
Body mass index	$\dfrac{\text{weight (kilograms)}}{\text{height}^2 \text{ (meters)}}$	See the tool *Body Mass Index*, pp. 162–164
Estimated body weight	Measured in cm Calf circumference (calf C) Knee height (Knee H) Midarm circumference (MAC) Subscapular skinfold thickness (subsc SF)	Men $(0.98 \times$ calf C$) + (1.16 \times$ Knee H$) + (1.73 \times$ MAC$) + (0.37 \times$ subsc SF$) - 81.69$ Women $(1.27 \times$ calf C$) + (0.87 \times$ Knee H$) + (0.98 \times$ MAC$) + (0.4 \times$ subsc SF$) - 62.35$
Midarm circumference (MAC)	Measure in cm Use flexible measuring tape	Increase in norm ages 22–70 Women about 6% Men only slightly
Triceps skinfold thickness (TSF)	Measure in mm Use calipers	More reliable predictor of body fat in women than in men
Subscapular skinfold thickness (Subsc SF)	Measure in mm Use calipers	More reliable predictor of body fat in men than in women
Arm muscle circumference	MAC TSF	AMC (cm) = MAC (cm) $-$ [$3.14 \times$ TSF (mm)]

References

Bowan B, Rosenberg I. Assessment of the nutritional status of the elderly. Am J Clin Nutr 1982; 35:1142.

Chernoff R, Lipschitz D. Nutrition and aging. In: Shils M, Young V, eds. Modern nutrition in health disease. 7th ed. Philadelphia: Lea & Febiger, 1988:982.

Chumlea W, Roche A, Mukherjee D. Nutritional assessment of the elderly through anthropometry. Columbus, OH: Ross Laboratories, 1987.

Karkeck J. Assessment of nutritional status of the elderly. Nutritional Support Services 1984; 4:23.

Masters A, Lasser R, Beckman G. Tables of average weight and height of Americans aged 65 to 95 years. Relationship of weight and height to survival. JAMA 1960; 172:658.

Morley J, Glick Z, Rubenstein L, eds. Geriatric nutrition: A comprehensive review. New York: Raven Press, 1990.

Average Weight in Pounds per Inch of Height in Women Aged 65–94

Height (inches)	Age (years) 65–68	69–74	75–79	80–84	85–89	90–94
58	133	125	123	—	—	—
59	134	127	124	116	110	—
60	135	129	126	118	113	—
61	137	131	128	121	116	—
62	139	134	131	124	120	119
63	141	137	134	128	124	119
64	144	140	137	132	133	120
65	147	144	140	136	138	124
66	151	147	143	140	142	129
67	155	151	146	144	—	—
68	159	155	—	—	—	—
69	164	160	—	—	—	—

Average Weight in Pounds per Inch of Height in Men Aged 65–94

Height (inches)	Age (years) 65–69	70–74	75–79	80–84	85–89	90–94
61	142	139	137	—	—	—
62	144	141	139	135	—	—
63	146	143	141	136	133	—
64	149	146	143	138	135	—
65	151	149	145	141	139	130
66	154	152	148	144	142	133
67	156	155	151	147	145	136
68	159	158	154	150	148	140
69	163	162	158	154	152	144
70	167	165	162	159	156	149
71	172	169	166	164	160	154
72	177	173	171	170	165	—
73	182	178	175	—	—	—

From O'Hanlon P, Kohrs M. Dietary studies of older Americans. Am J Clin Nutr 1978; 31:1257; with permission.

Average Weight in Pounds per Inch of Height in Persons Aged 65–94 in 5-year Age Groups

Height (inches)	Age (years) 65–69		70–74		75–79		80–84		85–89		90–94	
	M	F	M	F	M	F	M	F	M	F	M	F
58	—	133	—	125	—	123	—	—	—	—	—	—
59	—	134	—	127	—	124	—	116	—	110	—	—
60	—	135	—	129	—	126	—	118	—	113	—	—
61	142	137	139	131	137	128	—	121	—	116	—	—
62	144	139	141	134	139	131	135	124	—	120	—	119
63	146	141	143	137	141	134	136	128	133	124	—	119
64	149	144	146	140	143	137	138	132	135	128	—	120
65	151	147	149	144	145	140	141	136	139	133	130	124
66	154	151	152	147	148	143	144	140	142	138	133	129
67	156	155	155	151	151	146	147	144	145	142	136	—
68	159	159	158	155	154	—	150	—	148	—	140	—
69	163	164	162	160	158	—	154	—	152	—	144	—
70	167	—	165	—	162	—	159	—	156	—	149	—
71	172	—	169	—	166	—	164	—	160	—	154	—
72	177	—	173	—	171	—	170	—	165	—	—	—
73	182	—	178	—	175	—	—	—	—	—	—	—

M, males; F, females.
From Masters A, Lasser R, Beckman G. Tables of average weight and height of Americans aged 65 to 95 years. Relationship of weight and height to survival. JAMA 1960; 172:658; with permission. Copyright 1960, American Medical Association.

Body Mass Index
(Applies to tools on pp. 163 and 164)

Calculation/Interpretation

Underweight: BMI <20.7 for men and <19.1 for women.

Acceptable weight: BMI 20.7–27.8 for men and 19.1–27.3 for women. (*Note:* Intervention is indicated for men at BMI levels of 26.4 or more and for women at levels of 25.8 or more if they have a family history or current indications of diseases or risk factors complicated by obesity.)

Overweight: BMI ≥27.8 for men and ≥27.3 for women.

Severe overweight: BMI ≥31.1 for men and ≥32.3 for women.

Morbid obesity: BMI ≥45.4 for men and ≥32.3 for women.

From Rowland M. Dietetic currents, a Ross timesaver. Vol 16, No. 2. 1989. Columbus, OH: Ross Laboratories, 1989; with permission.

Body Mass Index

Males

Height, m (in.)

Weight kg(lb)	1.47 (58)	1.50 (59)	1.52 (60)	1.55 (61)	1.57 (62)	1.60 (63)	1.63 (64)	1.65 (65)	1.68 (66)	1.70 (67)	1.73 (68)	1.75 (69)	1.78 (70)	1.80 (71)	1.83 (72)	1.85 (73)	1.88 (74)	1.90 (75)	1.93 (76)
39 (85)	17.8	17.2	16.6	16.1	15.5	15.1	14.6	14.1	13.7	13.3	12.9	12.6	12.2	11.9	11.5	11.2	10.9	10.6	10.3
41 (90)	18.8	18.2	17.6	17.0	16.5	15.9	15.4	15.0	14.5	14.1	13.7	13.3	12.9	12.6	12.2	11.9	11.6	11.2	11.0
43 (95)	19.9	19.2	18.6	18.0	17.4	16.8	16.3	15.8	15.3	14.9	14.4	14.0	13.6	13.2	12.9	12.5	12.2	11.9	11.6
45 (100)	20.9	20.2	19.5	18.9	18.3	17.7	17.2	16.6	16.1	15.7	15.2	14.8	14.3	13.9	13.6	13.2	12.8	12.5	12.2
48 (105)	21.9	21.2	20.5	19.8	19.2	18.6	18.0	17.5	16.9	16.4	16.0	15.5	15.1	14.6	14.2	13.9	13.5	13.1	12.8
50 (110)	23.0	22.2	21.5	20.8	20.1	19.5	18.9	18.3	17.8	17.2	16.7	16.2	15.8	15.3	14.9	14.5	14.1	13.7	13.4
52 (115)	24.0	23.2	22.5	21.7	21.0	20.4	19.7	19.1	18.6	18.0	17.5	17.0	16.5	16.0	15.6	15.2	14.8	14.4	14.0
54 (120)	25.1	24.2	23.4	22.7	21.9	21.3	20.6	20.0	19.4	18.8	18.2	17.7	17.2	16.7	16.3	15.8	15.4	15.0	14.6
57 (125)	26.1	25.2	24.4	23.6	22.9	22.1	21.5	20.8	20.2	19.6	19.0	18.5	17.9	17.4	17.0	16.5	16.0	15.6	15.2
59 (130)	27.2	26.3	25.4	24.6	23.8	23.0	22.3	21.6	21.0	20.4	19.8	19.2	18.7	18.1	17.6	17.2	16.7	16.2	15.8
61 (135)	28.2	27.3	26.4	25.5	24.7	23.9	23.2	22.5	21.8	21.1	20.5	19.9	19.4	18.8	18.3	17.8	17.3	16.9	16.4
64 (140)	29.3	28.3	27.3	26.5	25.6	24.8	24.0	23.3	22.6	21.9	21.3	20.7	20.1	19.5	19.0	18.5	18.0	17.5	17.0
66 (145)	30.3	29.3	28.3	27.4	26.5	25.7	24.9	24.1	23.4	22.7	22.0	21.4	20.8	20.2	19.7	19.1	18.6	18.1	17.7
68 (150)	31.4	30.3	29.3	28.3	27.4	26.6	25.7	25.0	24.2	23.5	22.8	22.2	21.5	20.9	20.3	19.8	19.3	18.7	18.3
70 (155)	32.4	31.3	30.3	29.3	28.4	27.5	26.6	25.8	25.0	24.3	23.6	22.9	22.2	21.6	21.0	20.4	19.9	19.4	18.9
73 (160)	33.4	32.3	31.2	30.2	29.3	28.3	27.5	26.6	25.8	25.1	24.3	23.6	23.0	22.3	21.7	21.1	20.5	20.0	19.5
75 (165)	34.5	33.3	32.2	31.2	30.2	29.2	28.3	27.5	26.6	25.8	25.1	24.4	23.7	23.0	22.4	21.8	21.2	20.6	20.1
77 (170)	35.5	34.3	33.2	32.1	31.1	30.1	29.2	28.3	27.4	26.6	25.8	25.1	24.4	23.7	23.1	22.4	21.8	21.2	20.7
79 (175)	36.5	35.3	34.2	33.1	32.0	31.0	30.0	29.1	28.2	27.4	26.6	25.8	25.1	24.4	23.7	23.1	22.5	21.9	21.3
82 (180)	37.6	36.4	35.2	34.0	32.9	31.9	30.9	30.0	29.1	28.2	27.4	26.6	25.8	25.1	24.4	23.7	23.1	22.5	21.9
84 (185)	38.7	37.4	36.1	35.0	33.8	32.8	31.8	30.8	29.9	29.0	28.1	27.3	26.5	25.8	25.1	24.4	23.8	23.1	22.5
86 (190)	39.7	38.4	37.1	35.9	34.8	33.7	32.6	31.6	30.7	29.8	28.9	28.1	27.3	26.5	25.8	25.1	24.4	23.7	23.1
88 (195)	40.8	39.4	38.1	36.8	35.7	34.5	33.5	32.4	31.5	30.5	29.6	28.8	28.0	27.2	26.4	25.7	25.0	24.4	23.7
91 (200)	41.8	40.4	39.1	37.8	36.6	35.4	34.3	33.3	32.3	31.3	30.4	29.5	28.7	27.9	27.1	26.4	25.7	25.0	24.3
93 (205)	42.8	41.4	40.0	38.7	37.5	36.3	35.2	34.1	33.1	32.1	31.2	30.3	29.4	28.6	27.8	27.0	26.3	25.6	25.0
95 (210)	43.9	42.4	41.0	39.7	38.4	37.2	36.0	34.9	33.9	32.9	31.9	31.0	30.1	29.3	28.5	27.7	27.0	26.2	25.6
98 (215)	44.9	43.4	42.0	40.6	39.3	38.1	36.9	35.8	34.7	33.7	32.7	31.8	30.8	30.0	29.2	28.4	27.6	26.9	26.2
100 (220)	46.0	44.4	43.0	41.6	40.2	39.0	37.8	36.6	35.5	34.5	33.5	32.5	31.6	30.7	29.8	29.0	28.2	27.5	26.8
102 (225)	47.0	45.4	43.9	42.5	41.2	39.9	38.6	37.4	36.3	35.2	34.2	33.2	32.3	31.4	30.5	29.7	28.9	28.1	27.4
104 (230)	48.1	46.5	44.9	43.5	42.1	40.7	39.5	38.3	37.1	36.0	35.0	34.0	33.0	32.1	31.2	30.3	29.5	28.7	28.0
107 (235)	49.1	47.5	45.9	44.4	43.0	41.6	40.3	39.1	37.9	36.8	35.7	34.7	33.7	32.8	31.9	31.0	30.2	29.4	28.6
109 (240)	50.2	48.5	46.9	45.3	43.9	42.5	41.2	39.9	38.7	37.6	36.5	35.4	34.4	33.5	32.6	31.7	30.8	30.0	29.2
111 (245)	51.2	49.5	47.8	46.3	44.8	43.4	42.1	40.8	39.5	38.4	37.3	36.2	35.2	34.2	33.2	32.3	31.5	30.6	29.8
113 (250)	52.3	50.5	48.8	47.2	45.7	44.3	42.9	41.6	40.4	39.2	38.0	36.9	35.9	34.9	33.9	33.0	32.1	31.2	30.4
116 (255)	53.3	51.5	49.8	48.2	46.6	45.2	43.8	42.4	41.2	39.9	38.8	37.7	36.6	35.6	34.6	33.6	32.7	31.9	31.0
118 (260)	54.3	52.5	50.8	49.1	47.6	46.1	44.6	43.3	42.0	40.7	39.5	38.4	37.3	36.3	35.3	34.3	33.4	32.5	31.6
120 (265)	55.4	53.5	51.8	50.1	48.5	46.9	45.5	44.1	42.8	41.5	40.3	39.1	38.0	37.0	35.9	35.0	34.0	33.1	32.3
122 (270)	56.4	54.5	52.7	51.0	49.4	47.8	46.3	44.9	43.6	42.3	41.1	39.9	38.7	37.7	36.6	35.6	34.7	33.7	32.9
125 (275)	57.5	55.5	53.7	52.0	50.3	48.7	47.2	45.8	44.4	43.1	41.8	40.6	39.5	38.4	37.3	36.3	35.3	34.4	33.5
136 (300)	62.7	60.6	58.6	56.7	54.9	53.1	51.5	49.9	48.4	47.0	45.6	44.3	43.0	41.8	40.7	39.6	38.5	37.5	36.5
159 (350)	73.2	70.7	68.4	66.1	64.0	62.0	60.1	58.2	56.5	54.8	53.2	51.7	50.2	48.8	47.5	46.2	44.9	43.7	42.6
181 (400)	83.6	80.8	78.1	75.6	73.2	70.9	68.7	66.6	64.6	62.6	60.8	59.1	57.4	55.8	54.3	52.8	51.4	50.0	48.7

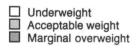

□ Underweight
▨ Acceptable weight
▨ Marginal overweight
▨ Overweight
▨ Severe overweight
■ Morbid obesity

Body Mass Index

Females

Height, m (in.)

Weight kg(lb)	1.47 (58)	1.50 (59)	1.52 (60)	1.55 (61)	1.57 (62)	1.60 (63)	1.63 (64)	1.65 (65)	1.68 (66)	1.70 (67)	1.73 (68)	1.75 (69)	1.78 (70)	1.80 (71)	1.83 (72)	1.85 (73)	1.88 (74)	1.90 (75)	1.93 (76)
39 (85)	17.8	17.2	16.6	16.1	15.5	15.1	14.6	14.1	13.7	13.3	12.9	12.6	12.2	11.9	11.5	11.2	10.9	10.6	10.3
41 (90)	18.8	18.2	17.6	17.0	16.5	15.9	15.4	15.0	14.5	14.1	13.7	13.3	12.9	12.6	12.2	11.9	11.6	11.2	11.0
43 (95)	19.9	19.2	18.6	18.0	17.4	16.8	16.3	15.8	15.3	14.9	14.4	14.0	13.6	13.2	12.9	12.5	12.2	11.9	11.6
45 (100)	20.9	20.2	19.5	18.9	18.3	17.7	17.2	16.6	16.1	15.7	15.2	14.8	14.3	13.9	13.6	13.2	12.8	12.5	12.2
48 (105)	21.9	21.2	20.5	19.8	19.2	18.6	18.0	17.5	16.9	16.4	16.0	15.5	15.1	14.6	14.2	13.9	13.5	13.1	12.8
50 (110)	23.0	22.2	21.5	20.8	20.1	19.5	18.9	18.3	17.8	17.2	16.7	16.2	15.8	15.3	14.9	14.5	14.1	13.7	13.4
52 (115)	24.0	23.2	22.5	21.7	21.0	20.4	19.7	19.1	18.6	18.0	17.5	17.0	16.5	16.0	15.6	15.2	14.8	14.4	14.0
54 (120)	25.1	24.2	23.4	22.7	21.9	21.3	20.6	20.0	19.4	18.8	18.2	17.7	17.2	16.7	16.3	15.8	15.4	15.0	14.6
57 (125)	26.1	25.2	24.4	23.6	22.9	22.1	21.5	20.8	20.2	19.6	19.0	18.5	17.9	17.4	17.0	16.5	16.0	15.6	15.2
59 (130)	27.2	26.3	25.4	24.6	23.8	23.0	22.3	21.6	21.0	20.4	19.8	19.2	18.7	18.1	17.6	17.2	16.7	16.2	15.8
61 (135)	28.2	27.3	26.4	25.5	24.7	23.9	23.2	22.5	21.8	21.1	20.5	19.9	19.4	18.8	18.3	17.8	17.3	16.9	16.4
64 (140)	29.3	28.3	27.3	26.5	25.6	24.8	24.0	23.3	22.6	21.9	21.3	20.7	20.1	19.5	19.0	18.5	18.0	17.5	17.0
66 (145)	30.3	29.3	28.3	27.4	26.5	25.7	24.9	24.1	23.4	22.7	22.0	21.4	20.8	20.2	19.7	19.1	18.6	18.1	17.7
68 (150)	31.4	30.3	29.3	28.3	27.4	26.6	25.7	25.0	24.2	23.5	22.8	22.2	21.5	20.9	20.3	19.8	19.3	18.7	18.3
70 (155)	32.4	31.3	30.3	29.3	28.4	27.5	26.6	25.8	25.0	24.3	23.6	22.9	22.2	21.6	21.0	20.4	19.9	19.4	18.9
73 (160)	33.4	32.3	31.2	30.2	29.3	28.3	27.5	26.6	25.8	25.1	24.3	23.6	23.0	22.3	21.7	21.1	20.5	20.0	19.5
75 (165)	34.5	33.3	32.2	31.2	30.2	29.2	28.3	27.5	26.6	25.8	25.1	24.4	23.7	23.0	22.4	21.8	21.2	20.6	20.1
77 (170)	35.5	34.3	33.2	32.1	31.1	30.1	29.2	28.3	27.4	26.6	25.8	25.1	24.4	23.7	23.1	22.4	21.8	21.2	20.7
79 (175)	36.6	35.3	34.2	33.1	32.0	31.0	30.0	29.1	28.2	27.4	26.6	25.8	25.1	24.4	23.7	23.1	22.5	21.9	21.3
82 (180)	37.6	36.4	35.2	34.0	32.9	31.9	30.9	30.0	29.1	28.2	27.4	26.6	25.8	25.1	24.4	23.7	23.1	22.5	21.9
84 (185)	38.7	37.4	36.1	35.0	33.8	32.8	31.8	30.8	29.9	29.0	28.1	27.3	26.5	25.8	25.1	24.4	23.8	23.1	22.5
86 (190)	39.7	38.4	37.1	35.9	34.8	33.7	32.6	31.6	30.7	29.8	28.9	28.1	27.3	26.5	25.8	25.1	24.4	23.7	23.1
88 (195)	40.8	39.4	38.1	36.8	35.7	34.5	33.5	32.4	31.5	30.5	29.6	28.8	28.0	27.2	26.4	25.7	25.0	24.4	23.7
91 (200)	41.8	40.4	39.1	37.8	36.6	35.4	34.3	33.3	32.3	31.3	30.4	29.5	28.7	27.9	27.1	26.4	25.7	25.0	24.3
93 (205)	42.8	41.4	40.0	38.7	37.5	36.3	35.2	34.1	33.1	32.1	31.2	30.3	29.4	28.6	27.8	27.0	26.3	25.6	25.0
95 (210)	43.9	42.4	41.0	39.7	38.4	37.2	36.0	34.9	33.9	32.9	31.9	31.0	30.1	29.3	28.5	27.7	27.0	26.2	25.6
98 (215)	44.9	43.4	42.0	40.6	39.3	38.1	36.9	35.8	34.7	33.7	32.7	31.8	30.8	30.0	29.2	28.4	27.6	26.9	26.2
100 (220)	46.0	44.4	43.0	41.6	40.2	39.0	37.8	36.6	35.5	34.5	33.5	32.5	31.6	30.7	29.8	29.0	28.2	27.5	26.8
102 (225)	47.0	45.4	43.9	42.5	41.2	39.9	38.6	37.4	36.3	35.2	34.2	33.2	32.3	31.4	30.5	29.7	28.9	28.1	27.4
104 (230)	48.1	46.5	44.9	43.5	42.1	40.7	39.5	38.3	37.1	36.0	35.0	34.0	33.0	32.1	31.2	30.3	29.5	28.7	28.0
107 (235)	49.1	47.5	45.9	44.4	43.0	41.6	40.3	39.1	37.9	36.8	35.7	34.7	33.7	32.8	31.9	31.0	30.2	29.4	28.6
109 (240)	50.2	48.5	46.9	45.3	43.9	42.5	41.2	39.9	38.7	37.6	36.5	35.4	34.4	33.5	32.6	31.7	30.8	30.0	29.2
111 (245)	51.2	49.5	47.8	46.3	44.8	43.4	42.1	40.8	39.5	38.4	37.3	36.2	35.2	34.2	33.2	32.3	31.5	30.6	29.8
113 (250)	52.3	50.5	48.8	47.2	45.7	44.3	42.9	41.6	40.4	39.2	38.0	36.9	35.9	34.9	33.9	33.0	32.1	31.2	30.4
116 (255)	53.3	51.5	49.8	48.2	46.6	45.2	43.8	42.4	41.2	39.9	38.8	37.7	36.6	35.6	34.6	33.6	32.7	31.9	31.0
118 (260)	54.3	52.5	50.8	49.1	47.6	46.1	44.6	43.3	42.0	40.7	39.5	38.4	37.3	36.3	35.3	34.3	33.4	32.5	31.6
120 (265)	55.4	53.5	51.8	50.1	48.5	46.9	45.5	44.1	42.8	41.5	40.3	39.1	38.0	37.0	35.9	35.0	34.0	33.1	32.3
122 (270)	56.4	54.5	52.7	51.0	49.4	47.8	46.3	44.9	43.6	42.3	41.1	39.9	38.7	37.7	36.6	35.6	34.7	33.7	32.9
125 (275)	57.5	55.5	53.7	52.0	50.3	48.7	47.2	45.8	44.4	43.1	41.8	40.6	39.5	38.4	37.3	36.3	35.3	34.4	33.5
136 (300)	62.7	60.6	58.6	56.7	54.9	53.1	51.5	49.9	48.4	47.0	45.6	44.3	43.0	41.8	40.7	39.6	38.5	37.5	36.5
159 (350)	73.2	70.7	68.4	66.1	64.0	62.0	60.1	58.2	56.5	54.8	53.2	51.7	50.2	48.8	47.5	46.2	44.9	43.7	42.6
181 (400)	83.6	80.8	78.1	75.6	73.2	70.9	68.7	66.6	64.6	62.6	60.8	59.1	57.4	55.8	54.3	52.8	51.4	50.0	48.7

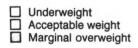

☐ Underweight
☐ Acceptable weight
☐ Marginal overweight

▨ Overweight
■ Severe overweight
■ Morbid obesity

Food Diary

Name _____   DOB _____

Physician _____   ID# _____

Directions for using food diary:
List all foods as soon as possible after eating.
Write only one food item on a line.
Include brand names when possible.

Record amounts in household measures.
Tell how food was packaged: fresh, frozen,
canned (include liquid: water, syrup).

Day	Date	Time	Food eaten	Amount	How prepared
Sun	6/2	Noon	canned tuna in oil	3 oz	with mayonnaise, pickles, olives
Mon	6/3	8AM	egg	2	scrambled in teflon pan, no oil
	6/3	10AM	peaches	2 halves	canned in heavy syrup

Nutritional Assessment

Parameter	Indicators	Use

Anthropometric measurements	Height/weight
	Arm circumference
	Skinfolds
	  Tricep
	  Subscapular
	BMI (body mass index)
		Calculate BMI
		Calculate ideal body weight
		Set weight goal

Biochemical assays	Serum albumin Hemoglobin/hematocrit Creatinine/height index (see box)	Determine nutritional status
Health history	Height/weight history Chronic diseases Appetite assessment Change in taste/smell Dental/oral health Digestive problems Laxative usage GI surgery Medications Vitamin/mineral supplements	Identify causative factors for intervention

Food intake analysis	Diet history
	  24-hour recall
	  Food frequency
	Problems associated with eating
		Assess nutrient content

Home life/meal preparation	Number in household Grocery shopping Food preparation Meals away from home Finances/food dollar source	Evaluate support systems and guide referrals

Creatinine/Height Index

Purpose	Predicted	Calculation	Interpretation
Used to evaluate muscle mass	Men 23 mg/kg IBW* Women 18 mg/kg IBW*	$$\dfrac{\text{actual urinary creatinine (mg)} \times 100\%}{\text{predicted urinary creatinine (mg)}}$$	Reduction in excretion with no renal disease present is a sign of a wasting disease

*IBW, Ideal body weight.

Stages of Skin Ulceration

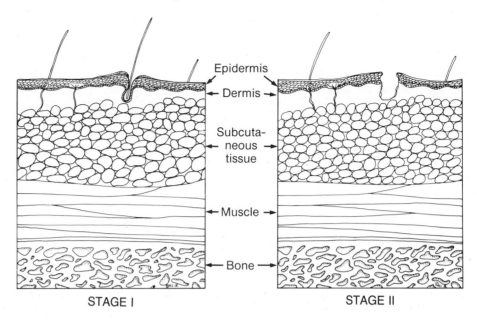

STAGE I

STAGE II

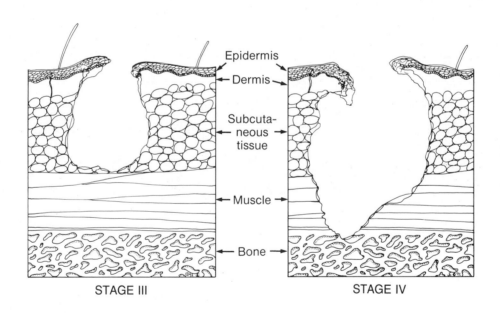

STAGE III

STAGE IV

Instructions for a High-Fiber Diet

Sources of dietary fiber	*fruits (raw or cooked) *vegetables (raw or cooked) *whole grains
High-fiber foods that may aggravate diverticulitis	*nuts *legumes *berries *foods with seeds
How to start a high-fiber diet	*gradually increase dietary fiber *drink 2–3 L of fluid a day *begin with as little as 10 g of fiber a day (2 slices of whole-grain bread, 2 bran biscuits, or 2 spoons of bran) *keep a food diary to help if referral to a dietitian is made
Problems following a high fiber diet	*difficulty ingesting enough food to get 20–60 g of fiber a day *limited ability to chew with ill-fitting dentures or poor dentition *increased cost of high fiber food *abdominal distention, flatulence or diarrhea

DIGESTION

POOR DENTITION/CARIES

Talar L. Glover

Caries is the most common chronic human disorder. Causes of poor dentition include poor oral hygiene, xerostomia (lack of saliva), and repeated vomiting.

A. History taking should focus on
   - oral hygiene practices (see Gum Irritation/Gingivitis, p. 172)
   - interference with eating or digestion of food
   - presence of
     - pain when eating cold, hot, or sweet foods
     - toothache
     - bad taste in the mouth
     - medical conditions that cause repeated vomiting
     - medications or conditions that reduce saliva output

   Nutritional questions include
   - nutrition diary (see Therapeutic Diet Compliance/Adherence, p. 156, and Nutritional Deficits Requiring Supplementation, p. 154)
   - changes in eating habits
   - changes in bowel and GI function
   - indications that food is not well chewed

B. Perform a complete oral examination (see p. 183 and the tool *Food Diary*, p. 165) and determine tooth mobility. Observe any color changes of the teeth where decay or cracks may be present. Check for halitosis. Assess for denture fit and condition
   - poor adherence and slippage in mouth
   - too tight and difficult to remove
   - causing gum irritation or mouth lesions (see Mouth Lesions/Ulcers, p. 174, and Gum Irritation/Gingivitis, p. 172)
   - surface cracks
   - missing teeth
   - poor hygiene

   If the patient describes changes in bowel and GI function, a further examination may help rule out motility problems or food intolerances.

C. Teach the patient
   - oral hygiene techniques (see Gum Irritation/Gingivitis, p. 172).
   - avoidance of sugar-containing foods.
   - how to select a toothbrush (see box).

D. Referrals may be needed for tooth extraction or treatment of caries. Unfortunately, resources for dental care are scarce for many patients. Investigate dental schools or dental hygiene schools in the area to determine whether they accept referrals.

How to Select a Toothbrush	
Feature	*Characteristic*
Bristles	Soft Rounded Flat brushing surface
Handle	Fit comfortably in hand
Head	Small enough to reach sides of all teeth

References

Bates JF, Adams D, Stafford GD. Dental treatment of the elderly. Bristol, England: John Wright, 1984.

Little JW, Falace DA. Dental management of the medically compromised patient. St Louis: CV Mosby, 1988.

POOR DENTITION/CARIES

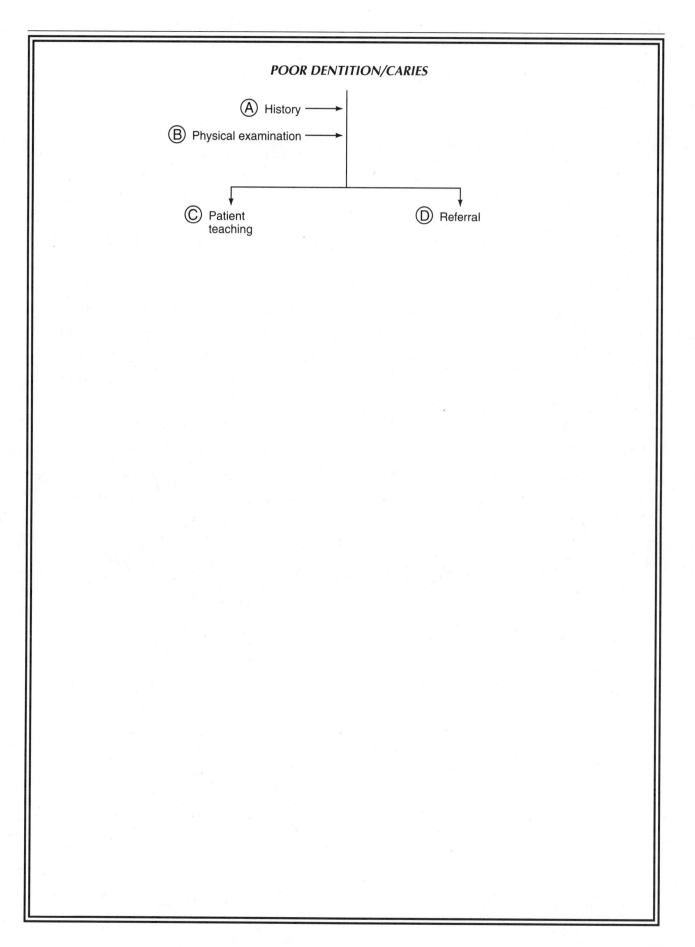

GUM IRRITATION/GINGIVITIS

Talar L. Glover

Gum irritation/gingivitis can result from inappropriate oral hygiene; intraoral injury; medications; or malnutrition, including vitamin and mineral deficiencies. Gingivitis is a common result of the interaction of food debris with enzymes and the mixed oral flora in the saliva (Table 1).

A. History taking for gum irritation/gingivitis elicits
    • onset
    • precipitating factors
    • type and duration of appliance/denture use
    • presence or absence of
      • bleeding
      • pain
      • swelling
    • habits
    • nutrition
    • medical history
    • medications
    Obtain exact details on oral hygiene practices and how much time dentures or appliances are worn.

B. Steps in a gingival examination are
    • put on gloves
    • perform visual inspection before removing appliances or dentures
    • safeguard appliances or dentures once removed
    • palpate gingiva
    • palpate gingival margins and observe for bleeding or expression of matter or exudate from beneath the gums (see the tool *Oral Examination,* p. 183).
    Observe the bite to determine whether chewing is causing pressure areas.

C. Adequate oral hygiene requires tools to remove food debris from tooth surfaces and the gingival margins, remove impacted particles, and stimulate circulation within the gingiva. The box shown above lists oral

Oral Hygiene Tools	
Tool	*Purpose*
Oral rinse	Remove loose debris
Toothbrush	Remove debris adhering to teeth
Dentifrice	Prolong brushing
	Impart pleasant aftertaste
Floss	Remove impacted particles
	Clean under gingival margins
Gum stimulator	Stimulate gingival circulation
Disclosing tablet	Determine effectiveness of oral cleaning
Oral irrigation device	Remove food particles by water pressure
Mouthwash	Freshen breath temporarily
Fluoride	Harden tooth enamel
	Prevent bacteria from becoming attached to teeth

hygiene tools and their uses. Evaluate tools used in oral hygiene. Mechanical injury to the mouth can result from inappropriate selection or use of tools. For tips on how to select a toothbrush, see the box on p. 170. Recommend
• oral rinses after meals
• brushing teeth at least once a day
• use of floss daily
• rinsing dentures/appliances thoroughly before reinserting in the mouth
• have teeth cleaned at least yearly
• change the toothbrush every 3–6 months
Review the techniques used in oral hygiene with the patient. Mechanical injury can result from learning a new technique. Chemical injury can result from contact with harsh denture-cleaning agents.

D. A lifestyle review looks at habits and medications that may cause gum irritation, such as
    • tobacco use
    • use of toothpicks
    • using teeth or mouth to open jars or bottles
    • alcohol use
    Medications such as aspirin may be caustic if chewed or held in the mouth. Dilantin causes painless gingival hypertrophy in some cases.

E. Reassessment of nutritional status may be necessary. Gum irritation can influence food choices or the amount of food eaten. A food diary (see p. 165) will help determine whether current food choices are deficient in protein, vitamins, or minerals.

F. Refer patients to the appropriate resource. Those with poor oral hygiene need professional prophylaxis if home measures are to be successful. Alternative

TABLE 1   Possible Causes of Gum Irritation/Gingivitis

Symptom	Finding	Causes to Consider
Bleeding	Spontaneous	Poor oral hygiene
		Malnutrition
		Periodontal disease
	With manipulation	Overzealous oral hygiene
		Inappropriate hygiene tools
		Mechanical irritation
Swelling	Painful	Mechanical injury
		Chemical injury
		Thermal injury
		Poor oral hygiene
		Overzealous oral hygiene
	Nontender	Drug-related hypertrophy

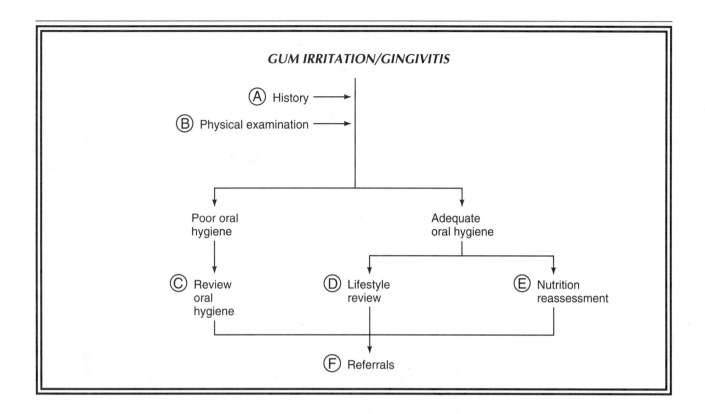

GUM IRRITATION/GINGIVITIS

Ⓐ History

Ⓑ Physical examination

Poor oral hygiene

Adequate oral hygiene

Ⓒ Review oral hygiene

Ⓓ Lifestyle review

Ⓔ Nutrition reassessment

Ⓕ Referrals

funding for professional dental services and appliances may be difficult to obtain. The patient's physician needs to determine whether changes can be made in the medication regimen if it is determined that drugs are contributing to the irritation. Patients with nutritional intake problems may need to be referred to a dietitian or to social service agencies that can assist with meal delivery, homemaker services, or financial assistance to purchase food.

References

Hatfield D. Tooth and gum care. Springhouse, PA: American Family Health Institute, 1986.

Shaver RO. Dentistry for the homebound, institutionalized and elderly. Lakewood, CO: Portable Dentistry Publisher, 1982.

Thompson J. Oral hygiene and dental care. Community Outlook 1990; January:10, 12, 15.

MOUTH LESIONS/ULCERS

Talar L. Glover

The oral mucosa is one of the most easily observed mucous membranes of the body. It is often evaluated as an indicator of systemic health. Any lesion or ulcer of the mouth is in constant contact with the saliva and the mixed oral flora, multiple bacteria and microorganisms, contained within. This increases the probability of infection when a lesion or ulcer develops.

A. The goal of history taking is to determine causative factors. Questions should focus on
   • onset
   • precipitating factor or injury
   • lifestyle
   • habits
   • nutrition
   • medical history
   • medications
   (See the tool *Components of Oral History*, p. 182.)

B. Wear gloves for all oral examinations because of the potential for saliva to transmit communicable disease. Equipment that may be needed includes gauze, tongue blade, penlight, and oral mirror; a soft toothbrush is optional. Perform an initial visual examination before removing dentures or appliances. Note the location of lesions for proximity to dentures or appliances, particularly edges. Help the patient remove dentures and appliances before proceeding, and note the ease with which this is done. Be sure to safeguard dentures or appliances by placing them in water in a labeled denture cup or emesis basin. Next, perform a complete intraoral examination without dentures or removable appliances in place (see p. 183). Evaluate the function and interaction of oral structures and look for characteristics of the lesion or ulcer that may delineate the cause (Table 1). Pain is present when a lesion is new; its absence may indicate a healing lesion or neuropathy. Dentures or appliances may have to be cleaned with tap water, using gauze or a soft toothbrush, before being inspected. Rubbing with dry gauze helps find rough edges once the dentures are clean.

C. If a denture or appliance is found to have rough edges, refer the patient to a dental professional; repair or replacement may be needed.

D. It may be difficult to change habits that contribute to mouth lesions and ulcers. Steps that may need to be recommended include
   • stopping the use of tobacco
   • taking medication differently
   • changing eating patterns
   • increasing fluid intake
   • taking vitamin/mineral supplements
   • changing denture cleaning routines

TABLE 1 Lesion/Ulcer Characteristics

Characteristic	Observation	Consider
Location of lesion(s)	Proximity to appliance edge	Mechanical
	Cheek	Tobacco use Chemical
	Tongue	Tobacco use Thermal Chemical
	Gums	Mechanical
	Lips	Mechanical
Number of lesions	Widespread	Immunocompromise Infection/illness Fluid-electrolytes Medication Diet
	Single	Chemical Thermal Mechanical
	Multiple, localized	Mechanical Thermal Medication
Appearance	Crater	Chemical Thermal
	Abrasion	Mechanical
	Laceration	Mechanical

Remind the patient that most denture cleaners should be used outside the mouth. Cleaning agents must be rinsed thoroughly from the denture or appliance before replacing, to prevent irritation or injury to the oral tissue.

E. Local treatment of mouth lesions and ulcers aims at maintaining an environment conducive to healing. The two major components are
   • oral hygiene
   • oral rinses
   Oral hygiene consists of
   • tooth brushing
   • flossing
   • routine professional prophylaxis
   Inappropriate tools for oral hygiene include toothpicks, toothbrushes with hard or worn-out bristles, and inappropriate dentifrice. These items may cause mechanical or chemical injury to intraoral structures. Oral rinses can be done with saline solution or dilute commercial mouthwash. Oral saline rinse (0.9%) is made by adding 1 teaspoon of table salt to 1 pint of tepid water. The mouth should be rinsed after meals and at bedtime.

MOUTH LESIONS/ULCERS

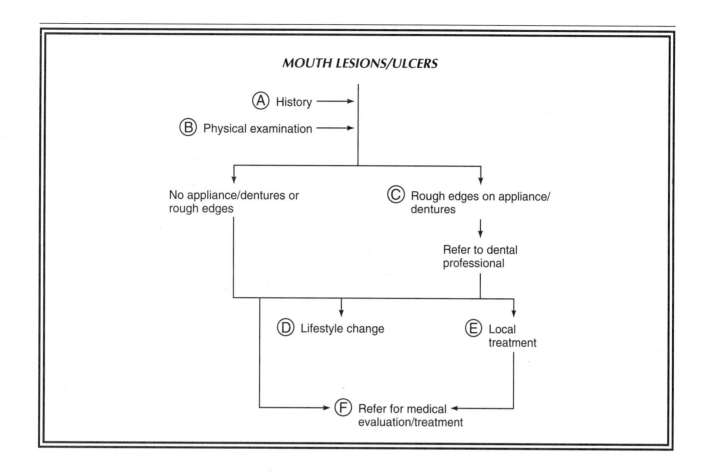

F. Reasons to refer the patient for medical evaluation or treatment include
- discovery of a systemic problem
- possibility of an iatrogenic problem
- possibility of cranial nerve neuropathy
- signs of infection
- compromised oral function

References

Bates JF, Adams D, Stafford GD. Dental treatment of the elderly. Bristol: John Wright and Sons, Ltd., 1984.

Bhaskar SN. A practical high yield mouth exam. Patient Care 1990; 24:53.

Jones JA. Integrating the oral examination into clinical practice. Hosp Pract 1989; 24:23.

Tryon AF. Oral health and aging: an interdisciplinary approach to geriatric dentistry. Littleton, MA: PSG Publishing Co., Inc., 1986.

MOUTH PAIN/DENTAL PAIN/JAW PAIN

Talar L. Glover

The health of the mouth can affect both physical and emotional well-being. Pain of the jaw or mouth structures can decrease oral intake and impair communication, leading to malnutrition and potential social isolation.

A. Questions to ask on history include
   • pain characteristics
     • onset
     • precipitating factors
     • location
     • alleviating/exacerbating factors
     • radiation
     • duration
   • oral hygiene practices
   • medical history
   • medications
   • presence of earache or tinnitus (see Tinnitus, p. 124)

Referrals for Mouth/Dental/Jaw Pain	
Professional	*Treatment*
Dentist	Grind tooth surfaces to redistribute pressure
	Refit dentures/appliances
	Treat oral lesions/injuries
Orthodontist	Realign teeth
	Refit dentures/appliances
	Make mouthguard for night wear
Oral surgeon	Treat temporomandibular joint syndrome
Physician	Prescribe muscle relaxants
	Relaxation/biofeedback therapy
Other health care workers	Relaxation therapy
	Biofeedback

• presence of clicking or popping sound when the jaw is moved
• habits
  • gum chewing
  • nail biting
  • bruxism (tooth grinding, jaw clenching)

B. Observe the face for asymmetry both at rest and in motion. Palpate the muscles of the face and neck, paying particular attention to the temporomandibular joint. Perform a complete oral examination (see p. 183). Observe teeth alignment and note how dentures or appliances fit. Observe for lesions or discoloration of the gingiva and oral mucosa.

C. Recommend lifestyle adjustments such as
   • changing habits that place stress on mouth/jaw structures
   • use of relaxation techniques, including biofeedback
   • avoidance of known irritants
   • use of heat or cold on face and intraorally
   • taking nonsteroidal anti-inflammatory drugs if not contraindicated

D. Referrals may be needed to help manage mouth/dental/jaw pain. The choice of medical/dental professional depends on the problem identified (see the box).

References

Guinn NJ. Hiding in plain sight: Detection of oral cancer. Today's OR Nurse 1990; 12:24.
Tyron AF. Oral health and aging: An interdisciplinary approach to geriatric dentistry. Littleton, MA: PSG Publishing, 1986.

MOUTH PAIN/DENTAL PAIN/JAW PAIN

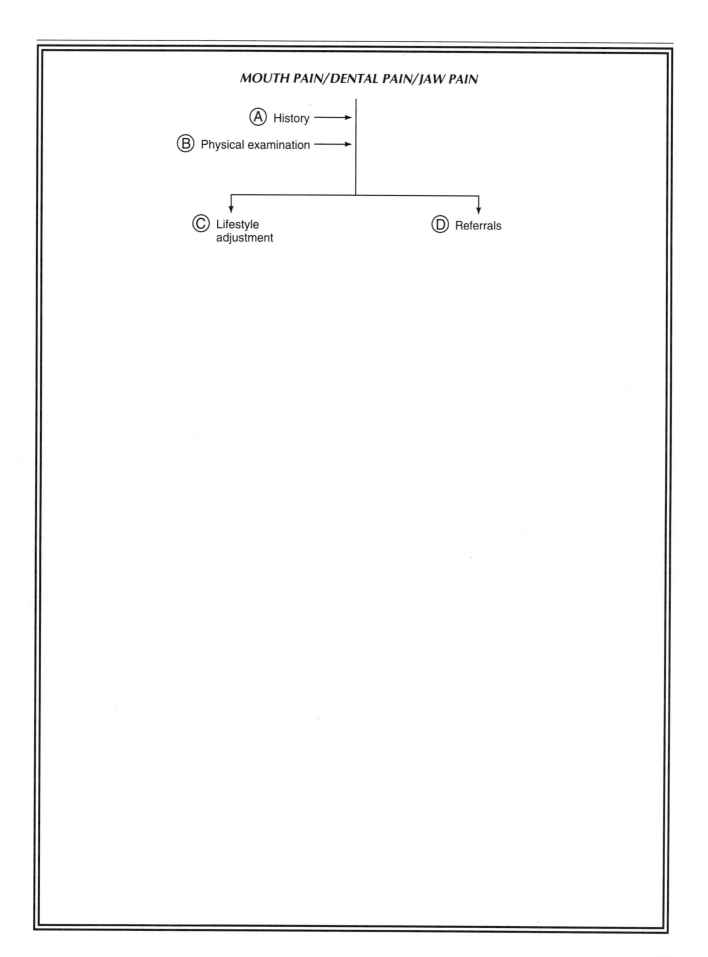

(A) History ⟶

(B) Physical examination ⟶

(C) Lifestyle adjustment

(D) Referrals

DIVERTICULAR DISEASE

Sara B. Wick

Diverticulosis is found predominantly in developed Western societies. The United States, United Kingdom, and Australian populations have a 10% occurrence rate. Diverticulosis is rarely seen before 40 years of age and increases to 50% or more in the ninth decade. A diverticulum is a herniation or sacculation of the mucosa of the colon through the first layer of muscle at the point of blood vessel penetration. Diverticulosis occurs primarily in the sigmoid portion of the left colon. Contributing factors may be atrophy of the musculature, a diet high in refined foods and low in fiber, constipation, and obesity causing alterations in GI motility with increased intraluminal pressures.

A. A thorough history ensures that patients give specific and detailed information about GI complaints (see box "What to Ask About Gastrointestinal Complaints"). Information needed includes occurrence of hemorrhoids, anal disease, bowel surgery, hernia, emotional problems, cancer, neurologic disorders, or thyroid problems. Determine whether there is a family history of polyps or colon cancer.

B. Physical examination should include a thorough abdominal and rectal evaluation (see Constipation, p. 184). This often reveals lower left quadrant tenderness. Obtain weight and temperature, and serial stools for occult blood. Evaluate dentition. Clinical features of pain, fever, leukocytosis, abdominal tenderness, palpable masses, fistulas, obstruction, perforation, and rectal bleeding can be presenting symptoms of colon cancer, Crohn's disease, ulcerative colitis, ischemic colitis, or diverticular disease. Alternative diagnoses can be confirmed on radiographic or endoscopic examination, with or without biopsy. Rarely, surgical interventions are indicated to make an accurate diagnosis.

C. Eighty percent of persons affected with diverticulosis are asymptomatic. The condition is most often recognized through radiographic studies or laparotomy. Treatment consists of patient education to prevent diverticulitis (inflammation in the diverticuli).

D. A total of 10–20% of patients with diverticular disease develop symptomatic diverticulitis. The chance of diverticulitis increases if the diverticuli are numerous, are widely distributed in the colon, appear at an early age, or have been present >10 years. Diverticulitis occurs when a single diverticulum becomes inflamed by fecal material. This local inflammation may progress to involve surrounding tissue, leading to necrosis, perforation, and fecal contamination of surrounding tissue. The most common presenting symptoms of diverticulitis are griping left lower quadrant pain with guarding and rebound tenderness. The pain is usually of acute onset, constant, worse after eating, and relieved somewhat after a bowel movement or passage of flatus. Fever and chills may be present. The patient may also report constipation, diarrhea, nausea, vomiting, abdominal bloating, or anorexia. Complications of diverticulitis are abscesses, fistulas, bowel obstruction, and peritonitis.

E. Bleeding diverticulosis is found in 10%–30% of persons with diverticular disease. Hemorrhage is often preceded by abdominal cramping and the urge to defecate. It occurs in otherwise asymptomatic individuals as sudden, painless, profuse rectal bleeding. The bleeding may be intermittent or constant and ceases spontaneously in 80% of cases.

F. Obtain a complete blood count, sedimentation rate, electrolyte panel, and serial stools for occult blood. These, in addition to radiologic and endoscopic procedures, are used to confirm the diagnosis of diverticular disease.

G. Therapy for diverticular disease is aimed at placing the bowel at rest. Measures should include decreased activity, clear liquids or nothing by mouth, and IV fluids.

H. Refer patients with symptoms to a primary care physician for evaluation. Medical diagnostic efforts

---

What to Ask About Gastrointestinal Complaints

- Patterns of elimination and any recent changes
- Characteristics of stools
- Toileting habits
- Weight changes
- Medication use
- Dietary patterns
- Fluid intake
- Exercise
- Presence and characteristics of abdominal pain or cramping
- Flatulence
- Anorexia
- Nausea/vomiting
- Heartburn
- Malaise
- Weakness
- Intolerance to heat or cold
- Recent losses or emotional crises

Diagnostic Sequencing for Bleeding Diverticulosis

Minimal	Severe
Endoscopy	Angiography
Barium studies	Endoscopy
Angiography, if other studies inconclusive	Barium studies

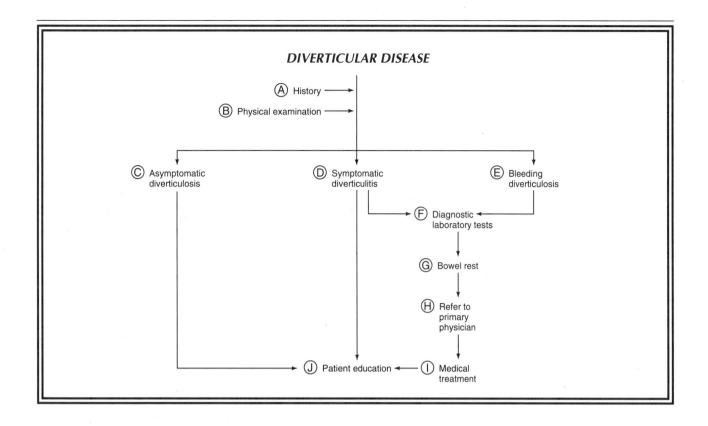

DIVERTICULAR DISEASE

(A) History
(B) Physical examination

(C) Asymptomatic diverticulosis
(D) Symptomatic diverticulitis
(E) Bleeding diverticulosis

(F) Diagnostic laboratory tests
(G) Bowel rest
(H) Refer to primary physician
(I) Medical treatment
(J) Patient education

concentrate on determining the source of the bleeding or pain and may include endoscopy, blood coagulation studies, and abdominal radiologic procedures and barium studies (see box "Diagnostic Sequencing for Bleeding Diverticulosis"). Noninvasive CT is a useful diagnostic tool, especially if barium studies are contraindicated. The invasive procedures of sigmoidoscopy and barium enema may be deferred until the acute flare has subsided because of the risk of perforation causing peritoneal contamination with feces and contrast material.

I. Less severe forms of symptomatic diverticular disease may be treated at home with a high-fiber diet, antispasmodics, and oral antibiotics (ampicillin or tetracycline). Inpatient treatment may include bed rest, IV fluids, nasogastric intubation and aspiration, blood transfusions, correction of blood coagulation abnormalities, sedation, and intra-arterial vasopressin. Reserve surgical intervention for cases with severe complications. Surgical procedures may include initial diversion and colostomy with subsequent resection and closure, or bowel resection.

J. Patient education target areas are diet, bowel management, and lifestyle changes. A diet high in fiber (20–60 g/day of fiber) is recommended (see the tool *High-Fiber Diet*, p. 168). Such a diet does not reduce the number or size of existing diverticuli. Fiber binds water, which acts to make stools heavier, bulkier, and softer, thus decreasing intracolonic pressure and reducing transit time through the colon.

Obesity is a probable precursor to diverticular disease. Instruct overweight patients about a low-calorie, weight reduction diet and an exercise program.

Bowel management includes a high-fiber diet, increased fluid intake of 2–3 L/day, increased exercise, and bowel retraining (see Constipation, p. 184). Bulk agents and stool softeners are advised. Bowel irritant laxatives and large-volume enemas should be avoided.

Lifestyle changes involve actions to reduce stress and promote a sense of well-being. Specific steps include
• regular exercise
• avoidance of alcohol
• smoking cessation
• stress management

References

Gioiella EC, Bevil CW. Nursing the client experiencing problems of fluids and electrolytes. In: Gioiella EC, Bevil CW, eds. Nursing care of the aging client: Promoting health adaptation. Norwalk, CT: Appleton-Century-Crofts, 1985:365.

Heitkemper M, Bartrol MA. Gastrointestinal problems. In: Carnevali DL, Patrick M, eds. Nursing management for the elderly. Philadelphia: JB Lippincott, 1986:431.

Naitove A, Almy TP. Diverticular disease of the colon. In: Sleisenger MH, Fordtran JS, eds. Gastrointestinal disease: Pathophysiology, diagnosis and management. Philadelphia: WB Saunders, 1989:1419.

Sklar M. Gastrointestinal diseases. In: Calkins E, Davis PJ, Ford AB, eds. The practice of geriatrics. Philadelphia: WB Saunders, 1986:566.

FLATULENCE

Sara B. Wick

Flatulence is often encountered by health care providers but has received very little scientific attention. Treatment is usually based on the patient's description of the problem. Diagnostic studies are seldom performed with an initial presentation of "excessive" intestinal gas. A total of 99% of rectal gas is composed of nitrogen, oxygen, carbon dioxide, hydrogen, and methane; the percentages of each gas vary, depending on the source. The sources of intestinal gas are air swallowing, diffusion of gas from blood to intestinal lumen, and food processing. Excessive flatulence may be a symptom of certain organic disorders such as colon cancer or diverticular disease.

A. The history of a patient with flatulence should include onset of symptoms; change in bowel function; pain, frequency, and intensity of gas passage; dietary history, attempting to identify foods that aggravate the problem; medications; family history of flatulence or GI problems; personal history of any GI problems, including rectal surgery; food intolerances; and anxiety. Explore symptoms such as bloating, abdominal pain, nocturnal discomfort, bleeding, and weight loss.

B. Physical examination should include inspection, auscultation, percussion, and palpation of the abdomen. Perform a rectal examination and obtain stool for occult blood. Pay attention to the dentition and evidence of air swallowing or gulping noted during conversation or ingestion of foods.

C. Intestines of normal individuals usually contain <200 ml of gas but may produce 200–2000 ml/day. A frequency of gas passage of 7–20 per day can be considered a normal flatulence pattern. Patients with this pattern should be reassured that this is normal.

D. Excessive gas production is frequently determined by the patient's subjective report. A crucial component in the diagnosis of excessive gas passage is that the patient should keep meticulous records of the frequency of gas passage and foods ingested to determine a relationship between diet and severity of flatulence. Malabsorption of lactose or ingestion of fructose and sorbitol in excessive amounts can produce excessive flatus.

E. Patient education mainly concerns changing diet habits. See the Box for foods to avoid to reduce gas production. Diets low in lactose, starches, and legumes help decrease intraluminal production of gas. Over-the-counter drugs that help to control flatus include simethicone and antacids.

F. If the patient is still bothered with flatulence, a referral for medical management is indicated. Medications such as antacids, anticholinergics, simethicone alone or with pancreatic enzymes, and metoclopramide have been used, but their effectiveness is less than persuasive. These agents help decrease transit time of intestinal gas, which, if prolonged, often makes a person more sensitive to the intestinal distention and discomfort caused by the presence of gas. Gas volume studies, gastric motility studies, and radiographic studies of the GI tract may be indicated.

Potential Gas-Producing Foods

Apples	Eggplant
Apricots	Lettuce
Bagels	Milk and milk products
Bananas	Onions
Beans	Pastries
Bread	Potatoes
Brussel sprouts	Pretzels
Cabbage	Prune juice
Carrots	Raisins
Celery	Wheat germ
Citrus fruits	

References

Levitt MD, Bond JH. Intestinal gas. In: Sleisenger MH, Fordtran JS, eds. Gastrointestinal disease: Pathophysiology, diagnosis and management. Philadelphia: WB Saunders, 1989:257.

Peterson W. Intestinal gas. Unpublished manuscript, University of Texas Southwestern Medical Center, Dallas, TX, 1984.

Sutalf LO, Levitt MD. Follow-up of a flatulent patient. Dig Dis Sci 1979; 24:652.

FLATULENCE

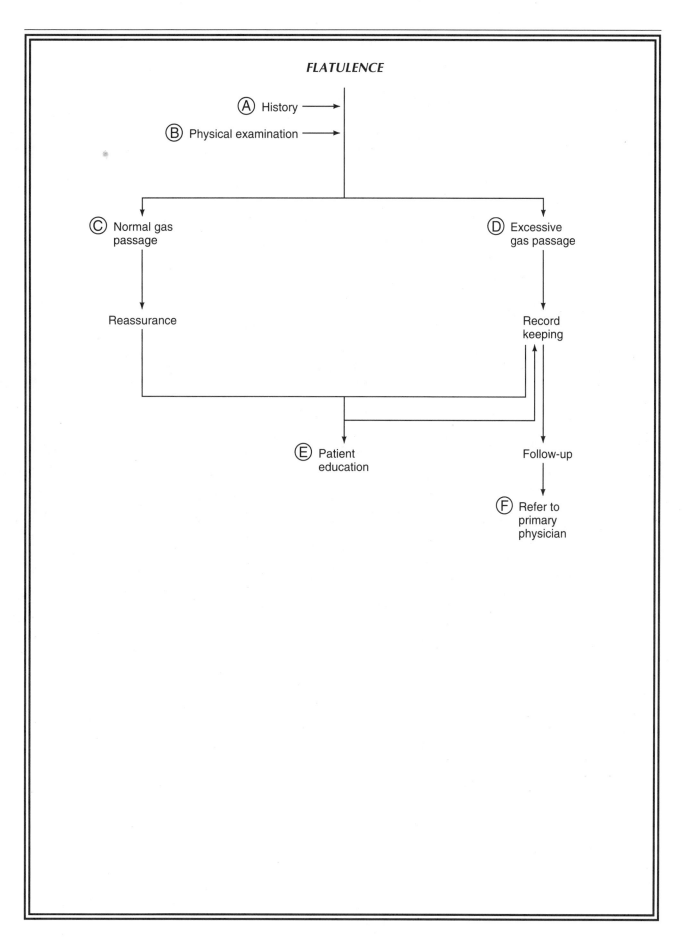

Components of Oral History

Component	Category	Possible Causes
Precipitating factor/injury	Thermal	Smoking Hot or cold foods
	Chemical	Tobacco/snuff Drugs Lozenges, mints
	Mechanical	Appliances Dentures Teeth Foreign objects (e.g., toothpicks)
Pain	Present	Recent injury Infection
	Absent	Old injury Neuropathy
Habits/lifestyle	Tobacco use Alcohol use Bruxism Oral hygiene Diet	Vitamin/mineral deficiency Malnutrition
Medical history	Immunocompromise	Chemotherapy
	Fluid-electrolytes	Dehydration
	Nutrition	Malabsorption Diminished nutrient storage and utilization
	Medications	Dilantin Lozenges/troches
	Infection/illness	Herpes

Oral Examination

Method	Structure	Normal Findings	Comments
Inspection	Mucosa	Intact Smooth Moist Pink/coral	May require use of tongue blade or oral mirror
	Gingiva	Well-defined margins	
	Tongue	Protrudes symmetrically	
	Lips	Symmetric Smooth	
	Teeth	Smooth Pearly 32 present	
	Dentures/appliances	Intact	
Palpation	Mucosa	Pliant	Wear gloves
	Gingiva	Adheres to teeth	May require use of gauze or tongue blade
	Tongue	Elastic	
	Lips	Elastic Change in texture at vermilion border	
	Teeth	Nonmobile	
	Dentures/appliances	Smooth edges Nonmobile	

ELIMINATION

CONSTIPATION

Pamela S. Ruby

Constipation is usually defined as abnormally infrequent or difficult evacuation of hard, dry feces. Failure to relieve constipation results in fecal impaction.

A. A history of a lifelong pattern of bowel function is necessary to establish an individual's "normal" function. Pay attention to frequency, consistency, and color of stool as well as factors that affect defecation (foods, activities, medications, mental outlook, stress). Perception of normal bowel habits/functions must also be established. History taking includes a detailed description of the symptoms, onset and duration, and associated conditions and pain, as well as identification of any contributory factors such as
- environmental changes or concerns (lack of privacy, inability to reach commode/bedpan, poor positioning on commode/bedpan, decreased exercise or mobility, poor dentition, neglecting the urge to defecate)
- inadequate bulk and fluids in the diet
- chronic enema/laxative use
- painful anorectal disorders
- history of pathology (colonic tumors, strictures, volvulus, neurologic degeneration)
- mental stress or depression
- certain medications (anticholinergics, narcotics, aspirin, aluminum hydroxide, calcium carbonate antacids, mineral oil, tranquilizers)
- belief that at least one bowel movement a day is necessary

B. Examination includes assessment of
- bowel sounds
- stool color and consistency and occult blood determination
- abdominal and rectal muscle tone that may play a significant role in the inability to defecate
- rectal examination to determine the presence of hemorrhoids (p. 192) as well as sphincter tone

C. Goals of treatment are to immediately relieve the constipation and its associated discomfort and prevent the complication of fecal impaction. Treatment may consist of suppositories, enemas, or laxatives. Suppositories are used for lubrication and digital stimulation (glycerin) or for neural stimulation to the intestinal wall (Dulcolax). Enemas act as irritants, lubricants, and softeners or to provide volume to stimulate defecation. Laxatives act (1) to stimulate peristaltic actions by increasing local irritation to the intestine or by selective action on the nerve complex of intestinal smooth muscle, (2) to increase bulk, (3) to increase wetting efficiency of intestinal water which prevents development of constipation but does not treat existing constipation or fecal impaction, or (4) to lubricate and soften stool.

D. Hypertonic constipation results from an increased transit time and a consequent increased reabsorption of water. It is characterized by hard, dry stools and occasionally lower abdominal pain. The aim of treatment is to decrease transit time of bowel contents, thus decreasing the amount of water reabsorbed. Pathologic conditions that contribute to hypertonic constipation are colonic atony, in which propulsive bowel contractions are impaired; tumors; and anorectal disorders, including hemorrhoids.

E. Habit constipation results from a decreased amount of bulk and fluids in the diet and a conscious or unconscious ignoring of the urge to defecate. The goal of treatment is to help the patient heed the urge to defecate; use the gastrocolic reflex that is stimulated when the stomach is stretched after eating; and provide a private, stress-free environment for relaxed toileting. A regular schedule of toileting also helps. Promoting a diet with increased bulk and fluids encourages a stool large enough to stimulate the urge to defecate and soft enough to be passed painlessly.

F. Hypotonic constipation is characterized by soft, putty-like stool in the rectum. It is the result of decreased intestinal segmental motility.

G. Medical evaluation for individuals >60 years of age should include a rectal and sigmoid examination every 1-2 years. Also, consult the primary physician to ascertain the cause of acute, unexplained constipation.

Components of a Bowel Program

- Provide a private, stress-free atmosphere
- Respond to urge to defecate; do not suppress
- Establish a specific time each day for bowel movement activity, e.g., after breakfast, to take advantage of gastrocolic reflex (which occurs a few minutes after eating)
- Increase fluids to 2-3 L/day (unless contraindicated)
- Provide a well-balanced diet with adequate bulk
- Increase activities, e.g., walking or isometric exercises for the bedfast patient
- Avoid long-term or habitual use of laxatives and cathartics; use stool softeners, laxatives, suppositories, or enemas on an intermittent or as needed basis
- Use psyllium seed stool-bulking agents on a regular basis

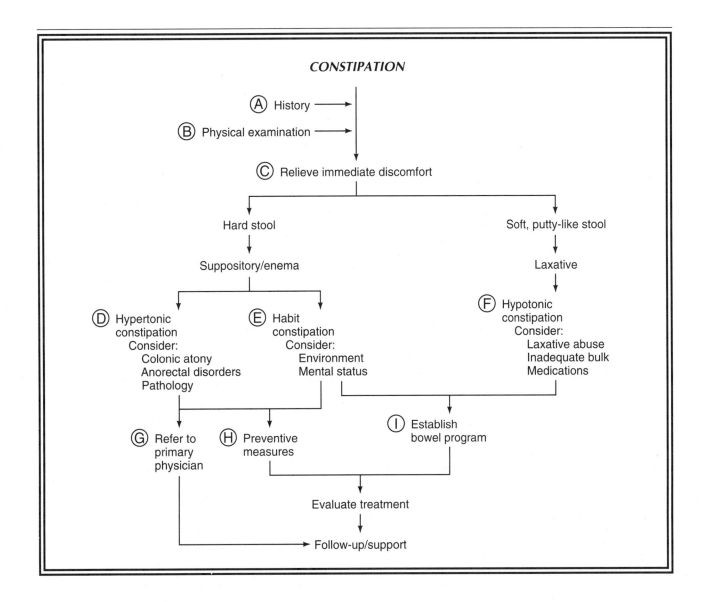

CONSTIPATION

A. History

B. Physical examination

C. Relieve immediate discomfort

Hard stool → Suppository/enema

Soft, putty-like stool → Laxative

D. Hypertonic constipation
Consider:
Colonic atony
Anorectal disorders
Pathology

E. Habit constipation
Consider:
Environment
Mental status

F. Hypotonic constipation
Consider:
Laxative abuse
Inadequate bulk
Medications

G. Refer to primary physician

H. Preventive measures

I. Establish bowel program

Evaluate treatment

Follow-up/support

H. Constipation is best prevented by eliminating or minimizing contributing factors and establishing a bowel program to maintain proper bowel function. Discourage regular use of laxatives and cathartics because of the risk of dependency.

I. A bowel program should take into account environment, diet, hydration, activity, and the gastrocolic reflex (see box).

References

Carnevali D, Patrick M. Nursing management for the elderly, 2nd ed. Philadelphia: JB Lippincott, 1986:435.

Kane R, Ouslander J, Abress I. Essentials of clinical geriatrics. New York: McGraw-Hill, 1984:131.

Steffl B. Handbook of gerontological nursing. New York: Van Nostrand Reinhold, 1984:331.

Thompson JM, ed. Mosby's manual of clinical nursing. 2nd ed. St. Louis: CV Mosby, 1989:1656.

DIARRHEA

Pamela S. Ruby

Diarrhea is defined as the frequent passage of unformed stool due to increased bowel motility, or interference with the normal absorption of water and nutrients from the bowel. Usual water loss in stools is 150 ml a day; severe diarrhea can amount to 5–10 L of water loss daily. Diarrhea is a serious occurrence in geriatric patients owing to the rapid sequelae of dehydration and electrolyte imbalance, which may prove fatal (Table 1).

A. Diarrhea may result from laxative abuse, intestinal infections, food poisoning, medications, food allergies, diverticulitis, inflammatory bowel disease, malignancies, emotional stress, or fecal impaction (see Fecal Impaction, p. 188). Fecal impaction may be the underlying factor causing diarrhea of any duration and should always be suspected on initial assessment. History should include the onset and duration of diarrhea; frequency and consistency of stools; associated symptoms; stress; foods eaten; changes in dietary habits or activities; and medications recently ingested, including over-the-counter drugs. An often overlooked cause of diarrhea is sugar-free candy containing mannitol or sorbitol, both potent osmotic agents.

B. Concern for complications related to diarrhea and dehydration should initially focus the examination on signs and symptoms of volume depletion, dehydration, and electrolyte imbalances. Symptoms of saline depletion include furrowed brown tongue, sunken cheeks, loss of skin turgor, orthostatic hypotension, increased hematocrit with stable hemoglobin, flat neck veins, and thirst. Symptoms of hypokalemia include apathy, malaise, lassitude, cardiac arrhythmias, profound weakness, and even general paralysis.

Symptoms of hyponatremia include fatigue, muscle weakness, apprehension, and abdominal cramps. Take vital signs to evaluate orthostatic changes (see Dehydration/Volume Depletion, p. 150). Also, assess mucous membranes and serum electrolytes. Skin turgor is not typically a reliable indicator of hydration in the elderly. Determine fecal impaction on rectal examination. Assess sphincter competency by the anal wink (see Fecal Incontinence, p. 190). Send stool for bacterial culture and ova and parasites. Stool for occult blood is taken on rectal examination.

C. Acute diarrhea can occur as a result of fecal impaction; food poisoning; infection; medications, especially antibiotics; or emotional stress. Acute onset of diarrhea is likely to cause acute dehydration and electrolyte imbalance. In most instances the underlying problem can be identified and resolved.

D. Chronic diarrhea can occur as a result of fecal impaction, laxative or enema abuse, food allergies, or emotional stress. Determining the cause of chronic diarrhea depends on thorough history taking.

E. Intermittent diarrhea may indicate fecal impaction, some type of neuropathy, inflammatory bowel disease, malignancy, diverticulosis, or stress. Intermittent diarrhea, unless caused by diverticulosis or stress, generally requires referral to a physician for evaluation and treatment.

F. Immediate action to resolve acute diarrhea begins with determining the presence of impaction and removing the impacted stool. If a medication is causing the diarrhea, discuss alternatives with the prescribing physician. Adequate hydration and fluid and electrolyte balance can be maintained with oral supplements (Table 2).

G. Nutrition intervention for diarrhea includes a nonirritating diet. Consider common food allergies when dealing with chronic diarrhea (see box below).

H. Education for the patient with diarrhea should cover nutrition changes, skin care (see Rectal Itching [Pruri-

TABLE 1 Classification of Diarrhea

Type	Cause	Result
Secretory	Excessive stimulation or irritation of intestinal mucosa	Stool pH neutral (approx 7.0) Increased secretion of electrolytes, especially sodium
Osmotic	Unabsorbed solute in intestine draws water into intestinal lumen	Water load exceeds colon capacity Stool pH acidic (<7.0) Loss of potassium Risk of hypokalemia for patients on potassium-losing diuretics
Mixed	Difficult to categorize	Exhibits symptoms of both secretory and osmotic diarrhea

---

Foods to Avoid in Chronic Diarrhea	
Spices	Chocolate
Caffeine	Wheat
Alcohol	Milk, milk products
Gas-forming vegetables (beans, cabbages)	Eggs
	Nuts
Corn	Yeast
Fish (especially shellfish)	Chicken

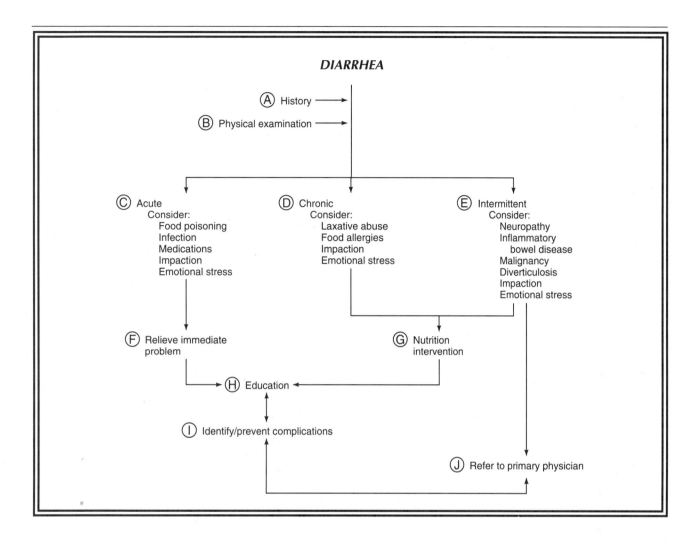

DIARRHEA

- (A) History ⟶
- (B) Physical examination ⟶

(C) **Acute**
Consider:
Food poisoning
Infection
Medications
Impaction
Emotional stress

(D) **Chronic**
Consider:
Laxative abuse
Food allergies
Impaction
Emotional stress

(E) **Intermittent**
Consider:
Neuropathy
Inflammatory
bowel disease
Malignancy
Diverticulosis
Impaction
Emotional stress

(F) Relieve immediate problem

(G) Nutrition intervention

(H) Education

(I) Identify/prevent complications

(J) Refer to primary physician

---

tus Ani], p. 196) to prevent skin breakdown, and stress reduction. Warn patients to report

- thirst
- weakness
- cardiac irregularities
- dizziness on changes in position
- abdominal cramping
- fatigue

I. Complications of diarrhea are dehydration and electrolyte imbalances, especially sodium and potassium. Careful monitoring of laboratory values (hematocrit, hemoglobin, sodium, potassium) may provide early

warning of complications. Treatment consists of maintaining adequate hydration and restoring electrolyte balance. IV replacement of fluids and electrolytes may be necessary (see Table 1). A *Monilia* infection in the perineal area can be treated with an antifungal powder. An immediate bowel program (see Constipation, p. 184) should be started, especially to prevent recurrence of a fecal impaction.

J. Referral to a primary physician may be necessary for definitive diagnosis, pharmacologic management, or IV fluid and electrolyte replacement. Once the cause of the diarrhea is established by stool culture and fiberoptic or radiologic examination (barium enema, upper GI, KUB), antidiarrheal medications may be used. When medications are used, it is more important to undertreat than overtreat the diarrhea.

TABLE 2 Nutritional Management of Acute Diarrhea

Food	Purpose
Clear liquids	Bowel rest for 12–24 hours
Carbonated or electrolyte-containing beverages	Provide sodium and phosphorus
Orange juice	Replace potassium
Potatoes	Replace potassium
Low-fiber, low-fat foods	Allow bowel rest
Yogurt or buttermilk	Replace intestinal flora destroyed by antibiotic therapy

References

Carnevali D, Patrick M. Nursing management for the elderly. 2nd ed. Philadelphia: JB Lippincott, 1986:433.

Steffl B. Handbook of gerontological nursing. New York: Van Nostrand Reinhold, 1984:239.

Thompson JM, ed. Mosby's manual of clinical nursing. 2nd ed. St. Louis: CV Mosby, 1989:1656.

FECAL IMPACTION

Pamela S. Ruby

Fecal impaction is the severest form of constipation and is caused by gradual loss of water from prolonged retention of fecal mass in the bowel.

A. Fecal impaction initially presents as symptoms of constipation, followed by diarrhea or fecal incontinence caused by leakage of liquid stool around the fecal mass. The history may include abdominal discomfort, nausea and vomiting, mental status changes, and a loss of appetite. Urinary incontinence may be the primary complaint.

B. Fecal impaction is diagnosed by detecting alterations in bowel sounds or abdominal distention. Digital rectal examination will reveal a hard, dry mass in the rectal vault.

C. Treatment of the existing impaction is the immediate concern. Digital removal of the fecal mass is not recommended because of vagal stimulation, which may result in cardiac arrhythmia. A warm oil retention enema, followed by a cleansing detergent or soap suds enema, can facilitate impaction removal. Hydrogen peroxide, instilled in small amounts, may help break up the impaction. Agency or institutional policy may dictate treatment.

D. Prevention of fecal impaction is best achieved by prevention of constipation. Prevention of constipation is best obtained by eliminating or minimizing contributing factors and establishing a bowel program to maintain proper bowel function (see Constipation, p. 184).

E. Medical evaluation may be indicated for recurrence or if a physiologic or pathologic problem is suspected.

References

Carnevali D, Patrick M. Nursing management for the elderly. 2nd ed. Philadelphia: JB Lippincott, 1986:435.

Kane R, Ouslander J, Abress I. Essentials of clinical geriatrics. New York: McGraw-Hill, 1984:131.

Steffl B. Handbook of gerontological nursing. New York: Van Nostrand Reinhold, 1984:331.

Thompson JM, ed. Mosby's manual of clinical nursing. 2nd ed. St. Louis: CV Mosby, 1989:1656.

FECAL IMPACTION

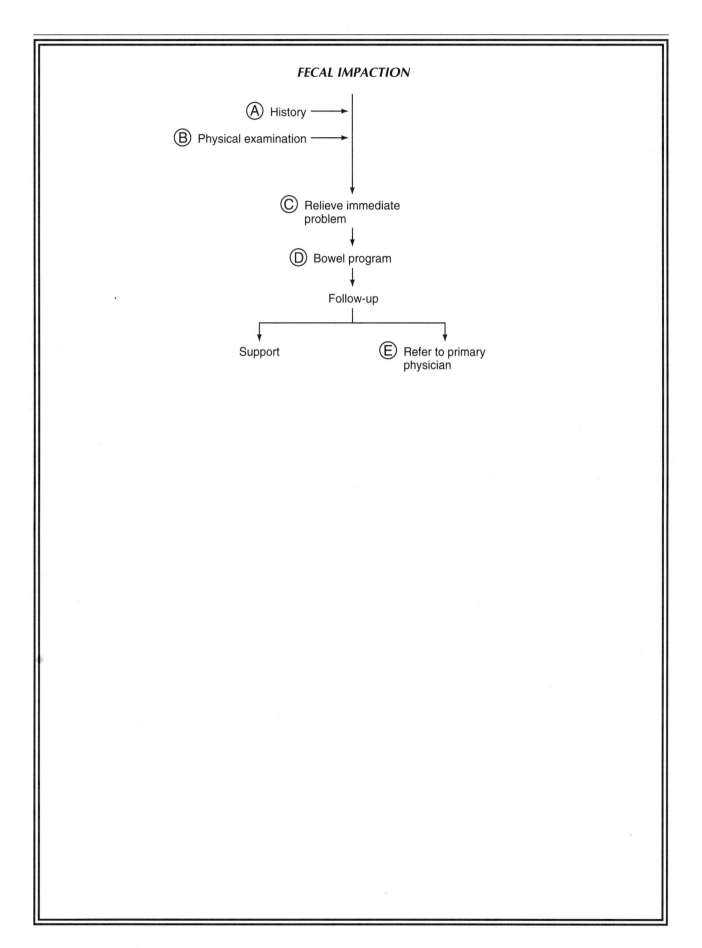

FECAL INCONTINENCE

Pamela S. Ruby

Fecal incontinence is defined as the involuntary passage of stool. It is common for individuals with incontinence to have a fecal odor, stained clothing and bed linens, embarrassed conduct, and decreased social interactions, as well as perineal excoriation. Fecal incontinence may also be accompanied by a high level of anxiety.

A. History taking should ascertain the onset and duration of the incontinence and any previous rectal surgery or pathology. Ascertain bowel habits, including laxative/enema use, diet and fluid intake, and bowel function history. Also, determine any present or past history of anal intercourse, which may have damaged the sphincter tone.

B. Physical assessment includes evaluating sphincter competency and recognizing perineal excoriation. Assess sphincter competency on anal examination. With a finger in the anus, ask the patient to squeeze the anal area as if attempting to stop a bowel movement.

C. Acute fecal incontinence may result from fecal impaction, colorectal disease, stress, and medications, including over-the-counter drugs (see box below).

D. Chronic fecal incontinence may be seen in diabetics with neuropathy or patients with neurologic disease or deficits, a low level of awareness, chronic diarrhea, trauma to the lumbosacral area, or a history of rectal surgery (especially hemorrhoidectomy). Laxative and enema abuse or overuse may also contribute to chronic fecal incontinence.

E. Assess sphincter competency by the anal wink, which results when the skin surrounding the anus is gently stimulated, causing a winking or puckering. This simple test will indicate whether there is innervation at the external anal sphincter.

F. Perineal excoriation results from a combination of skin maceration from moisture and protolytic action of the bacteria found in the stool. Meticulous care must be provided to maintain good skin integrity and prevent further skin breakdown.

G. Interventions include (1) removal of impaction, if present; (2) establishing a bowel program (see the box on p. 184), (3) establishing proper diet with adequate fluid and bulk intake; and (4) stress reduction.

H. Skin care should include cleansing and drying of the area and protection from ensuing incontinence. A number of incontinent kits are available. A fecal incontinent pouch may be applied over the anus to collect the stool and protect the skin if the incontinence is particularly severe.

I. Medical evaluation is required to differentiate among medical conditions that contribute to incontinency (e.g., colorectal disease, neurologic deficits, sphincter incompetency). Such evaluation may include anal manometry and defecrography.

J. The emotional repercussions of fecal incontinence can be more devastating to patients than the physical effects. Referrals to a local support group will help patients cope with the emotional stress produced by the incontinence and provide updated information on this condition. If no local support group is available, patients can be referred to Help for Incontinent People (HIP), PO Box 544, Union, SC 29379.

Drugs that Can Contribute to Fecal Incontinence	
Antibiotics	Mineral oil
Cholinergics	Home remedies
Laxatives	Blackstrap molasses
Geritol	Sulfur/molasses

References

Carnevali D, Patrick M. Nursing management for the elderly. 2nd ed. Philadelphia: JB Lippincott, 1986:440.

Steffl B. Handbook of gerontological nursing. New York: Van Nostrand Reinhold, 1984:240, 331.

Thompson JM, ed. Mosby's manual of clinical nursing. 2nd ed. St. Louis: CV Mosby, 1989:1656.

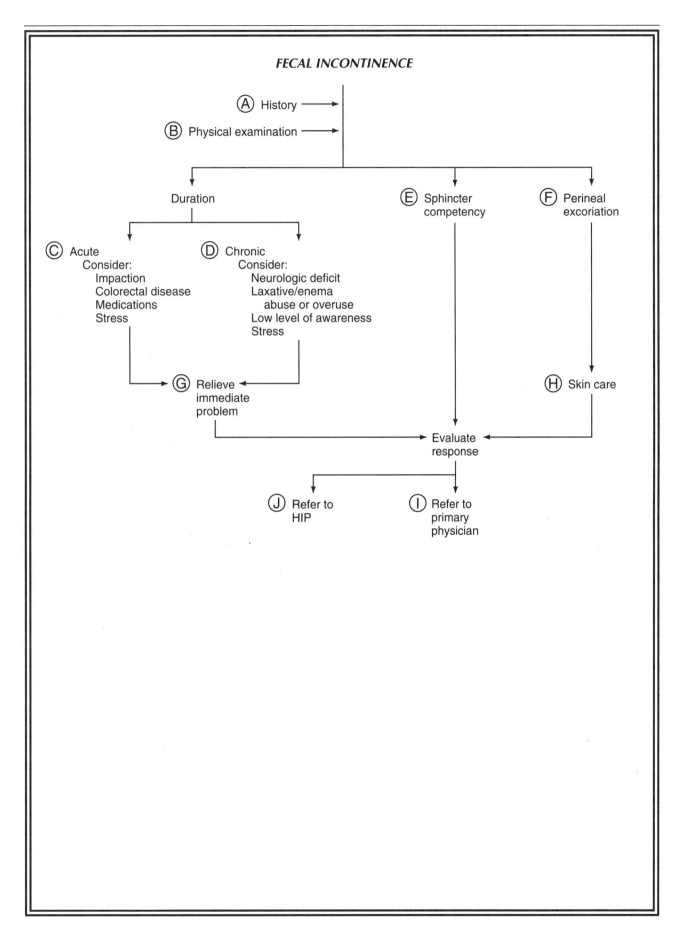

FECAL INCONTINENCE

(A) History →

(B) Physical examination →

Duration

(E) Sphincter competency

(F) Perineal excoriation

(C) Acute
Consider:
  Impaction
  Colorectal disease
  Medications
  Stress

(D) Chronic
Consider:
  Neurologic deficit
  Laxative/enema
    abuse or overuse
  Low level of awareness
  Stress

(G) Relieve
immediate
problem

(H) Skin care

Evaluate
response

(J) Refer to
HIP

(I) Refer to
primary
physician

HEMORRHOIDS/PILES

Diana N. West

Hemorrhoids or piles are a mass of dilated veins in swollen tissue near the anal sphincter. Although hemorrhoids can develop at any age, they usually cause more problems in older age groups.

External hemorrhoids may be asymptomatic. Non-thrombosed hemorrhoids do not cause pain. Internal hemorrhoids occasionally undergo massive prolapse and thrombosis, which results in excruciating pain or inability to sit or to defecate.

The low-fiber, highly refined diet typical of Western countries contributes to the development of hemorrhoids. Often this diet is combined with inadequate fluid intake, which contributes to constipation and hemorrhoid development.

Patients often worry unnecessarily about their bowels and work too hard at forcing sphincter muscles to do what they do naturally if given enough time. Factors contributing to hemorrhoids are
- avoiding the urge to defecate
- straining with bowel movements
- sitting on the toilet for long periods

Hemorrhoids can be caused or aggravated by
- heavy lifting
- obesity
- occupations requiring long periods of sitting or standing such as hair styling, dentistry, nursing, or computer operation

In addition women who have had one or more pregnancies also tend to develop hemorrhoids.

A. Ask questions about
- occupation and hobbies
- bowel habits
  - chronic constipation
  - straining at stool
  - amount of time spent sitting on toilet
  - use of laxatives or stool softeners
- nutrition
  - amount of fluids taken each day
  - fiber content of diet (consider 24-hour recall)

Try to determine how long the patient has had hemorrhoids and accompanying symptoms, such as
- passage of bright red blood with bowel movements
- spotting on toilet tissue
- a spurt of blood when constipated stool is expelled
- perianal itching (see Rectal Itching, p. 196)
- bulging in the rectal area
- mucous discharge
- protrusion of hemorrhoids from the rectum
- undergarments being soiled with mucus or blood

Teaching Plan for Patient with Hemorrhoids	
Subject	*Content*
Bowel program (see also Constipation, p. 184)	Avoid straining or sitting on toilet for long periods Defecate when the urge is felt Avoid constipation Plan toileting time
Nutrition/Hydration	Avoid irritating foods like mangos, fresh pineapple, and some nuts Avoid calcium-rich foods if they harden stools and lead to constipation Eat plenty of fresh fruit, vegetables, whole grain or bran cereals or breads Increase intake of liquids to 2000 ml daily (8 to 10 glasses), if not contraindicated Avoid liquids such as tea, coffee, alcohol, and grapefruit juice that cause diuresis
Hygiene	Clean perianal area morning, evening, and after each bowel movement Use warm water, NOT hot Wash thoroughly, using soft paper or cotton Dry carefully afterward

Symptom management	Control discomfort and pruritis with warm compresses
	Discourage hot sitz or tub baths because of increased risk of circulatory changes, hypotension, falls, and injuries
	During acutely painful episodes
	   decrease amount of time standing
	   elevate feet and legs when lying down or sitting

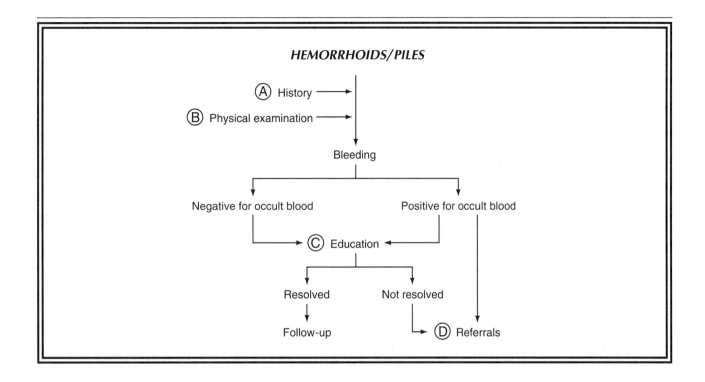

HEMORRHOIDS/PILES

Ⓐ History ⟶

Ⓑ Physical examination ⟶

Bleeding

Negative for occult blood → ← Positive for occult blood

Ⓒ Education

Resolved → Follow-up

Not resolved → Ⓓ Referrals

B. Examine the abdomen to exclude masses or evidence of abnormal distention. Encourage the patient to relax by breathing through the mouth prior to assessment of the anal area. Have the patient lie in the left lateral position for examination. Inspect perianal area and surrounding skin for
    • rashes
    • lesions
    • tumors
    • fissures
    • inflammation
    • bulging in the rectal area
    • swollen, dilated perianal veins
    • bleeding
    Gently part the buttocks to reveal hemorrhoids, which appear as a painless, moist, red mass protruding from the anus. The anal canal should be parted and examined for abnormalities, especially fissures, anteriorly and posteriorly.
        Perform a digital rectal examination with a well-lubricated, gloved finger. Palpate for
    • sphincter spasm
    • fissures
    • masses
    It is rarely possible to palpate internal hemorroids. Perform a stool for occult blood. Anemia may be present but is usually unrelated to the insignificant blood loss from hemorrhoids (see Rectal Bleeding, p. 194).

C. Patient teaching includes development of a bowel program, appropriate nutrition/hydration, hygiene,

and symptom management (see the box). Almost 50% of patients will respond to diet therapy alone.

D. Referral should be made for
    • positive occult blood
    • painful hemorrhoids
    • anemia
    Diagnosis of internal hemorrhoids requires proctoscopy or anoscopic exam using a flexible sigmoidoscope. Colonoscopy is recommended for a positive fecal occult blood, iron deficiency anemia, and in patients at high risk for development of colorectal cancer.
        If the patient continues to bleed and other studies are negative, rubber-band ligation or scleral therapy may be indicated. Scleral therapy causes fibrosis within the submucosa above the hemorrhoidal group, which prevents prolapse and stops the bleeding. Surgical hemorrhoidectomy may also be performed.

References

Abrams WB, Berkow R. The Merck manual of geriatrics. Rahway, NJ: Merck, 1990:490, 581.

Birkett DH. Hemorrhoids—diagnostic and treatment options. Hosp Prac 1988; 23(1):99.

Bohman HR. Trouble in the anorectal zone: 2. Hemorrhoids. Emerg Med 1986; 18(3):195.

Leibach JR, Cerfa JJ. Practical points on outpatient management of hemorrhoids. Hosp Med 1986; 22(6):75.

RECTAL BLEEDING

Pamela S. Ruby

Rectal bleeding is defined as the presence of blood in the stool or in the rectal area. Rectal bleeding is a symptom of an existing medical problem (hemorrhoids, rectal fissure/tear, carcinoma, or inflammatory bowel disease) that should be fully evaluated and treated as soon as possible.

A. Obtain a careful and detailed description of the symptoms, including onset and duration of bleeding, associated conditions (diarrhea, constipation), accompanying pain, and feeling of fullness/bloating. Take a drug and food history for the previous 5 days because of the possible effect on the results of the stool occult blood test and feces discoloration (see box below and Table 1). High-dose ascorbic acid can yield a false-negative stool occult blood test. Determine current use of medications, including over-the-counter drugs such as salicylates and nonsteroidal anti-inflammatory agents. Elicit a history of any activities causing rectal trauma (rectal intercourse, enema, laxative abuse).

B. Perform an anorectal examination to determine the presence of hemorrhoids or rectal tears/fissures. A

TABLE 1 Drugs that Discolor Feces

Drugs	Color Changes
Antacids (aluminum hydroxide)	Whitish or speckling
Antibiotics (oral)	Greenish-gray
Anticoagulants	Pink to red to black*
Bismuth-containing preparations	Black
Charcoal	Black
Ferrous salts	Black
Heparin	Pink to red to black*
Indomethacin (Indocin)	Green
Phenazopyridine (Pyridium)	Orange-red
Phenylbutazone (Butazolidin)	Pink to red to black*
Pyrvinium pamoate (Povan)	Red
Salicylates, especially aspirin	Pink to red to black*
Senna	Yellow

*These colors may indicate intestinal bleeding.

stool specimen for occult blood is indicated, and a CBC to determine the extent of bleeding.

C. Rectal bleeding represents a primary indicator of pathology and medical referral is imperative. Obtain medical evaluation for the definitive diagnosis and treatment of the underlying cause(s) of the rectal bleeding. The evaluation may include a digital rectal examination, anoscopy, flexible sigmoidoscopy, and barium enema.

D. Nursing interventions include preparation and support of patients for diagnostic procedures. Patients may need to be taught to obtain serial stool specimens for occult blood. Once diagnosis is made, the nurse must teach lifestyle changes needed to care for hemorrhoids, ostomies, or surgical sites.

E. The patient and family may be anxious before receiving test results because of the possibility of cancer. If cancer is diagnosed additional support may be appropriate, including referral to the American Cancer Society or a local I Can Cope Group.

Factors that Can Yield a False-Positive Stool Occult Blood Test		
Foods		Drugs
Horseradish	Lemon rind	Laxatives
Red meat	Grapefruit	Iron
Gelatin	Carrot	Cimetidine
Turnips	Cabbage	Nonsteroidal
Broccoli	Potato	anti-inflammatory
Cantaloupe	Pumpkin	agents
Cauliflower	Fig	Aspirin
Red radish	Peach	
Parsnips	Celery	
Bean sprouts	Lettuce	
Cucumber	Spinach	
Green beans	Pickles	
Mushrooms	Uncooked fruits	
Parsley	Uncooked	
Zucchini	vegetables	

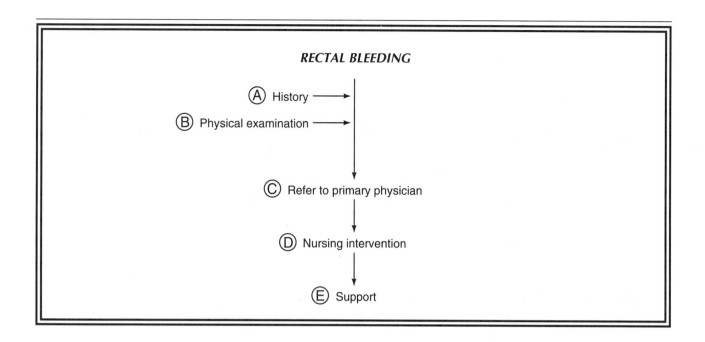

RECTAL BLEEDING

Ⓐ History ⟶

Ⓑ Physical examination ⟶

Ⓒ Refer to primary physician

Ⓓ Nursing intervention

Ⓔ Support

References

Alpers DH, et al. Manual of nutritional therapeutics. 2nd ed. Boston: Little, Brown, 1988.

Handbook of Nonprescription Drugs. 9th ed. American Pharmaceutical Association, National Professional Society of Pharmacists, Washington DC 1990.

Knoben JE, Anderson PO. Handbook of clinical drug data. 6th ed. Hamilton, IL: Drug Intelligence Publications, 1989.

Knodel LC, et al. University of Texas drug information services. Micromedics 1989; Vol 65.

RECTAL ITCHING (PRURITUS ANI)

Diana N. West

Rectal itching commonly results when the skin becomes drier and less elastic. It may be associated with burning or pain. Rectal itching is approximately four times more common in men than women. Over 50% of the patients complaining of pruritus have idiopathic disease and are best treated symptomatically. Rectal itching may be caused by
- metabolic and systemic disorders
- anorectal and genital disease
- foods and beverages (see the box "Foods and Beverages Commonly Associated with Pruritus Ani").

A. Determine specific symptoms that the patient has
  - pruritus with subsequent rubbing and scratching
  - pruritus especially bothersome at night
  - symptoms that start insidiously
  Are there contributing factors?
  - exposure to heat and sweating
  - urinary or fecal incontinence
  - infections such as moniliasis
  - antibiotic therapy causing bacterial or fungal overgrowth
  - medical history
    - metabolic or systemic disorders
      - diabetes
      - gout
      - uremia
      - jaundice
      - Hodgkin's disease
      - polycythemia
    - anorectal/genital diseases
      - hemorrhoids (see Hemorrhoids/Piles, p. 192)
      - anal fissure
      - rectal or vaginal prolapse
      - vaginitis
      - proctitis
    - hygienic factors
      - overvigorous cleaning of anal area causing trauma
      - inadequate cleaning
      - diarrhea
    - dietary habits (see the box "Foods and Beverages Commonly Associated with Pruritus Ani")

B. Examine rectal area looking for
  - hemorrhoids

Foods and Beverages Commonly Associated with Pruritus Ani

• coffee	• nuts
• chocolate	• tea
• citrus fruits	• cola
• tomatoes	• alcoholic drinks

Classification of Rectal Skin Changes

Class	Description
First degree	Normal or reddened skin with minimal excoriation
Second degree	Ridged and slightly edematous skin or thinning of skin with friability, blistering, and ulceration
Third degree	Either white, thickened, and ridged skin or raw and oozing skin

- fissures
- obvious scratch marks

Skin changes can be classified using the descriptions in the box "Classification of Rectal Skin Changes." Obtain blood chemistry to determine if systemic or metabolic disorders are contributing to the problem.

Patient Instruction Guide

Topic	Content
Dietary habits	Eliminate foods known to cause irritation for about 7 weeks (see the box "Foods and Beverages Commonly Associated with Pruritus Ani")
	After 7 weeks reintroduce one food at a time to determine which foods cause itching
	Completely eliminate foods that cause itching once they are identified
	Drink at least 8 cups of water per day, unless contraindicated
Hygiene	Clean the area each morning and evening and after each bowel movement using a soft cloth and warm water
	Keep the area dry
	Avoid abrasive towels
Reduction of local irritation	Do NOT use ointments, soaps, or medications unless they are prescribed
	Avoid the use of harsh soaps and laundry detergents to wash undergarments
	Do NOT use perfumed powders or talcs on the perianal area
	Avoid scratching or rubbing
	Wear loose-fitting cotton underwear rather than synthetics

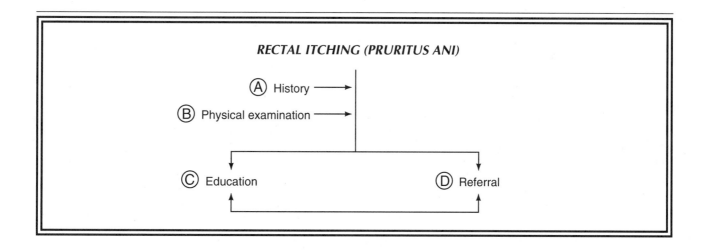

RECTAL ITCHING (PRURITUS ANI)

- Ⓐ History
- Ⓑ Physical examination
- Ⓒ Education
- Ⓓ Referral

C. Patient teaching focuses on dietary habits, hygiene, and reduction of local irritation (see the box "Patient Instruction Guide"). Patients must be warned that it may take considerable time to obtain relief from burning and itching.

D. Referral should be made to a primary physician for
- second- and third-degree skin changes
- prescription of oral antipruritics if necessary
- control of metabolic or systemic disorders
- treatment of anorectal or genital diseases
A dietitian may be helpful for dietary counseling.

References

Kunz, J, Finkel, AJ. The American Medical Association family medical guide. New York: Random House, 1987.

Rossman I. Clinical Geriatrics. 2nd ed. Philadelphia: JB Lippincott, 1979.

Ulanow RM. Trouble in the anorectal zone: 1. Pruritus ani. Emerg Med 1986; 18(2):134.

RECTAL PAIN

Leslie C. Trischank Hussey

Rectal pain is a symptom that can represent many underlying diseases or conditions. The cause of the pain must be identified and treated promptly. Rectal pain may be accompanied by other bowel habit changes that may be due to colorectal cancer or other factors such as diet, fluid intake, lack of exercise, medication, or benign disease.

A. Obtain a thorough description of the pain, including onset, duration, exacerbating factors, and accompanying signs and symptoms. The history should also include
   • usual bowel habits
   • existence of hemorrhoids
   • recent changes in character of stool
   • laxative use
   • type and amount of fluid intake
   • amount of bulk and fat intake in the diet
   • amount of daily activity
   • current medications
   • past or present GI disease
   • personal or family history of colorectal cancer

B. Physical assessment should include a rectal examination to determine the presence of hemorrhoids, rectal prolapse, rectal fissure, masses that may indicate abscesses, fecal impaction, and stool consistency and color. Stool should be tested for occult blood (see Rectal Bleeding, p. 194). An abdominal examination should note bowel sounds, masses, or tenderness. Rectal pain may be caused by bowel habit changes such as constipation resulting from poor diet, inadequate fluid intake, lack of exercise, or medications. Rectal pain accompanied by bleeding and itching may indicate hemorrhoids (see Hemorrhoids/Piles, p. 192). If rectal pain is accompanied by incontinence, a red mass protruding from the anus, and a feeling of incomplete evacuation and bleeding, a rectal prolapse is present. Bleeding, pain, and a change in bowel habits may also indicate colorectal cancer or an anal fissure. Inflammation and pain may indicate anal fistulas or abscesses.

C. Symptomatic treatment of rectal pain includes
   • warm sitz baths three to four times a day
   • over-the-counter preparations, which may help decrease pain
   • witch hazel soak (Tucks)
   • dibucaine ointment

Bulk-producing agents such as psyllium hydrophilic mucilloid (Metamucil) are recommended for hemorrhoids and anal fissures. The application of cold packs to hemorrhoids or an anorectal abscess for 3–4 hours at the onset of pain, followed by warm sitz baths, may be beneficial. A high-fiber diet and fluids are recommended to promote regular bowel movements without straining. (For more complete discussion, see Hemorrhoids/Piles, p. 192).

D. Lifestyle changes include
   • adherence to a high-fiber, high-fluid diet to promote regular bowel patterns
   • avoiding straining at stool
   • instituting a regular exercise program such as walking daily
   • avoidance of enema or laxative dependency
   Remind patients that adding high-fiber foods to the diet may initially increase flatulence or a feeling of fullness. Stress the importance of adequate fluids. Drug absorption from the gut may also be affected, so medication schedules may need to be changed.

E. A physician referral may be necessary for further diagnosis and treatment, including prescription analgesia and possible surgery. Rectal bleeding may signal cancer and should be referred to a physician immediately (see Rectal Bleeding, p. 194). If itching or inflammation is present, the physician may prescribe a steroid preparation.

References

Gillies D. Nursing care for aged patients with rectal prolapse. J Gerontol Nurs 1985; 11:29.

Hoexter B, Labow S, Moseson M. Common diseases of the anus and rectum. Hosp Med 1985; 21:119.

Ignatavicius D, Bayne MV. Medical-surgical nursing—a nursing process approach. Philadelphia: WB Saunders, 1991:1403.

Phipps S, Long B, Woods N. Medical-surgical nursing: Concepts and clinical practice. St. Louis: CV Mosby, 1987:1539.

Weinrich S, Blesch K, Dickson G, et al. Timely detection of colorectal cancer in the elderly: Implications of the aging process. Cancer Nurs 1989; 12:170.

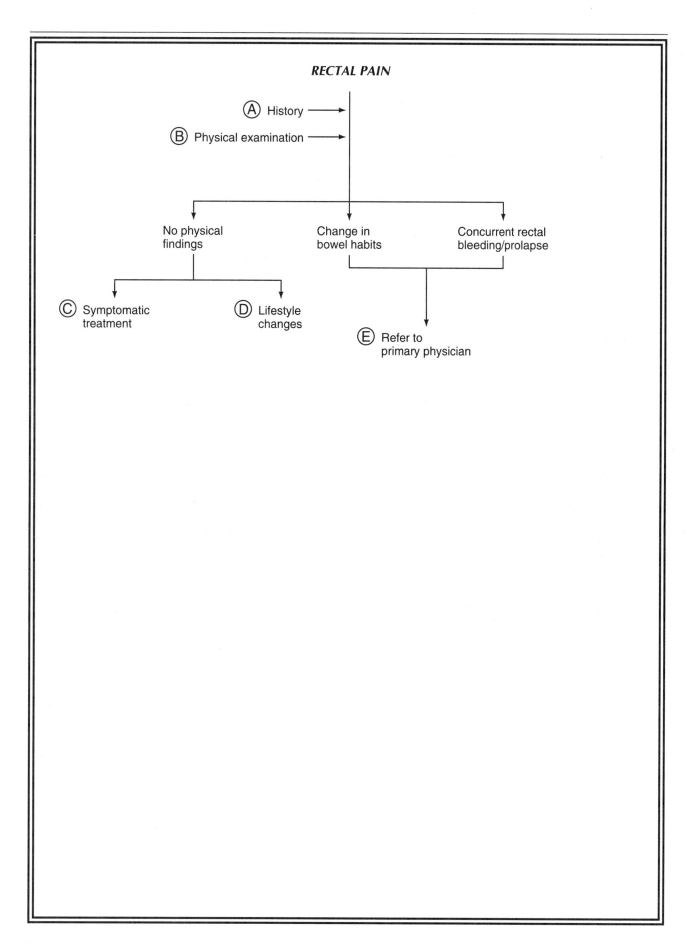

RECTAL PAIN

(A) History

(B) Physical examination

No physical findings

Change in bowel habits

Concurrent rectal bleeding/prolapse

(C) Symptomatic treatment

(D) Lifestyle changes

(E) Refer to primary physician

HEMATURIA

Estelle Kincaid

Microscopic or gross blood in the urine is a warning sign that cannot be ignored. Bleeding without pain is always considered related to urinary tract neoplasm until proved otherwise. Hematuria is alarming to the patient and always deserves a complete work-up as well as reassurance.

A. When obtaining a history, ask about
   • frequency
   • discharge
   • dysuria
   • flank or abdominal pain
   • when bleeding occurs: at the start of voiding, at the end, or throughout

   The site of bleeding in the urinary tract may be determined by the time bleeding occurs. If bleeding is at the start of the stream and clears, the site is often the anterior urethra, prostate, or seminal vesicles, and prostatitis and/or obstruction is suspected. If bleeding occurs at the end of the stream, this is usually at the posterior urethra, bladder neck, or trigone. If bleeding persists throughout the stream, this indicates the bladder, ureters, or kidneys, as in calculi or sickle cell anemia or trait. Rule out a family history of stones, renal disease, or sickle cell anemia. Determine the drug history, because anticoagulants can cause bleeding, and some drugs may cause chemical cystitis, papillary necrosis, or an allergic hematuria.

B. Physical assessment includes examination of
   • urine for microscopic hematuria by
     • clean-catch sample or
     • (in women with vaginal bleeding) a catheterized specimen
   • urine culture
   • the urethral meatus for a foreign body, condyloma, caruncle, or papilloma
   • abdomen, back, scrotum, and prostate for tenderness or masses
   • serum for sickle cell trait and hemoglobin electrophoresis in patients of African or Mediterranean descent
   • serum for renal function testing
   • urination for the point in the stream in which bleeding occurs

   Obtain urine culture and sensitivity and 24-hour urine for protein and creatinine. Serum chemistries should include BUN and creatinine, used to calculate creatinine clearance.

C. Dysuria (painful urination) may indicate infection such as cystitis, urethritis, prostatitis or infection associated with the passage of a stone. Renal colic (cramping pain) is most often associated with renal calculi or obstruction, including obstruction caused by a renal mass. Renal trauma may be associated with painful hematuria.

D. When no pain is involved, always consider urinary tract neoplasm. Genitourinary bleeding may be the first manifestation of papillary necrosis, a renal inflammation that causes sloughing of the papilla. Also, rule out sickle cell trait and blood dyscrasias as a cause of painless hematuria.

E. To decrease pain and recurrence of some stones, teach the patient to
   • decrease excessive use of caffeine (coffee, tea, carbonated beverages, chocolate)
   • increase water intake to flush the kidneys, especially when infection may be the cause of hematuria
   • rest with feet elevated to reduce strain

   Reassure the patient. Advise that if fever, chills or hematuria persist, a urologic consultation for definitive urodynamic testing is warranted. If the type of stone or the urine has been analyzed, specific dietary or pharmaceutical intervention may help. A more acid urine may decrease precipitation of particles, called nidus, which become the center of the stone.

F. Hematuria requires a complete work-up even if no pain is associated with the bleeding. The primary physician or urologist can use the laboratory results from renal function studies, urine cultures, and blood tests to determine which diagnostic procedures are indicated. Patients with a creatinine clearance <1.5 may have IV pyelography (IVP) (see the tool *Urodynamic Studies*, p. 219), CT scan, or ultrasonography. Retrograde pyelography (RGPG) may be used to rule out neoplasm, and may be indicated when there is an elevated creatinine clearance. A urologist may be consulted if cystoscopy is indicated.

G. Assistance with diagnostic studies may include
   • administering bowel cleansing agents
   • explaining procedures
   • participating in the informed consent process
   • offering necessary reassurance

   When contrast media is used, a patent IV is recommended. Monitor for allergic reactions (nausea, vomiting, itching, hives, changes in respiratory status, cardiac changes). Administer diphenhydramine (Benadryl) or epinephrine if prescribed.

References

Brunner L, Suddarth D. Medical-surgical nursing. 4th ed. Philadelphia: JB Lippincott, 1980.

Hanno P, Wein A. A clinical manual of urology. Norwalk, CT: Appleton-Century-Crofts, 1987.

Smith DR. General urology. 10th ed. San Mateo, CA: Lange Medical Publications, 1981.

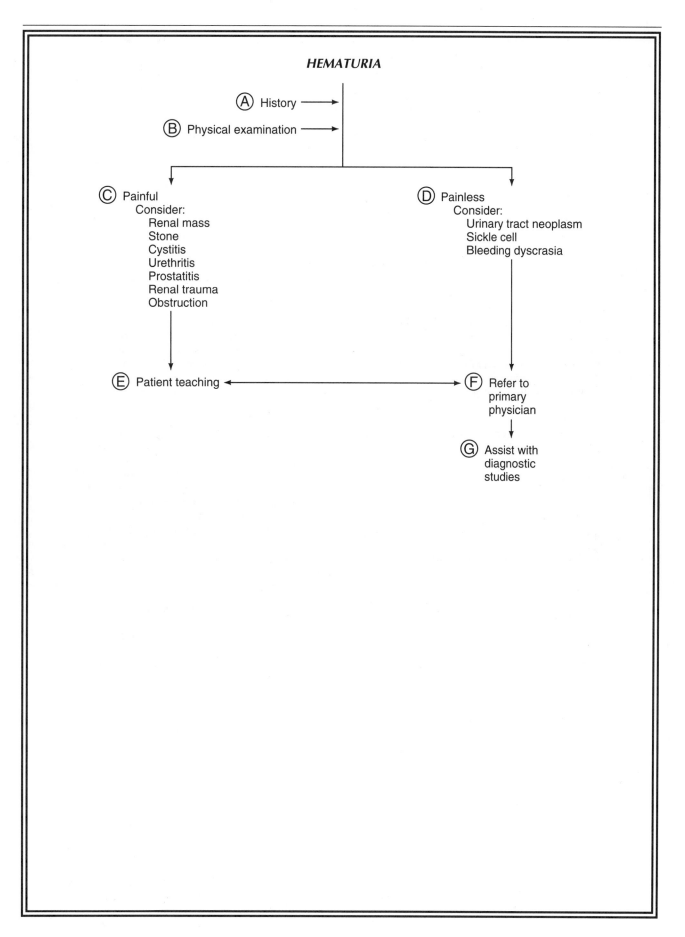

HEMATURIA

Ⓐ History ⟶

Ⓑ Physical examination ⟶

Ⓒ Painful
  Consider:
    Renal mass
    Stone
    Cystitis
    Urethritis
    Prostatitis
    Renal trauma
    Obstruction

Ⓓ Painless
  Consider:
    Urinary tract neoplasm
    Sickle cell
    Bleeding dyscrasia

Ⓔ Patient teaching ⟵

Ⓕ Refer to
   primary
   physician

Ⓖ Assist with
   diagnostic
   studies

IRRITATIVE VOIDING SYMPTOMS (DYSURIA, FREQUENCY, URGENCY, PAIN)

Estelle Kincaid

Irritative voiding symptoms are associated with inflammation of the lower genitourinary tract, radiation or chemotherapy, neoplasms, and neurogenic bladder dysfunction. See Table 1 for definitions of irritative voiding symptoms.

A. The history should determine
   • onset and duration of urinary symptoms
   • sensation
   • urine appearance: presence of blood or pus
   • nausea or vomiting
   • weight change
   • chronic disease such as hypertension, heart failure, diabetes, or neurologic disorders
   • change in urinary stream or initiation of stream
   • fever, chills
   • sexual activity
   • sexually transmitted diseases
   • urethral or penile discharge
   • malaise
   • pain
      • onset
      • location
      • duration
      • description
      • exacerbating and alleviating factors
      • presence with full or empty bladder
      • relation to activity or rest
      • positional changes

B. Physical examination may show
   • fever
   • weight loss
   • prostate enlargement
   • vaginitis (see Vaginal Dryness or Itching, p. 246)
   Examine the external genitalia for erythema, masses, lesions, cystocele, and urethral discharge. Palpate the abdomen to evaluate bladder distention and pelvic tenderness. Collect a clean-catch midstream or catheterized specimen to avoid a false-positive urinalysis because of the bacteria and pus cells present in the urethra. A postvoid catheterized specimen not only provides an uncontaminated specimen for urinalysis, but allows evaluation of the urethra for stenosis and the bladder for a postvoid residual. Urinalysis and microscopic and urine cultures can be performed. Use of a urine reagent test strip can screen for nitrite, leukocytes, specific gravity, pH, blood, protein, glucose, ketones, and urobilinogen (Table 2). For attempts to localize a lower urinary tract infection (UTI) in males, segmented cultures are helpful (Table 3).

C. Patient education should include
   • adequate fluid intake of six to eight 8-ounce glasses of water daily (studies have shown that bacteria introduced into a beaker can be removed by flushing with water; therefore, water intake will similarly help alleviate bladder bacteria).
   • reduce citrus juices and carbonated beverages with dysuria to decrease burning symptoms
   • proper hygiene for

Males	Females
• clean the glans penis	• shower instead of tub soaks
• if the foreskin is intact, retract and clean the glans penis	• clean the perineum from front to back so as not to introduce bacteria from the anus or vagina into the urethra
	• wear white cotton underwear
	• void immediately after intercourse

   • seek medical attention for fever ≥100.8°F.
   • void by the clock to decrease the potential for incontinence or urinary retention
   • use panty liners for sense of security if suffering from urgency
   • use the Kegel maneuver (see p. 216) to promote bladder emptying

D. Patients with recurrent irritative symptoms and/or a UTI warrant a complete medical work-up (see pp. 217 and 219) to determine the appropriate course of action. Prescribed medications may be antibiotics, antimicrobial agents, or stone-reducing drugs. Most renal stones consist of calcium salts, struvite (magnesium ammonium phosphate), cystine, or uric acid, causing nephrolithiasis.

E. The nurse may be involved in initiating interventions based on physician orders. These include ensuring that medication regimens are followed, obtaining needed specimens, and providing catheterization or catheter care when necessary. Assess for adaptative equipment needed in the environment to promote continence (see Urinary Incontinence, p. 206). In patients with diabetes, cerebrovascular accident (CVA), or neurologic deficits, the bladder does not empty to completion. Clean, intermittent catheterization (see the tool Self-Catheterization Instructions, p. 218) may help unless the urethra is irritated. Use of an indwelling catheter for up to 1 month will allow healing and decrease bladder size. Insertion of an

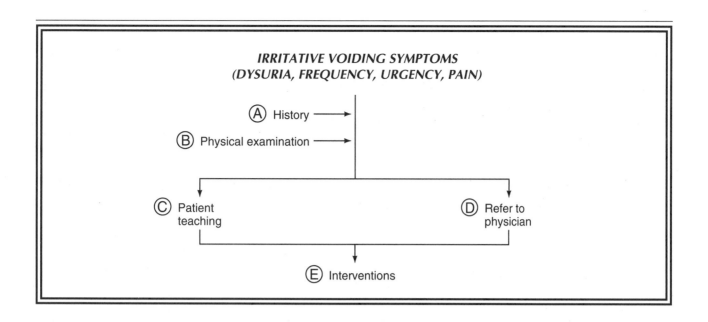

IRRITATIVE VOIDING SYMPTOMS
(DYSURIA, FREQUENCY, URGENCY, PAIN)

- (A) History
- (B) Physical examination
- (C) Patient teaching
- (D) Refer to physician
- (E) Interventions

TABLE 1 Irritative Voiding Symptoms

Term	Definitions	Causes
Dysuria	Burning sensation during or on completion of urination	Inflammation of urethra, bladder, or prostate
Frequency	Increased need to urinate Feeling of need to urinate	Decreased bladder capacity due to: decreased elasticity inflammatory edema ineffective bladder emptying
Urgency	Sudden severe need to urinate	Bladder irritability Inflammation Prostatic hypertrophy
Pain	Discomfort originating in urinary structures or adjacent organs	Distention Inflammation
Nocturia	Urination in the night	Decrease in effective bladder capacity Diuretic effect of caffeine and alcohol Excessive fluid consumption Osmotic diuresis

TABLE 2 Urinalysis Findings

Finding	Indicates	Rule Out
White cells/pyuria	Urinary tract disorder	Vaginitis with Gram's stain and *Chlamydia* culture
Positive culture	Cystitis	Genitourinary tuberculosis
pH (normal 4.5–7.5)		
Alkaline (above 6.0)	Risk for struvite stones Potassium depletion Hyperventilation, respiratory alkalosis Certain bacterial infections, e.g., *Proteus*	Calculi Excess bicarbonate intake Urinary tract infection
Acid (below 6.0)	Risk for uric acid stones Metabolic acidosis Respiratory acidosis	Excess vitamin C intake Gout Metabolic disorders Pyrexia Methyl alcohol poisoning

Text continued on page 204.

TABLE 3 Segmented Urine Culture in Males

Designated Label	Anatomic Source	Instructions	Findings
VB_1	Urethra	Collect initial 5–10 ml voiding	$VB_1 > VB_3$ = urethritis
VB_2	Bladder	Collect midstream specimen	Positive VB_2 = cystitis
VB_3	Prostate	Have patient void 200 ml, perform prostatic massage, then collect specimen	$VB_3 > VB_1$ = prostatitis

indwelling catheter can reduce prostate swelling, decrease urethral irritation, and promote bladder emptying. Obstruction of the urethra by stenosis, stricture, or an enlarged prostate may make it difficult to insert a catheter. The following procedure may help:

• mix 10 ml 1% lidocaine injectable with 30 ml lubricating jelly
• instill 10 ml of lidocaine/lubricating jelly into the urethra
• attempt to pass the catheter

If the catheter still cannot be inserted, refer the patient to the physician or a urologist to ensure bladder emptying. Parkinsonism, CVA, arthritis, and many other conditions affect ambulation, which governs the choice of the bathroom versus bedside commode or catheterization. Evaluate the patient's lifestyle in choosing equipment. Patients with nocturia and/or decreased mobility may benefit from a bedside commode or urinal. If the patient drives, is socially active, and has out-of-home activities, intermittent catheterization may be preferred to an indwelling catheter and bag. If an indwelling catheter is necessary, the patient may be able to wear a leg bag while active and change to a bedside bag at night or when napping to prevent urine backflow into the bladder (see the tool *Guidelines for Foley Catheter Care in the Home*, p. 215).

References

Hanno P, Wein A. A clinical manual of urology. Norwalk, CT: Appleton-Century-Crofts, 1987.

Stamm WE. Protocol for diagnosis of urinary tract infection: Reconsidering the criterion for significant bacteria. Urology (Suppl) August 1988.

URINARY INCONTINENCE

Estelle Kincaid
Paula A. Loftis

Urinary incontinence (UI) is the involuntary loss of urine resulting in social and/or hygienic consequences. The impact of UI on relationships and social activities can be devastating and lead to isolation and institutionalization. UI is a symptom, not a disease. It may be transient and reversible due to infection, delirium, atrophic vaginitis, stool impaction, or medications. UI is not a normal consequence of aging, but concomitant illnesses and age-related changes may predispose an older adult to urinary incontinence. Proper evaluation, diagnosis, and treatment is imperative and can ameliorate or at least improve the condition. Types of UI are identified in Table 1.

A. Ask open-ended questions such as
   • Do you have problems with your bladder?
   • Do you have difficulty getting to the bathroom on time?
   Elicit history of
   • urinary tract infections
   • multiparity
   • activities of daily living (ADL) or social activity impairment
   • constipation or fecal incontinence
   • alterations in sexual function
   • characteristics and symptoms such as
     • dribbling
     • urgency
     • straining
     • hesitancy
     • nocturia
     • stress
     • pain
     • frequency
     • interrupted urinary stream
     • hematuria
     • dysuria
     • sensation of incomplete bladder emptying
   • fluids: type, amount, and before bedtime use (e.g., use of caffeine or alcohol before bedtime)
   • medications: over-the-counter and prescribed, especially diuretics, sedative hypnotics, anticholinergic agents, calcium channel blockers, alpha-adrenergic agents. Are any new?
   • genitourinary tract or gynecologic surgery
   • cardiovascular, neurologic, or endocrine disease, osteoarthritis, or depression
   • previous UI treatment and its outcome

General inquiries determine
• onset and duration
• amount of urine loss
• frequency and timing of incontinent episodes using a voiding diary (see the tool *Bladder Record*, p. 214)
Identify environmental and social concerns including
• access to toilets or toilet substitutes
• toilet features such as elevation, arms, and supports
• living arrangements, caregiver availability, and socialization

B. Physical examination includes
   • functional level—can the patient toilet independently?
   • mental status—does the patient have adequate cognitive ability to self-toilet?
   • neurologic evaluation
     • lower extremity weakness?
     • posture?
     • tremor or rigidity?
     • mobility and dexterity?
   • abdominal assessment
     • masses, impaction?
     • obesity?
     • bladder or bowel distention?
     • suprapubic tenderness/fullness?
   • rectal/pelvic examination
     • adequate sphincter tone?
     • perineal skin condition?
     • masses, prostate size? (prostate size estimation on rectal examination may be misleading as a contributor to urinary obstruction)
     • impaction?
     • presence of cystocele, rectocele?
   Labs recommended on all UI patients include
   • clean catch urinalysis (enzymatic urine testing/dipstick)
   • creatinine/blood urea nitrogen
   • postvoid residual (PVR) volume estimation (Table 2)
   Useful additional tests include
   • blood glucose
   • urine culture, if bacteria or white blood cells present or nitrite positive
   • urinary cytology
   • bladder filling and provocative stress testing (see Table 2)
   • observation of voiding (see Table 2)

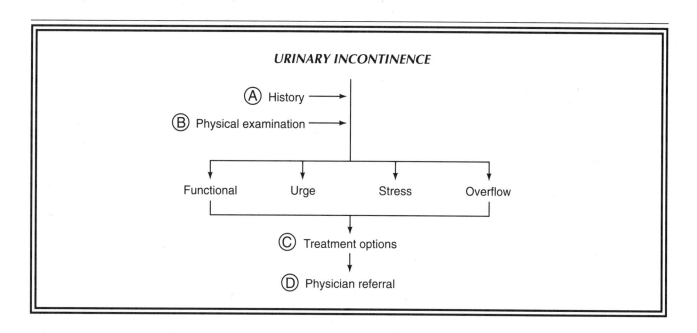

URINARY INCONTINENCE

Ⓐ History ⟶

Ⓑ Physical examination ⟶

Functional   Urge   Stress   Overflow

Ⓒ Treatment options

Ⓓ Physician referral

TABLE 1   Types of Urinary Incontinence

Type	Definition	Physiology	Characteristics/Findings
Stress	Urine loss occurring during activities that increase abdominal pressure—i.e., sneezing, laughing, coughing, lifting or bending	Dysfunction of bladder outlet (structure weakness around bladder and urethra) Anatomic damage of urethral sphincter (sphincter insufficiency)	Most common in women >75 yr Modest volume leakage Residual volume is low Occurs in men only if there is sphincter injury (following prostate surgery, radiation)
Urge	Loss of urine associated with an abrupt and strong desire to void, "unable to get to bathroom in time"	Uninhibited bladder contractions Urethral instability Detrusor hyperactivity with impaired bladder contractility	Neurologic findings may be normal or abnormal Usually CNS impairment Urinary tract infection Bladder tumor Moderate volume of urine loss Leakage occurs at intervals of several hours Residual volume is low Most common in persons >75 yr
Overflow	Bladder becomes overdistended, unable to empty normally with resultant frequency and nearly constant urine loss	Obstruction of outflow (tumors, benign strictures, prostate hypertrophy and pharmaceuticals) Impaired detrusor contractile capacity	Neurologic abnormalities (i.e., spinal cord injury) Severe pelvic prolapse Complication of anti-incontinence surgery Bladder fullness sensation absent Usually small amount of urine leakage Residual volume >100 ml
Functional	Urine loss results from factors other than the lower urinary tract	Intact lower urinary tract function	Cognitive impairment Immobility Environmental barriers Psychological unwillingness
Mixed	Combination of other types of UI		

Text continued on page 208.

TABLE 2   Assessment Procedures of Lower Urinary Tract Function

Procedure	Purpose	Steps	Interpretation of Findings
Postvoid residual (PVR) determination	Determine if bladder is emptying completely	Have patient void, record amount Within a few minutes catheterize patient with a straight catheter or assess by pelvic ultrasound Record catheterized urine amount	Residual volume <50 ml = adequate bladder emptying Residual volume >200 ml = inadequate emptying 50–199 ml is interpreted based on other clinical data
Bladder filling and simple cystometry	Fill bladder prior to stress testing Determine bladder capacity Assess for uninhibited detrusor contractions	Place female patient on fracture bedpan, for males have urinal or collection device available Insert straight catheter Hold 50 ml catheter tip syringe approx 15 cm above pubic symphysis Fill bladder with sterile water in 50 ml increments via catheter and syringe until patient has strong urge to void (attempt to instill at least 200–250 cc) Observe for fluctuation/rise in water level in syringe during filling Remove catheter	Normal bladder capacity is approximately 300 ml Soft abdomen (indicating no Valsalva) with rise in water level in syringe during filling = bladder contraction
Provocative stress testing (direct visualization)	Determine presence of stress incontinence	Patient with full bladder (see bladder filling procedure) Have patient relax in lithotomy position Place pad under the urethral area Instruct patient to cough vigorously Observe for urethral urine loss Have patient stand and cough again with pad in place Observe for urine loss	Instantaneous leakage = stress UI Delayed or persistent leakage after cough = detrusor overactivity
Voiding observation	Detect hesistancy, straining, slow or interrupted stream by clinical observation	Encourage patient to relax Observe voiding Ask patient to interrupt urine flow, begin stream	Determine ability of patient to interrupt urine flow and therefore ability to implement pelvic muscle exercises Voiding difficulty may suggest obstruction or bladder contractility problem

C. The four major classifications of treatment include (Table 3):
   • behavioral
   • surgical
   • pharmacologic
   • supportive
Treatment is dictated by the type of UI, risks, benefits, and patient choice. The least invasive and life-threatening treatment, such as behavioral interventions (Table 4), is the initial choice. Preserve skin integrity by
   • keeping the skin clean and dry
   • washing and changing undergarments or pads daily or when wet
   • monitoring skin for redness

TABLE 3 Common Therapeutic Options by Urinary Incontinence Type

UI Type	Behavioral	Pharmacologic	Surgical	Supportive
Urge	Bladder training Habit training (timed voids)	Bladder relaxant drug (anticholinergic agent)		
Overflow			Obstruction removal	Intermittent or chronic catheterization (see pp. 215 and 218)
Stress	Pelvic muscle (Kegel) exercises, with or without biofeedback (see the tool *Modified Kegel* *Exercises,* p. 216) Voiding schedule Vaginal cone retention Bladder training	Alpha-adrenergic agent Estrogen therapy (topical or oral)	Bladder neck suspension	Penile clamp Artificial sphincter Pessary
Functional	Scheduled toileting Prompted voiding	Modify medication regimen based on patient activities		Reduce environmental barriers (signs, privacy) Adjust fluid intake schedule, restrict fluids after 6 PM Caregiver education Undergarments/pads Toilet access and substitutes Chronic indwelling catheter External catheters

D. Indicators for urology referral are identified in the box. Referral is necessary to obtain urodynamic evaluation (see pp. 217 and 219 for roentgenographic procedures and urodynamic studies). Testing can determine what occurs in the bladder and bladder outlet during filling, storage, and emptying phases of voiding. Pharmacist and/or medical consultation is indicated if prescribed drugs are thought to be a contributing factor to UI. Poorly controlled diabetes warrants a medical referral.

Text continued on page 210.

TABLE 4   Behavioral Techniques

Technique	Purpose	Steps
Bladder training	Empty the bladder completely Increase sphincter contractility Decrease the number of urinary tract infections Improve bladder tone Enhance self-image/feeling of control	Instruct patient to delay voiding and resist urge Schedule voiding times Initiate voiding at every 30 minutes Increase time between voidings to 2–3 hours Do not enforce voiding schedule during sleep
Habit training (timed voiding)	Keep patient dry by voiding at variable intervals based on individual patient pattern and positive reinforcement	Encourage staff/caregiver participation Determine toileting schedule (voiding diary may help, see p. 214) Intervals between toileting should coincide with patient's natural urinating pattern
Prompted voiding	Supplement habit training in a dependent or cognitively impaired patient	Caregiver checks if patient is wet or dry on a routine basis (every 1–2 hours) Ask or prompt the patient to use toilet Praise patient for maintaining continence and using toilet
Scheduled toileting	Prevent wetting	Staff and/or caregiver availability and motivation Adhere to a fixed toileting schedule

---

Indicators for Urological Referral

- difficulty passing catheter
- sterile hematuria
- recent genitourinary operation
- recurrent symptomatic urinary infections
- physical abnormality (prostate mass, significant pelvic prolapse)
- retention, postvoid residual >100 ml.
- no improvement in social or hygiene circumstances with present interventions or therapy
- signs and symptoms of obstruction
- diagnostic uncertainty

References

Jeter K, Faller N, Norton C. Nursing for continence. Philadelphia: WB Saunders, 1990.

Ouslander J. Geriatric urinary incontinence. Diseases-A-Month #2, Vol. XXXVII, St. Louis: Mosby-Year Book, 1992.

Urinary incontinence. Clin Geriatr Med 1986; 2:639–885.

Urinary Incontinence Guideline Panel. Urinary incontinence in adults: Clinical practice guideline. AHCPR Pub. No. 92-0038. Rockville, MD: Agency for Health Care Policy and Research, Public Health Service, U.S. Department of Health and Human Services. March 1992.

URINARY RETENTION

Estelle Kincaid

Urinary retention can be defined as failure to expel urine from the bladder and can be classified as chronic or acute. Obstruction of urinary outflow can be caused by urethral strictures, bladder neck contracture, urethral diverticulum, cystourethrocele, or prostatic hypertrophy. Table 1 details pathologic processes leading to urinary retention.

A. Elicit the presence of
   * straining to start the urinary stream
   * bifurcation of stream in males
   * slow or weak stream
   * constant dribbling
   * suprapubic pain
   * change in color or odor of urine
   Ask questions to determine onset, duration, and precipitating or palliative factors. Obtain a complete medical history to include
   * sexually transmitted diseases
   * drug and alcohol use
   * urinary tract infections
   * genitourinary surgeries
   * childbirth history
   Review current and previous medications. Drug side effects from anticholinergics, such as over-the-counter cold preparations, include urinary retention.

B. Assess abdominal distention by palpation of the abdomen and bladder. A digital examination of the prostate can determine whether hypertrophy or nodules are present that may indicate cancer of the prostate. Electrolytes, BUN, and creatinine can reveal if retention has caused renal insufficiency or damage, although creatinine depends on glomerular filtration and may be misleading in the elderly. Acid phosphatase and prostatic specific antigen may be elevated in men with prostatic hypertrophy or cancer. Take care to draw these tests before prostatic examination or urethral catheterization, because such instrumentation may cause levels to rise.

C. Perform an aerogram to assess the need for chronic catheterization. The bladder is filled with sterile water via the catheter until the patient feels the urge to urinate, but use no more than 250 ml water; then instill 50 ml air into the bladder. Remove the catheter and tell the patient to urinate. If the air is not passed, reinsert the catheter into the bladder. If the air is passed with the water, the patient does not need a catheter. If residual urine volume is greater than 100 ml, intermittent catheterization is indicated.

D. Patients with urinary retention may decrease the amount of fluids they drink because of the discomfort they feel when their bladder is distended. This may be appropriate if they must go long periods between catheterizations or after 6 PM. Adequate hydration must be maintained, however, particularly when roentgenographic studies using contrast media are scheduled to reduce the risk of renal damage. Patients who have residuals ≥100 ml after a urogram are candidates for in-and-out catheterization. Done as a chronic procedure at home, this is not a sterile procedure. Female patients can be taught to catheterize themselves by touch rather than by sight, although some women can use a mirror to view the procedure (see the tool *Self-Catheterization Instructions*, p. 218). Generally a red rubber catheter is used, which can be boiled between catheterizations and reused many

TABLE 1 Urinary Retention Profile

Obstructive Process	Causative Factors	Pathophysiology	Occurrence and Prevalence
Bladder neck contracture	Transurethral resection of prostate Trauma	Concentrically narrowed bladder neck	Males
Urethral diverticulum	Infection Trauma secondary to vaginal delivery Vaginal surgery Urinary stasis	Pouches form in musculature of urethra holding urine	Diabetes Females
Cystourethrocele	Multiple vaginal deliveries Posthysterectomy	Relaxation of pelvic muscles	Females
Acquired urethral strictures	Gonococcal urethritis Urethral injury	Stenosis of lower urinary tract	Nonspecific
Prostatic hypertrophy	Aging	Causes mechanical obstruction of urethra	Males >45 yr old

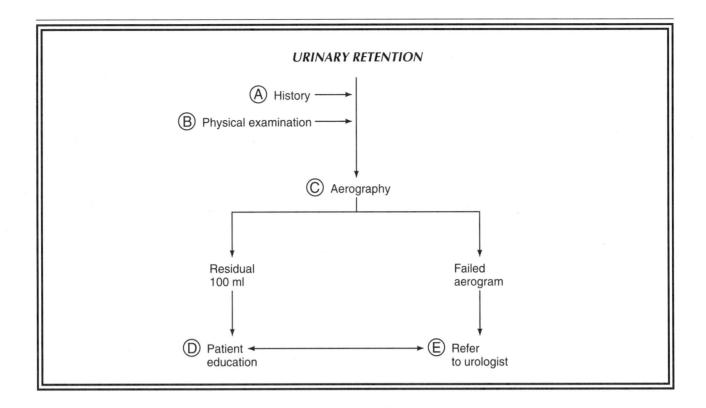

URINARY RETENTION

(A) History →

(B) Physical examination →

(C) Aerography

Residual 100 ml

Failed aerogram

(D) Patient education ←→ (E) Refer to urologist

times. To avoid injury or discomfort, patients should be taught to
• allow the catheter to cool to room temperature before use
• inspect the catheter for cracks and overall integrity
A cracked catheter may actually separate in the urethra. Making kits of catheters, povidone-iodine (Betadine) swabs, gloves, and lubricating jelly in sealed plastic bags allows patients to continue a routine of daily living. The bags of supplies can be carried in a pocket or purse, and any restroom can be used. The dirty catheter can then be taken home for cleaning. Also, instruct patients about urodynamic or other tests that may be performed by the urologist. These tests require preparation ranging from fasting to full bowel prep. Some patients need help understanding the instructions. Support systems (family or friends) may be essential to help patients with intermittent catheterization because of reluctance or problems with dexterity. Home health care nursing education and follow-up may be necessary until patients or caregivers become confident and their ability to perform catheterization is confirmed.

E. Referral to a urologist for urodynamic testing is warranted for comprehensive diagnostic evaluation.

Generally, a retrograde urethrogram (RGUG) is performed in males. A voiding cystourethrogram (VCUG) is done to assess for strictures or diverticulum (see the tool *Roentgenographic Urologic Procedures*, p. 217) and a cystoscopy to visually explore the bladder anatomy. Assisting with x-ray studies will necessitate catheterization, placing the patient in the lithotomy position, and preparing and draping for cystoscopy. It is essential to reassure and inform the patient what to expect during the procedures. Review and scrutiny of all prescribed and over-the-counter medications is important to eliminate agents potentially causing urinary retention. Medications particularly suspect include anticholinergics, beta-adrenergics, and narcotics.

References

Hanno P, Wein A. A clinical manual of urology. Norwalk, CT: Appleton-Century-Crofts, 1987.
Smith DR. General urology. 10th ed. San Mateo, CA: Lange Medical Publications, 1981.

Bladder Record

Name _____ Date _____

Day	Date	7AM	8AM	9AM	10AM	11AM	12PM	1PM	2PM	3PM	4PM	5PM	6PM	7PM	8PM	9PM	10PM	11PM	12AM	1AM	2AM	3AM	4AM	5AM	6AM
M																									
T																									
W																									
TH																									
F																									
S																									
S																									
M																									
T																									
W																									
TH																									
F																									
S																									
S																									

Bladder Record Instructions

To use as assessment tool
1. Write a "D" for Dry each time you urinate and do not find yourself wet.
2. Write a "W" for Wet each time you find yourself wet.

To use as bladder training tool
1. Write "D" for Dry each time you urinate and do not find yourself wet.
2. Write "W" for Wet any time during the day you find yourself wet.

To use as self-catheterization tool
1. Write the amount of residual measured during the hour you perform self-catheterization.

Guidelines for Foley Catheter Care in the Home

Change Foley once a month or PRN
  To evaluate need for change, roll catheter between thumb and index finger; if catheter feels "gritty" (this indicates calcium deposits in catheter lumen), change catheter

18Fr 5-ml catheter is appropriate size for most patients; do not change to larger Foley if there is spasm of urine around Foley
  Use only distilled water to inflate balloon, never normal saline; a 5-ml balloon can be hyperinflated to 30 ml

Disconnect catheter from tubing only if absolutely necessary
  Instruct patient/primary caregiver how to empty bag without disconnecting tubing
  If connection is broken, carefully clean both ends with alcohol and reconnect

Always keep drainage bag and tubing below level of bladder
  Avoid loops over side rails or patient's legs

Use leg bag only for short periods; do not wear while in bed or recliner
  Full leg bags cause back pressure in bladder and kidneys, which can result in infection

Maintain adequate fluid intake every day
  1–2 quarts

If catheter is clogged, nurse may irrigate with 60 ml normal saline; if unable to irrigate or flush tubing, readjust catheter and try again

Patients with indwelling Foley catheters who develop a fever should always be seen and evaluated by a physician
  Temperatures over 100.8°F may indicate a bladder infection
  Consult with primary care physician before collecting urine specimen

Bedside urinary drainage bags can be changed weekly. Bags may be reused by rinsing with a solution of 1:1 vinegar and water, and then air drying

Modified Kegel Exercises
Pelvic Muscle Exercises for the Incontinent

The purpose of the following exercises is to strengthen the pelvic floor muscles, which perform the squeezing action that helps hold back the flow of urine. It is important that these exercises be done faithfully for 3–4 months to see improvement. If no improvement is seen in this time, consultation with a urologist is suggested.

A. FOLLOW THESE INSTRUCTIONS TO IDENTIFY THE MUSCLES YOU WILL BE EXERCISING
1. Sit or stand. Without tensing the muscles of your legs, buttocks, or abdomen, imagine that you are trying to hold back a bowel movement by tightening the ring of muscle around the anus. Do this exercise only until you identify the back part of the pelvic floor.
2. When you are passing urine, try to stop the flow, then restart it. This will help you identify the front part of the pelvic floor. Now you are ready to do the complete exercise.

B. DO THIS EXERCISE FOR 2 MINUTES AT LEAST THREE TIMES DAILY (AT LEAST 100 REPETITIONS)
1. Working from back to front, tighten the muscles while counting to four slowly, then release them. You can do this exercise anywhere—while sitting or standing, watching TV, or waiting for a bus. There is no need to interrupt your normal daily activity. Do not tighten the abdominal, thigh, or buttock muscles or cross your legs, in order to feel only the pelvic muscles. Their movement is distinct and separate from that of the other muscles and can be checked by women while in the bath or shower, by placing one finger inside the vagina and contracting the muscles. Men can check success only through improved urinary control.

C. DO THIS EXERCISE EVERY TIME YOU URINATE
1. Start and stop your stream five times each time you urinate: i.e., start the flow of urine, squeeze, hold back, and let go to resume the flow. Hold back, let go, etc. Remember, do this every time you urinate. You probably will notice that you have much more control of the flow of urine in the morning than in the afternoon. This is because your muscles are not so tired.

HIP Report, HIP Help for Incontinent People, Inc, PO Box 544, Union, SC 29379; with permission.

Roentgenographic Urologic Procedures

Type	Purpose	Indications	Contraindications
KUB (kidney, ureter, bladder)	1. To determine size, congenital absence, position, shape, and calcifications 2. To differentiate between gastrointestinal and genitourinary diseases	Nonspecific abdominal pain	
IVP (intravenous pyelogram)	1. To visualize the genitourinary tract with the use of contrast media 2. To determine obstruction or nonobstructive tumors, cysts, or calcifications of the genitourinary tract 3. To determine malformation or duplication of the genitourinary tract	Hematuria, flank pain, and impaired renal function	1. Allergy to contrast 2. Elevated creatinine ≥4 mg/day 3. Dehydration 4. Use caution in patients with diabetes mellitus 5. Pregnancy
RGPG (retrograde pyelogram)	To visualize the genitourinary tract with the use of contrast media via ureteral catheter done in conjunction with cystoscopy	1. When creatinine ≥1.5 2. When allergic to contrast media, minimal absorbed via the bladder 3. Drained via a ureteral catheter; therefore, decreased risk to patients with chronic renal insufficiency 4. To visualize when attempting to pass an internal ureteral catheter to allow urine flow from kidney to bladder	1. Untreated urinary tract infection 2. In patients who cannot or should not be cystoscoped
VCUG (voiding cystourethrogram)	1. To visualize the bladder and demonstrate the anatomy of the lower urinary tract during micturition 2. To evaluate the urethra for diverticula, voiding dysfunction, or ectopic ureter, which commonly results in reflux	Recurrent lower tract infections due to reflux	
RGUG (retrograde urethrogram)	1. To visualize the anterior urethra in a male by retrograde flow of contrast 2. To evaluate for urethral stricture or trauma	1. When a catheter cannot pass 2. Traumatic removal of a catheter	None
Ultrasonography	1. To visualize structures not able to be seen by other techniques (e.g., prostate) 2. To evaluate perinephric fluid collection 3. To evaluate the scrotum and external genitalia to differentiate solid from fluid	1. When palpation cannot be done 2. In patients with impaired renal function 3. To visualize filling defects 4. Renal surveillance without undue exposure to x-ray 5. Prostate and seminal vesicle evaluation not visualized by other means	1. Limitation as some structures cannot be visualized (e.g., nondilated ureters) 2. Inferior resolution compared with IVP

Self Catheterization Instructions

Supplies needed:
  Clean straight catheter 14 or 16Fr
  Hot soapy water and rinse water
                    or
  Brown paper bag and microwave with microwavable bowl of water
  Povidone-iodine (Betadine) preps
  Water-soluble lubricant

How to perform catheterization:
1. Urinate before catheterization, but do not strain to start stream
2. Wash hands with soap and water
3. Clean labia and urethra front to back (women); glans penis, pulling back foreskin (men) with Betadine preps
4. Lubricate catheter; finding meatus, place through urethra into bladder
5. Allow urine to drain until flow stops; advance and retract to make sure all urine has been expelled
6. Remove catheter
7. Wash in hot soapy water, rinse well, drain dry on clean cloth; may reuse catheter until it becomes hard or color of catheter begins to change (about 30 uses)
Note: If there is a wish to sterilize by home microwave, after washing, place in brown paper bag and microwave for up to 30 minutes. A bowl of water must be in the microwave. The mean time to microwave is 13 minutes when the catheter is being sterilized, to preserve the integrity of the catheter. The bowl should contain one cup, or 8 oz, of water. To sterilize more than one catheter, increase microwave time by 13 minutes per catheter. Store in closed paper bag.

From Silbar EC, et al. Microwave sterilization: A method for home sterilization of urinary catheters. J Urol 1989; 141:88. Reproduced with permission.

Urodynamic Studies

Type	Purpose	Indications	Pertinent Information
Flow rate	To measure detrusor contraction harmony with sphincter activity	Primarily done in males who demonstrate weak, slow stream; hesistancy; or straining to start stream	The bladder may be full to the point of urgency. The quantity, peak pressure exerted, and length of time to empty are measured. A peak of less than 10 cm is highly suggestive of obstruction or dysfunction
CMG (cystometrogram)	1. To measure intravesical pressure during filling and storing phase of micturition 2. To evaluate dysfunction of detrusor muscles and urethra, especially when the pressure or volume need measuring	In patients with decreased tone (diabetes, neurologic injury, or neurogenic disease). In women with multiple vaginal trauma due to births, surgery, or cystourethrocele	The bladder is filled via a catheter until the patient has the urge to void. The rate is known and the intravesical pressure is measured simultaneously. The compliance, tone, volume capacity, and irritability are evaluated
UPP (urethral pressure profile)	1. To measure pressure sphincter activity by determining the efficiency of sphincteric elements around the urethral canal 2. To detect any weakness or hyperactivity in the smooth and voluntary components	Noncontractility of the sphincter to hold urine	Caution against voluntary straining during testing. Summation is of true intravesical pressure and intra-abdominal pressure
EMG (electromyogram)	To measure sphincter muscles and assess if working with bladder muscle	Dyssynergic bladder	Usually done in conjunction with CMG and flow rate. When the bladder muscle contracts to empty, the sphincter muscle should relax, allowing urination. Wire electrodes are placed into perineal sphincter muscles to perform the test
Marshall test	To measure ability to retain urine when the bladder is suspended	In women with stress urinary incontinence	Determining whether bladder suspension will be successful

METABOLIC

ANEMIA

Donna A. Bachand

Hemoglobin and hematocrit levels remain relatively constant throughout life. Subnormal levels in the elderly do not occur with aging but are due to insufficient dietary intake of iron, impaired iron or vitamin B_{12} absorption, or bleeding.

A. Elicit symptoms of
   - syncope or palpitations
   - fatigability
   - weakness
   - dyspnea
   - pallor
   - headache
   - sleep disturbances

   Determine which over-the-counter and prescription drugs the patient is taking. Long-term aspirin or nonsteroidal anti-inflammatory drug use may cause gastric irritation and chronic blood loss from the GI tract. Medications such as potassium chloride and oral hypoglycemics inhibit vitamin B_{12} absorption and lead to pernicious anemia. A 24-hour record of actual food intake is useful to determine whether iron deficiency is secondary to insufficient intake. Additional data pertinent to the nutrition history include frequency of meals, snacks, and amount of "junk food" consumed; food storage and preparation facilities (canned or fresh); alcohol consumption; medically prescribed diet restrictions; and recent changes in food habits. Inquire whether the patient has noticed any changes in taste or smell. To determine socioeconomic issues ask the following questions:
   - Who does your grocery shopping?
   - How often do you or someone else get to the store?
   - How much money do you spend on food? (Determine what proportion of monthly income is spent on food).
   - Do you eat meals on a regular schedule?
   - Who do you eat with?

   Elderly persons who live alone may be less inclined to prepare or eat regular meals. Food choices may be restricted by income or inability to travel to and carry groceries from the market. Determine whether GI problems affect appetite, food retention, or elimination. Ask if there is a history of GI disorders such as diverticular or peptic ulcer disease, hemorrhoids, or malignancy.

B. Assess vital signs, including blood pressure for orthostasis, pulse for tachycardia, and respirations for rate and effort. Observe dentition, denture fit, and ability to chew and swallow. Test sensations of taste and smell, if materials are available. Examine mucous membranes (see the tool *Oral Examination*, p. 183), conjunctiva, and nailbeds for capillary refill. Perform abdominal, rectal, and genitourinary examinations. Test for fecal occult blood. Obtain a complete blood count. If indicated, additional testing may include
   - sickle cell trait
   - vitamin B_{12}
   - iron
   - folate
   - methylmalonic acid

C. Community resources are available in many areas and include senior citizen/nutrition centers, home-delivered meals, food banks, financial support such as food stamps or supplemental income, and aging information and referral. A social service referral may be indicated.

D. Educate individuals to increase consumption of iron-rich foods such as green leafy vegetables, meat, fish, poultry, dried fruits, and enriched breads and cereals. Increasing vitamin C intake (citrus fruits and juices, berries) promotes iron absorption. The texture, palatability, and presentation of foods can be altered to meet individual needs. Consider a nutrition consultation if the patient has multiple food intolerances or restrictions. Educate patients to obtain serial stools for occult blood testing (see Rectal Bleeding, p. 194) and to decrease the use of aspirin and nonsteroidal anti-inflammatory drugs.

E. Medical evaluation includes diagnostic work-up of the GI tract, interpretation of laboratory findings, and assessment for malignancy. Referral to a medical subspecialty may be necessary. Medical management and further nursing interventions will be dictated by the diagnostic outcome. Specific oral supplements may be recommended to augment therapy. Vitamin B_{12} injections are indicated only for pernicious anemia. Dietary and bowel management changes may be required on the basis of definitive diagnosis.

Reference

Libow LS, Sherman FT. The core of geriatric medicine: A guide for students and practitioners. St. Louis: CV Mosby, 1981:280.

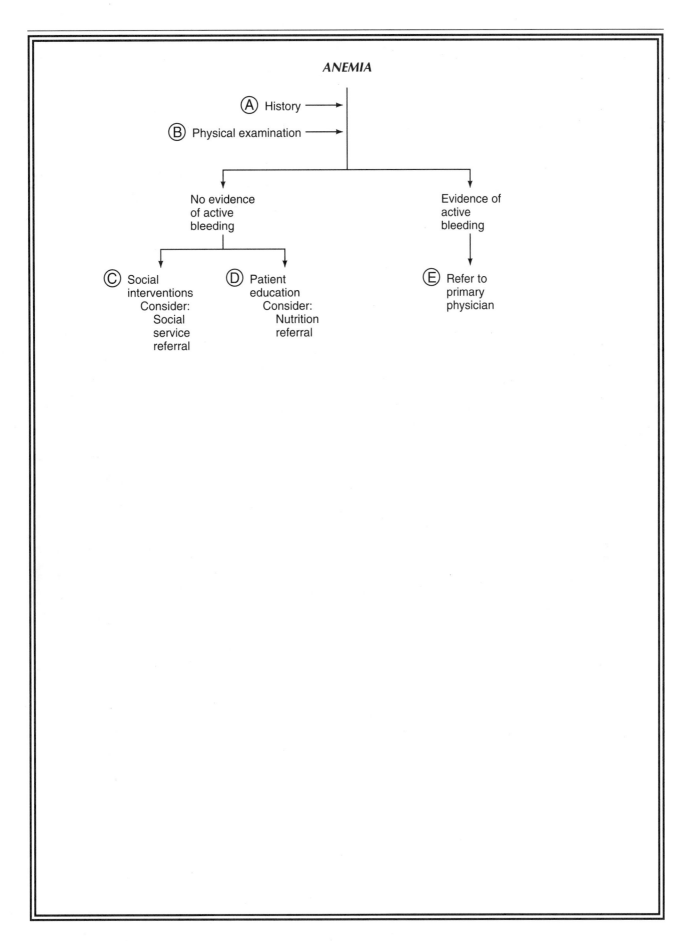

ANEMIA

Ⓐ History ⟶

Ⓑ Physical examination ⟶

No evidence
of active
bleeding

Evidence of
active
bleeding

Ⓒ Social
interventions
Consider:
Social
service
referral

Ⓓ Patient
education
Consider:
Nutrition
referral

Ⓔ Refer to
primary
physician

CHEST PAIN

Aline C. Schwob

Chest pain is a nonspecific complaint that may indicate a variety of health problems. Because the most frequent cause of death in the elderly is coronary artery disease, consider this first when chest pain occurs. In patients older than 80 years of age, the risk of heart disease is equal in males and females. Angina pectoris may occur as a premonitory symptom in 30–60% of patients who have a myocardial infarction (MI). The pain is associated with reduced blood supply to the heart muscle secondary to obstruction of the coronary arteries. Angina pectoris, in its classical presentation, lasts <5 minutes and is relieved by rest and nitroglycerin (NTG). It is described as constriction, tightness, and/or suffocating pressure. Other conditions may mimic the symptoms of angina and present as chest pain, but do not present the same pain pattern. Chest pain may be referred from other systems. GI, pulmonary, or musculoskeletal conditions may present as chest pain. Complaints of chest pain must be thoroughly investigated.

A. A careful history helps establish whether the pain is of cardiac or some other origin. *It is important to remember that the elderly frequently have an atypical presentation.* Pain should be evaluated for
- Character
  - pressure
  - squeezing
  - tightness
  - suffocating or constricting
- Location
  - neck
  - jaw
  - arms
  - back
  - shoulders
  - epigastric
  - substernal
  - radiation
- Duration of less or more than 5 minutes
Symptoms associated with the pain may include
- shortness of breath
- a feeling of suffocation
- diaphoresis
- confusion or giddiness
- syncope
Question the patient about factors that aggravate or alleviate the pain. Does it occur at rest or only with activity? What type of activity? Is there an emotional component? In addition to evaluating symptoms, obtain information on current medications; family history; current lifestyle; and any history of cardiac, gastric, pulmonary, or musculoskeletal problems. Symptoms may vary in the elderly. The significant factor is their effect on the patient's level of functioning. Be alert to changes in activities of daily living (ADL) or independent functioning.

B. Rule out significant systemic problems by physical examination, including
- vital signs, especially blood pressure, sitting, lying, and standing when possible
- height and weight
- general appearance
  - color
  - physical signs of pain such as
    - rigidity
    - grimace
- funduscopic examination of the eyes
- cardiac examination
  - jugular vein distention
  - bruits
  - adventitious heart sounds
- chest
  - rales
  - wheezes
- abdomen
  - bruits
  - guarding
- extremities
  - pulses
  - edema
  - clubbing
  - capillary refill
- mental status for an acute change
Ask the patient to localize the pain. Palpate the identified site for tenderness, masses, and temperature. Other differential evaluation should include an electrocardiogram (ECG), laboratory studies, and (if indicated), a chest film. The ECG is usually normal at rest but may show a sagging S-T segment and a flattened or inverted T wave during an anginal episode. Use laboratory studies to rule out such factors as anemia and hyper- and hypothyroidism. Cardiac enzymes are usually not elevated in angina. Electrolyte imbalances such as hyperkalemia and hyponatremia may affect the patient's presentation and symptoms. A chest film may be indicated to discriminate among pneumonia, congestive heart failure (CHF), and other acute conditions (see Shortness of Breath p. 232). GI studies such as upper GI or esophagoduodenoscopy (EGD) may be needed to discover hiatal hernia, incompetent cardiac sphincter, or gastric/duodenal ulcer.

C. Chest pain that does not interfere with independent functioning may respond to risk factor reduction, which should include programs for
- smoking cessation
- diet modification
- dealing with anxiety
- weight loss

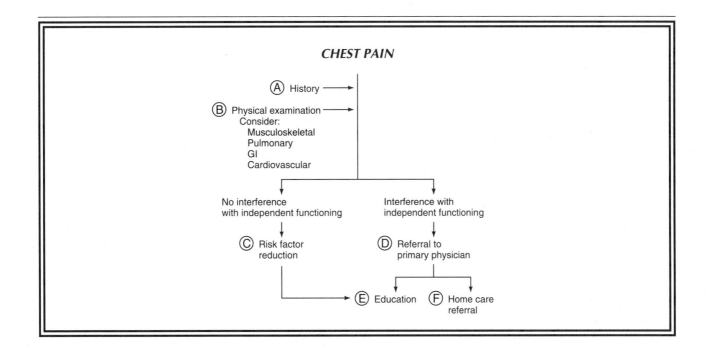

CHEST PAIN

A History →

B Physical examination →
Consider:
Musculoskeletal
Pulmonary
GI
Cardiovascular

No interference
with independent functioning

Interference with
independent functioning

C Risk factor
reduction

D Referral to
primary physician

E Education

F Home care
referral

Symptomatic treatments such as the following may help reduce chest pain
- not lying flat after meals
- elimination of gas-producing foods
- not exercising too soon after eating
- muscle massage
- careful application of heat or cold
- removal of restrictive garments

D. Patients with chest pain require physician referral for evaluation of a potentially life-threatening or acute condition. The diagnostic outcome will dictate subsequent interventions and treatment plans, including choice of medications.

E. Nursing management involves teaching patients the signs and symptoms of complications and side effects of drug therapy. Management of angina includes NTG by one or more routes: sublingual, longer-acting oral, or transdermal. Sublingual NTG may be used prophylactically before activity (one tablet) or at the onset of angina (one every 3–5 minutes); these should be kept in a dark container and replaced every 6 months. Instruct the patient to obtain emergency care if the angina is unresolved after three sublingual NTG tablets. Beta blockers such as propranolol, atenolol, and timolol, as well as newer agents, are frequently used with NTG to treat stable angina. These agents carry a greater risk of side effects in the elderly, the most common being bradycardia, heart block, CHF, fatigue, depression, and postural hypotension. Dosages should be increased and decreased gradually, since abrupt withdrawal may precipitate unstable angina or MI. The calcium channel blockers are the newest class of drugs used to treat angina as well as hypertension. Verapamil, diltiazem, and nifedipine all have a vasodilatory effect. Fewer side effects have been reported, but these include flushing, dizziness,

headaches, palpitations, ankle edema, constipation, and facial pains. Additional nursing interventions for angina should focus on
- cardiac rehabilitation
- therapeutic exercise as allowed
- supportive care (essential so that the patient does not become a "cardiac cripple")

F. Referral for home care may require physician orders. Essential self-care elements that home care can address with patient education concern
- the disease process
- medication purpose and administration
- activity
- energy conservation measures
- emergency precautions/home safety
- dietary changes

Supportive home health services that may be provided include
- personal hygiene
- assistance with chores
- delivered meals

References

Opie LH. Drugs for the heart. 2nd ed. Orlando: Grune & Stratton, 1987.

Pietro DA. Coronary disease in the elderly. In: Walshe TM, ed. Manual of clinical problems in geriatric medicine. Boston: Little, Brown, 1985:128.

Thompson CE, Jones JM, Cox AR, Levy EY. Adult health management: Guidelines for nurse practitioners. Reston, an imprint Simon and Schuster, VA: Reston, 1983.

Wright C. Managing stable angina pectoris: Nitroglycerin, beta blockers and risk factor reduction. Nurse Pract 1984; 2:54.

DECREASED HEIGHT, DORSAL KYPHOSIS, BACK PAIN (OSTEOPOROSIS)

Leslie C. Trischank Hussey

Osteoporosis is a degenerative bone problem particularly prevalent in postmenopausal women. It affects millions of people and results in 3 million fractures a year. Factors contributing to primary osteoporosis are
• calcium deficiency
• osteoclastic (bone resorption) activity greater than osteoblastic (bone formation) activity
• decreased vitamin D utilization
These cause structural weakness of both trabecular and cortical bone. Factors contributing to secondary osteoporosis include
• diabetes
• Cushing's syndrome
• multiple myeloma
• chronic obstructive pulmonary disease
• immobility
• alcohol abuse
• treatment with anticonvulsants and cortisone
Additional risk factors for the development of osteoporosis are
• low dietary calcium intake
• minimal sun exposure
• inadequate estrogen replacement

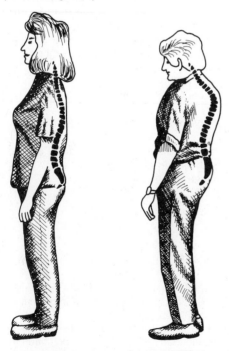

Figure 1 Loss of height from vertebral collapse. (Illustration courtesy of JoAnn Clemons Elliott, 1992.)

• fair skin
• female gender (up to six times greater risk than that of males)
• white race

A. Ask questions to determine the presence of risk factors for osteoporosis and possible subsequent treatment regimens
   • menstrual history
      • oophorectomy before age 45 years
      • age at menopause
   • medical history
      • hyperthyroidism
      • poorly controlled hypertension
      • diabetes
      • Cushing's syndrome
      • breast cancer
      • endometrial disease
      • pulmonary disease
      • rheumatoid arthritis
      • renal calculi
      • multiple myeloma
      • symptomatic cerebrovascular disease
      • thromboembolic disease
      • gastrectomy
      • seizures
   • medication history
      • use of anticonvulsants
      • estrogen replacement therapy
      • glucocorticosteroid use
   • nutrition history
      • malabsorption
      • lactose intolerance
      • vitamin and mineral supplementation
      • ingestion of calcium-containing foods
   • lifestyle
      • current and previous sun exposure
      • exercise patterns
   • family history
      • vertebral or hip fractures
      • osteoporosis
   Determine symptoms such as
   • pain
      • location
      • radiation
      • onset
      • exacerbating factors
      • alleviating factors
   • loss of height: ask how tall the patient was in high school (Fig. 1)

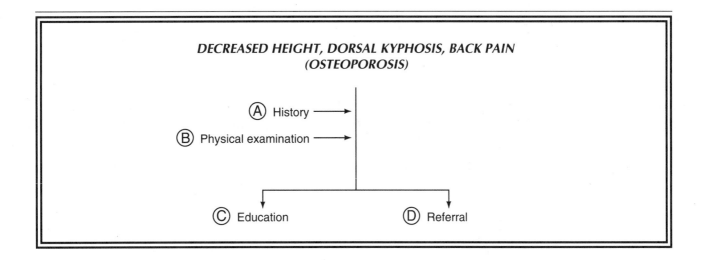

DECREASED HEIGHT, DORSAL KYPHOSIS, BACK PAIN (OSTEOPOROSIS)

Ⓐ History ⟶

Ⓑ Physical examination ⟶

Ⓒ Education   Ⓓ Referral

B. The most simple and indicative measurement of vertebral collapse related to osteoporosis is loss of height: a loss of 2–3 inches is not uncommon (Fig. 1). Be sure to measure height with the patient standing on a flat surface. It may be necessary to use a ruler placed on the patient's head to determine height, because spinal deformities may not allow the back to remain flat against the wall. Observe skin pigmentation and the presence of dorsal kyphosis. Pay particular attention to common fracture sites: vertebra, hip, wrist (ulna). Perform a neurologic examination to determine whether loss of sensation has occurred (see Decreased Sensation, p. 138). Laboratory tests that may be helpful include
- thyroid function
- parathyroid hormone (PTH)
- serum phosphorus
- serum magnesium
- alkaline phosphatase
- vitamin D level
- 24-hour urine for calcium
- creatinine clearance (requires 24-hour urine and serum creatinine)

The purpose of serum chemistry studies is to rule out other medical problems requiring intervention rather than to determine calcium balance. Serum calcium, phosphorus, magnesium, alkaline phosphatase, PTH, and thyroid functions should be normal in uncomplicated osteoporosis. Serum calcium is maintained by bone breakdown when necessary, so is not indicative of bone health or adequate therapeutic intervention.

Text continued on page 226.

Osteoporosis Education

Topic	Content	Topic	Content
Injury prevention	Home safety • Rearrange furniture to prevent falls • Do not string electrical cords across walkways • Anchor or remove area rugs Lifting • Do not lift more than 5 lb • Get help with groceries • Carry a small purse • Use bathroom scales to weigh purse Support • Use walker or cane to help support weight on arms Clothing • Wear sturdy, low-heeled, rubber-soled shoes for better balance • Avoid long, flowing clothing, which may become caught and cause a fall Exercise • Practice good body mechanics • Sit with knees above hips • Stand with your back at rest • Do not bend over at the waist to pick anything up • Perform muscle strengthening exercises daily • Pelvic tilt • Leg lifts • Cat's back • Weight-bearing exercise such as walking is beneficial	Medications (cont'd.) Nutrition/ nutrient supplemen- tation Pain manage- ment Bowel management program	Fluoride • Take with meals to prevent stomach irritation • Forms bone faster than calcium, but bone is not normal bone Calcium • Need to take 1000–1500 mg daily • May cause constipation initially • Take foods high in calcium if possible Vitamin D • Eat only as prescribed • Vitamin is fat soluble, and therefore stored; dose must be evaluated regularly Pharmacologic agent use • Analgesics • Muscle relaxants • Use to maintain soft stools • Drink adequate fluids • Take stool softeners as ordered • Exercise regularly • Do not rush when toileting Positioning • Use body positions that relieve pain • Avoid standing or sitting for long periods • Avoid movements or positions that cause strain or pain, such as • lifting • twisting • Bed rest may be prescribed at times Comfort measures • Use a bed board under a hard mattress • Apply heat (carefully) for acute pain • Wear a prescribed corset or back brace
Medications	Estrogen replacement • How to take cyclic regimen if ordered • Other precautions to take • monthly breast self-examination • pelvic examination at least yearly • Risks • endometrial or breast cancer • stroke • hypertension		

C. Education focuses on
- prevention of further injury
- altering lifestyle
- medication compliance
- nutrition and nutrient supplementation
- pain management (see box on p. 226).

D. Referral to a primary physician or bone and mineral metabolism specialist is in order for more definitive testing and prescription of medication. Tests that may be ordered include
- Radiography of involved areas (shows loss of bone mass but only after 35% loss of bone mass has occurred)
- photon absorptiometry (bone densitometry)
  - single photon measures wrist density
  - dual photon measures density usually of the lumbar vertebrae
- quantitative CT scan, to measure density of vertebral trabecular bone
- bone biopsy of iliac crest, to actually visualize bone cell activity

Treatment may include cyclic estrogen therapy (see Atrophic Vaginitis, p. 246), calcium supplementation, vitamin D supplements, and fluoride therapy. An elastic lumbosacral corset may be prescribed for daytime or for severe back pain episodes. A rigid back brace may be used after careful consideration for a limited time. Referral may also be made to physical and/or occupational therapy for an exercise program and assistance in developing new activity habits. Programs are geared to muscle strengthening, decreasing the risk of injury to weakened bone, and decreasing pain.

References

Chestnut C, Cummings S, Drinkwater B, Johnston C. New options in osteoporosis. Patient Care 1988; 160.

Marcus R. Understanding and preventing osteoporosis. Hosp Pract 1989; 24:189.

Miller G. Osteoporosis: Is it inevitable? J Gerontol Nurs 1985; 11:10.

ELEVATED BLOOD PRESSURE/HYPERTENSION

Aline C. Schwob

Hypertension is a significant health problem with about a 50% incidence rate after age 65 years. Prevention, detection, and treatment will take nursing time and effort as more and more Americans live longer. Contrary to folk beliefs, hypertension is asymptomatic until complications occur. In addition, there are no unequivocal formulas for the evaluation and management of hypertension in the elderly. Arterial stiffening increases with age and is considered a major factor for the age-related increase in systolic blood pressure (BP). Evidence suggests that aggressive treatment is beneficial in reducing the risk of a cardiovascular event.

A. Ascertain
- any family history of hypertension
- any history of elevated BP
- other acute or chronic illnesses
- medications, prescribed and over the counter
- presence of cardiac disease
- history of stroke
- dietary sodium intake
- symptoms of postural hypotension

A review of the patient's lifestyle is especially important in identifying factors that may be modified to decrease BP. Ask about the use of tobacco and alcohol, composition of diet, exercise, and level of stress indicated by recent life events.

B. Physical assessment is used to determine the presence of hypertensive complications as well as actual BP control. Specific evaluation elements are
- height and weight
- BP sitting, lying, and standing (both arms with a cuff of appropriate size)
- serial BP
- neck
  - bruits
  - jugular vein distention
  - thyroid size
- eyes (funduscopic)
  - papilledema
  - exudates
  - hemorrhages
  - nicking
- heart
  - rate
  - rhythm
  - murmurs
  - gallops
- chest
  - wheezes
  - crackles
- abdomen
  - bruits
  - pulsatile masses
- extremities
  - pulses
  - edema
- neurologic assessment
  - visual fields
  - accommodation
  - pupil reaction
- asymmetric muscle tone of extremities and face

Because atherosclerosis can account for a 10–15 mm Hg BP error, perform the Osler maneuver. Raise the cuff pressure above the systolic BP and palpate the radial artery. A palpable radial artery may indicate pseudohypertension. Extensive testing is usually not indicated unless the hypertension is severe and unresponsive to usual treatment methods. Studies that may be indicated are ECG, chest film, hemoglobin and hematocrit, urinalysis, K^+, Ca, creatinine, BUN, thyroid studies, lipids, and glucose. Second-level tests include creatinine clearance, IV pyelography or renal arteriography. The latter two are not indicated on initial evaluation, but rather for therapy-resistant patients.

C. Encourage patients with normal BP readings to maintain positive lifestyle patterns and modify those that may put them at risk in the future. Counseling should focus on factors that may exacerbate a tendency for an elevated BP (e.g., obesity, sedentary lifestyle, smoking, alcohol, stress). Sodium intake may be a significant factor in certain susceptible individuals. Exercise such as walking is beneficial; strenuous exercise is unnecessary.

D. Physician referral for medical management is recommended even in a case of isolated systolic hypertension (systolic elevation with no diastolic elevation). An initial reading that exceeds 190/104 should be referred immediately.

E. Medications such as thyroid preparations and antihistamines may elevate BP. Ongoing management should have as its goal a *gradual* decrease in BP with minimal side effects such as postural hypotension. Pay attention to the altered pharmacokinetics and increased risk of drug interactions. Second-step therapy is used when the first step does not control BP. A

Sequencing of Antihypertensives	
First Step	*Second Step*
Thiazide diuretic	Beta blocker, angiotensin converting enzyme (ACE) inhibitor, or calcium antagonist
Beta-blocking agent	Thiazide diuretic
ACE inhibitor	Thiazide diuretic
Calcium antagonist	Thiazide diuretic

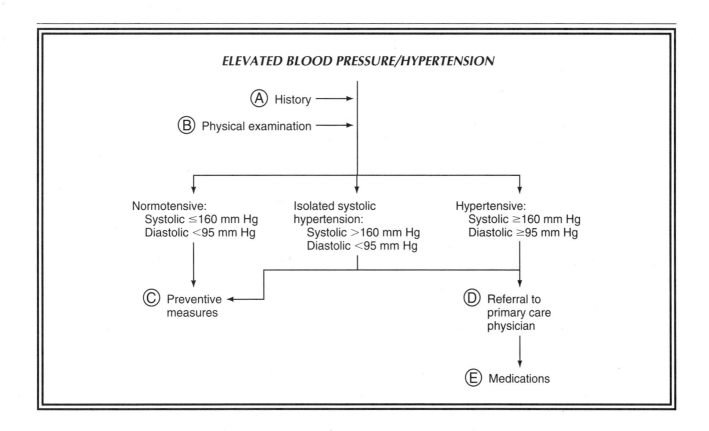

ELEVATED BLOOD PRESSURE/HYPERTENSION

(A) History

(B) Physical examination

Normotensive:
Systolic ≤160 mm Hg
Diastolic <95 mm Hg

Isolated systolic
hypertension:
Systolic >160 mm Hg
Diastolic <95 mm Hg

Hypertensive:
Systolic ≥160 mm Hg
Diastolic ≥95 mm Hg

(C) Preventive
measures

(D) Referral to
primary care
physician

(E) Medications

single drug (monotherapy) is preferred in any case. The box shows the accepted sequencing of antihypertensive agents. The cardinal rule with medications is to start with a low dose and titrate slowly. A simplified dosage schedule to avoid compliance problems is also indicated.

References

Carnevali DL, Patrick D. Nursing management for the elderly. 2nd ed. Philadelphia: JB Lippincott, 1986.

Fontana SA. Update on high blood pressure: Highlights from the 1988 National Report. Nurse Pract 1988; 12:8.

La Bresh KA, Peitro DA. Hypertension in the elderly. In: Walshe TM, ed. Manual of clinical problems in geriatric medicine. Boston: Little, Brown, 1985:119.

Lakatta EG. Geriatric hypertension: Aggressive therapy and its physiologic rationale. Geriatrics 1986; 41:44.

IMPAIRED PERIPHERAL CIRCULATION

Kay Bolding

Impaired peripheral circulation is associated with changes that result in narrowing of the arterial lumen and diminished blood flow from either normal aging or pathologic processes of arteriosclerosis or atherosclerosis. Peripheral vascular disease describes occlusion, vasodilation, vasoconstriction, or insufficiency of the arteries, veins, and lymphatic vessels of the extremities, resulting in ischemia to the area served by the vessel. Peripheral vascular disease can produce inconvenience, affect ability to perform activities of daily living, cause psychological problems such as depression, and even jeopardize the viability of the extremities in patients over the age of 50.

A. History elicits
   - presence of calf or leg pain or cramps
   - onset and duration of pain or cramps
   - thrombophlebitis
   - fractures
   - changes in temperature of extremities
   - nutrition and fluid intake
   - prolonged bed rest or inactivity
   - mental status changes (see Confusion/Cognitive Changes/Dementia, p. 254)
   - medical history: hypertension, diabetes mellitus, heart disease
   - medications: vasoconstrictors, vasodilators
   - use of hot water bottles, heating pads, hot foot soaks
   - family history of vascular disease
   - pain at rest
   - tobacco use
   - varicosities
   - surgery
   - delayed healing
   - falls
   - diminished mobility
   - psychosocial stressors

Self-Care for Patients with Vascular Problems

- stop smoking
- do NOT use hot foot soaks, hot water bottles, or heating pads on extremities
- test bath water temperature with fingers, elbow, or bath thermometer
- do NOT cross legs at the knee
- do NOT wear constricting clothing such as girdles or garters
- wear proper shoes (see the tool *Foot Care*, p. 60)
- avoid prolonged standing
- use support stockings
- protect against cold and chilling by keeping home thermostat at 70° to 72° F and wearing protective clothing when exposed to cold
- if chilled, take a warm bath, drink warm liquids, and place a hot water bottle on abdomen (NOT extremities)
- keep skin clean and dry
- watch for skin breakdown or infection
- maintain ideal body weight; lose weight if overweight
- follow a diet low in saturated fat
- follow a moderate, prescribed exercise and rest program
- elevate legs above heart frequently (see illustrations, pp. 237)
- sleep with foot of bed elevated on 6-inch blocks

Patients reporting leg pain should be questioned about specific conditions or activities that worsen or relieve the problem.

B. Physical examination focuses on
   - skin: temperature, texture, dryness, scaling and color, erythema, inflammation, local redness
   - hair patterns and decreased hair distribution or amount
   - circulation: pulse presence and amplitude, capillary refill, edema
   - sensation, motor strength and function
   - nails: thickened or brittle
   - pain or tenderness on palpation
   - leg ulcers, cellulitis, or gangrenous findings

Deep vein inflammation with clot formation is identified by
   - increased muscle turgor over an area of tenderness on affected vein
   - deep muscle tenderness
   - greater warmth of affected extremity than the other
   - positive Homans' sign, calf pain caused by dorsiflexion of foot
   - venous distention of extremity
   - cyanosis
   - occasional temperature <101° F

Noninvasive studies such as Doppler ultrasonography yield valuable information regarding blood flow and blood vessel patency. Other helpful tests may include isotope and venous pressure studies and phlebography.

TABLE 1 Acute Versus Chronic Circulation Impairment

Vessel	Acute	Chronic
Artery	Sudden onset of pain pallor, pulselessness, coldness, lack of sensation or movement	Resting pain Skin color and texture changes Sensation of coldness Paresthesias Ischemic ulcers or inflammation Diminished or absent pulses
Vein	Pain, tenderness, edema, erythema	Enlarged varicosities Edema

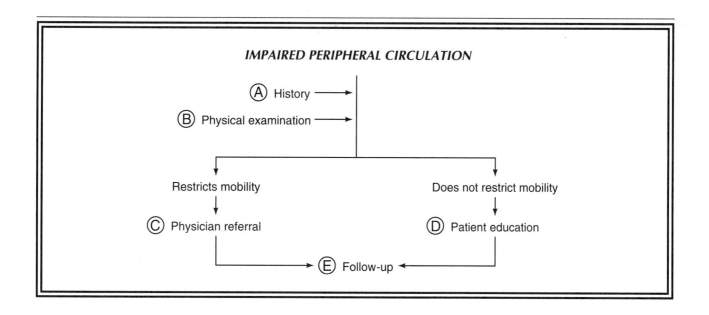

IMPAIRED PERIPHERAL CIRCULATION

(A) History

(B) Physical examination

Restricts mobility   Does not restrict mobility

(C) Physician referral   (D) Patient education

(E) Follow-up

C. Acute circulatory impairment requires immediate medical attention. Treatments selected are based on symptoms (Table 1) and may include
- anticoagulation or thrombolytic therapy
- vasodilators
- application of jalapeño pepper ointment for pain relief
- surgical intervention

D. Patient education focuses on improving peripheral circulation, increasing venous flow, and preventing extremity injury or complications of decreased blood flow (see box on facing page). Patients should be warned to immediately report
- sudden onset of severe pain
- changes in pulses; skin color, integrity, or temperature
- increase in pain, cramps, numbness, or tingling

E. Follow-up can monitor
- understanding of previous teaching
- appearance of extremities
- need for additional medical intervention
- level of mobility
- progress of lesions

References

Goiella EC, Bevil CW. Nursing care of the aging client. Norwalk, CT: Appleton-Century-Crofts, 1985:157.

Nurses Reference Library. Assessment Nursing '82 books. Springhouse, PA: Intermed Communication, 1982:358.

Swearingen PL. Manual of nursing therapeutics: Applying nursing diagnoses to medical disorders. St. Louis: Mosby–Year Book, 1986:76.

SHORTNESS OF BREATH

Marybeth Navas

Shortness of breath is a feeling of breathlessness that may be associated with physiologic or psychological symptoms such as fatigue, weakness, hyperventilation, or chest discomfort. Shortness of breath reduces the ability to perform activities of daily living and contributes to deconditioning and increased risk of respiratory infection, which is among the 10 leading causes of death in the over 65 age group.

A. History reflects data on
- history of chronic illnesses
  - chronic obstructive pulmonary disease
  - congestive heart failure
  - Guillain-Barré syndrome
  - amyotrophic lateral sclerosis
  - GI disorders causing poor nutrition
  - cardiomyopathy
  - anemia
  - myasthenia gravis
  - muscular dystrophies
  - malabsorption
- psychosocial factors
  - recent life stresses or losses
  - past coping methods
  - alcohol use
  - support systems
  - sleep disturbances
  - smoking
- medications, especially over-the-counter bronchodilators
- infectious diseases: pneumonia, flu, colds
- neuromuscular and skeletal symptoms
  - exercise intolerance
  - fatigue (see p. 14)
  - limitations on activity
  - changes in strength
- nutritional information
  - usual weight
  - weight changes
  - appetite
  - vomiting or diarrhea
- current symptoms
  - onset of shortness of breath
  - swelling of ankles
  - cough, sputum
  - ability to perform activities of daily living, including eating
  - associated activities
  - chest tightness
  - wheezing, congestion

B. Physical assessment focuses on
- general appearance: weight, muscle wasting, lackluster hair, skin color and texture
- vital signs: temperature; blood pressure; pulse rate and rhythm; respiratory rate, rhythm, volume, and timing of inspiration and expiration
- chest: use of accessory muscles, motion of chest wall and abdomen, anteroposterior chest diameter, bony deformities restricting lung expansion
- lung sounds and sputum color, amount, and character
- heart rhythm, adventitious sounds or bruits
- abdomen for ascites or prominent aortic pulsation
- extremities for peripheral edema and pulses
- mental status: cognition, mood, affect, level of consciousness
- chest radiograph: posteroanterior and lateral
- pulse oximetry for oxygen saturation
- arterial blood gases, particularly P_{CO_2} and P_{O_2}
- other laboratory tests
  - complete blood count with differential
  - albumin level
  - electrolytes
  - sputum cultures
  - blood cultures if indicated by fever

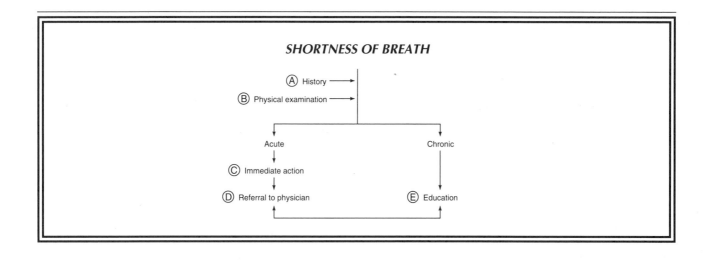

SHORTNESS OF BREATH

Ⓐ History
Ⓑ Physical examination

Acute — Ⓒ Immediate action — Ⓓ Referral to physician

Chronic — Ⓔ Education

Coughing and Breathing Exercises	
Pursed-lip breathing	Exhale against pursed lips to prolong exhalation and improve airway stability.
Abdominal/diaphragmatic breathing	Relax abdominal muscles during inspiration so that abdomen expands and allows diaphragm to descend.
Huff coughing	Say "huff" with forced expiration. Do with glottis open to prevent airway closure on expiration.
Respiratory muscle retraining	Breathe for 15 minutes at maximum ventilation.
Resistive breathing	Use a device that requires increased inspiratory force.

C. Acute shortness of breath requires immediate action to
- maintain a clear airway: remove secretions, open or insert airway
- facilitate breathing: position to promote chest expansion, remove constricting clothing
- promote gas exchange: encourage slow, deep breaths, consider oxygen if SaO_2 <90% or Po_2 <55 mmHg
- decrease anxiety

D. Medical intervention is often required for acute shortness of breath. Medications ordered depend on the pathology involved and may include
- antibiotics
- bronchodilators
- cardiac drugs
- oxygen therapy

Serial chest radiographs can be used to assess effectiveness of treatment. In severe instances, intubation and mechanical ventilation are necessary to sustain life. The patient and caregiver must receive information necessary to decide whether such treatment is consistent with their wishes and beliefs. Advocacy for patients' rights may become very important at this time.

E. Education should include that of both patient and caregiver. Topics include
- coughing and deep breathing (see box)
- nutrition and fluid intake
- signs and symptoms of respiratory infection
- avoidance of aggravating environmental factors
- energy conservation
- effective posture
  - sitting up
  - elbows on table
  - arms extended leaning forward
  - feet flat on floor
- signs and symptoms of cardiac decompensation
- medications: dosage and frequency, desired effects, side effects
- chest physiotherapy
- anxiety-reducing techniques

References

Hanley MV, Tyler ML. Ineffective airway clearance related to airway infection. Nurs Clin North Am 1987; 22:135.

Hoffman LA. Ineffective airway clearance related to neuromuscular dysfunction. Nurs Clin North Am 1987; 22:151.

Hopp LJ, Williams M. Ineffective breathing pattern related to decreased lung expansion. Nurs Clin North Am 1987; 22:193.

Kim MJ, Larson JL. Ineffective airway clearance and ineffective breathing patterns: Theoretical and research base for nursing diagnosis. Nurs Clin North Am 1987; 22:125.

Lareau S, Larson JL. Ineffective breathing pattern related to airflow limitation. Nurs Clin North Am 1987; 22:179.

Larson JL, Kim MJ. Ineffective breathing pattern related to respiratory muscle fatigue. Nurs Clin North Am 1987; 22:207.

Openbrier DR, Covey M. Ineffective breathing pattern related to malnutrition. Nurs Clin North Am 1987; 22:225.

Siskind NM. A standard of care for the nursing diagnosis of ineffective airway clearance. Heart Lung 1989; 18:5, 477.

VENOUS STASIS

Ruby Taylor

Venous stasis is slowing or stagnation of the flow of blood in the veins, a physiologic occlusion, caused by enlarged and inelastic veins that decrease functional blood volume and affect cardiac output, blood distribution, and tissue oxygenation. Venous flow, particularly from the lower extremities, is enhanced by the squeezing effect of muscles as they function. Lack of muscular activity or the presence of constricting garments allows blood to pool in dependent areas.

A. Determine whether the patient has experienced
    • itching
    • aching pain
    • sensation of heaviness
    • cramps
    • edema
    Ask the patient to describe actions that alleviate or exacerbate symptoms: e.g., does the edema resolve with elevation or overnight?

B. Physical examination should include observation of
    • redness
    • edema
    • dermatitis
    • skin temperature
    • dilated veins
    • shiny moist skin
    • peripheral cyanosis
    • peripheral pulses
    Dilatation and increased pressure of the veins in the upper extremities is observable because the neck veins do not collapse when the head is elevated. Monitor vital signs, noting the character of the pulses. A Doppler may be used for more accurate assessment of the pulse. Measure extremity girth with a tape measure.

C. Decrease systemic demand by
    • decreasing sodium intake
    • encouraging exercises that increase circulation in dependent areas
    • using elastic stockings
    • maintaining ideal body weight
    • avoiding caffeine, which constricts vessels and hampers blood flow
    • wearing clothes that are not too tight

D. Teach the patient
    • to report increase in symptoms
    • during periods of forced inactivity to
      • elevate the legs when possible
      • rest at intervals
      • avoid prolonged standing or sitting
      • exercise the calf muscles by flexing and extending the feet
    Teach the patient also to
    • exercise regularly
    • follow the medication regimen
    • wear therapeutic stockings
    • follow a prescribed diet

E. Physician referral is indicated for
    • pain unrelieved by nursing interventions
    • lack of pulses
    • open wounds

References

Bergen J, Yoa J. Venous problems. Chicago: Year Book, 1978.
Christ MA, Hohloch FJ. Gerontologic nursing: A study and learning tool. Springhouse, PA: Springhouse, 1988.
McCarthy ST. Peripheral vascular disease in the elderly. New York: Churchill Livingstone, 1983.

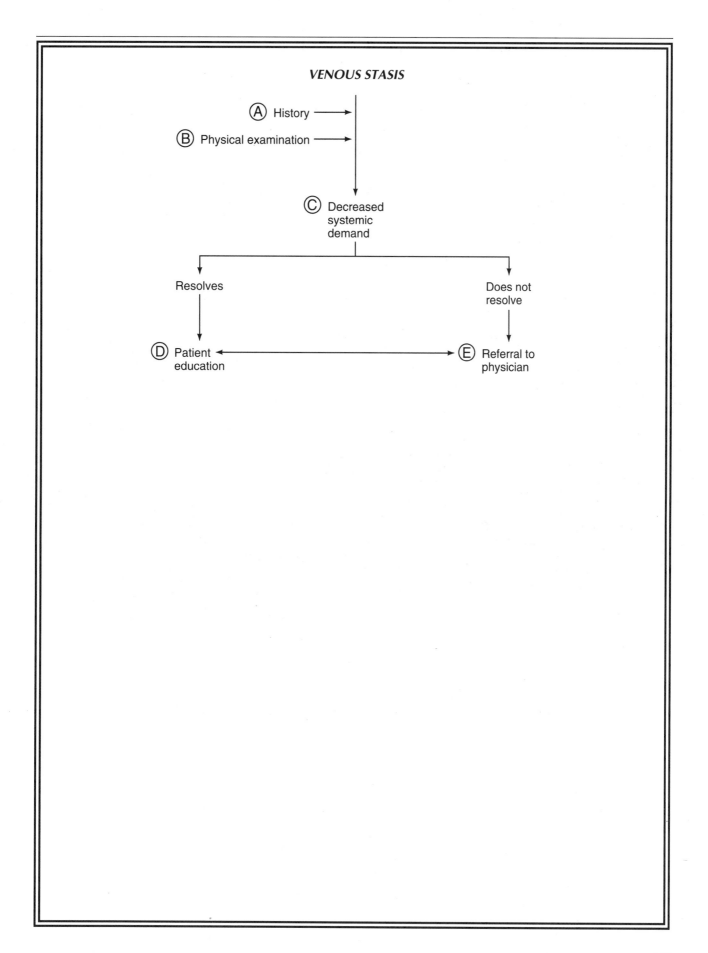

Placement and Interpretation of Doppler Procedure

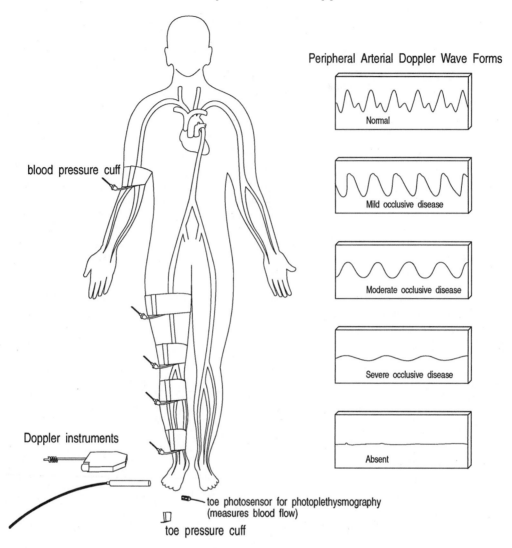

Peripheral Arterial Doppler Wave Forms

Normal

Mild occlusive disease

Moderate occlusive disease

Severe occlusive disease

Absent

blood pressure cuff

Doppler instruments

toe photosensor for photoplethysmography
(measures blood flow)

toe pressure cuff

Proper Elevation of Lower Extremities

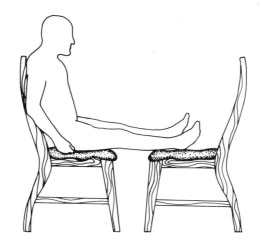

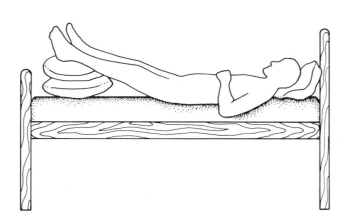

SEXUAL/REPRODUCTION

SEXUAL DYSFUNCTION

Jane H. Kass-Wolff

Sexuality is a central part of life. Because the most important sex organ is the brain, sexual pleasure and intimacy can be maintained, despite physical problems, at any age. Sexual activity in later years correlates with that during earlier years. The primary problem with sexual function for men is impotency and for women a lack of opportunity. Table 1 lists physiologic changes associated with aging.

A. Obtaining a history about sexual dysfunction requires sensitivity. Obtaining general health information before asking questions about sexual history may yield better information. Initial questions may rule out or identify physiologic, iatrogenic, or psychological contributors to sexual problems (see the box). Other questions include
   * for men:
     * when and where penile erections occur (In organic dysfunctions no nocturnal erections are present, whereas with psychogenic dysfunction, nocturnal erections occur.)
     * orgasm problems
     * description of what is meant by loss of erection
   * for women: pain during intercourse, occurrence of bleeding, orgasm problems

B. Physical examination focuses on
   * blood pressure
   * neurologic examination
   * genitourinary examination (see the box "Genitourinary Examination")

Contributors to Sexual Dysfunction	
Physiologic/Iatrogenic	*Psychological/Social*
Medications:	Partner relationship
Antihypertensives:	problems
thiazides, beta-blockers	Work-related stress
Central nervous system	Substance abuse
blocking agents	Emotional factors, such as
Psychotropic drugs:	anger, anxiety, fear,
antipsychotics, tricyclic	depression
antidepressants	Misconceptions regarding
Antiparkinsonians	sexual activity in later
Medical Problems:	years
Hypertension, diabetes	Ageism
mellitus, spinal cord	
disease or injury, heart	
disease, and rheumatoid	
arthritis or osteoarthritis	
Surgical Procedures:	
Prostatic resection,	
oophorectomy, and	
hysterectomy	
Fatigue	

---

   * rectal examination for masses and sphincter control
   * peripheral pulses
   * vibratory sense
   * range of motion

   Useful laboratory tests include
   * serum glucose level
   * complete blood count
   * liver panel
   * testosterone level
   * thyroid function tests
   * Pap smear

C. Medical evaluation by the primary care physician, urologist, gynecologist, or impotency specialist includes
   * diagnostic work-up
   * penile blood pressure with Doppler
   * evaluation of nocturnal penile tumescence, which measures erections occurring during sleep
   * exploration of surgical options, penile prosthesis
   * hormonal recommendations, i.e., testosterone or estrogen
   * investigation of alternative devices to achieve erection
   * medication review

   Additional testing can include arteriography, pulsed Doppler analysis, high-resolution ultrasonography, and direct neurophysiologic testing.

TABLE 1   Physiologic Changes with Aging

Sex	Aspect of Sexuality	Physiology
Male	Erection	Less full, decreased erectile angle
		Takes longer to achieve and disappears faster
		Manual stimulation necessary
		May require days to recover after orgasm
	Testicles	Do not fully elevate, decreased muscle tone
	Ejaculation	Lost sensation preceding ejaculation
	Sperm	Volume decreased
		May not be ejaculated
Female	Lubrication	May not occur due to lack of estrogen
Either sex	Position	Pathologic conditions may decrease range of motion

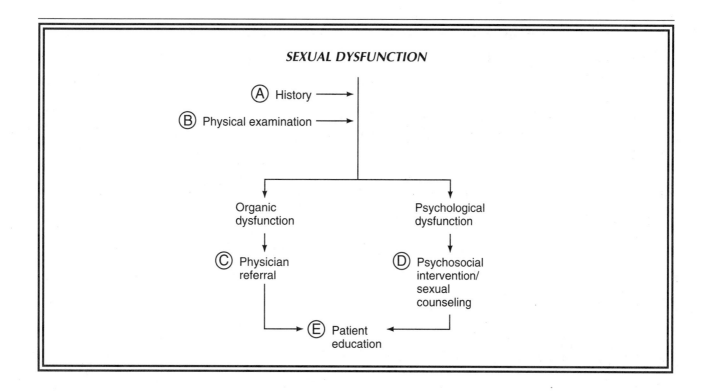

SEXUAL DYSFUNCTION

A. History
B. Physical examination

Organic dysfunction → C. Physician referral

Psychological dysfunction → D. Psychosocial intervention/ sexual counseling

E. Patient education

D. Support and reassurance in solving psychosocial contributors to sexual dysfunction are warranted. Referral to a social worker, sexual therapist, or counselor may be beneficial. Stress management and the development of communication techniques may provide useful skills toward ameliorating problems.

E. Patient and sexual partner education should include
- normal physiologic changes with aging
- importance of intimacy and ways to achieve satisfaction other than through sexual intercourse
- individual choice to be sexually active
- use of water-soluble lubricant during intercourse

Genitourinary Examination	
Female	*Male*
Cystocele	Testicular size
Rectocele	Hernia
Vaginal atrophy	Monilial infection of glans penis
Vaginal phimosis	Testes and epididymis: size, tenderness, inflammation
Vaginal discharge	Prostate
	Penile phimosis
	Hydrocele

References

Kolodny RC, Masters W, Johnson V, Biggs M. Textbook of human sexuality for nurses. Boston: Little, Brown, 1979.

Mason DR. Erectile dysfunctions: Assessment and care. Nurse Pract 1989; 14:23.

Sexual problems in the elderly: Men's vs women's. Geriatrics 1989; 44:75.

Thienhaus OJ. Practical overview of sexual function and advancing age. Geriatrics 1988; 43:63.

URETHRAL DISCHARGE

Jane H. Kass-Wolff

Urethral discharge may be associated with dysuria (see Irritative Voiding Symptoms [Dysuria, Frequency, Urgency, Pain], p. 202). The possibility of sexually transmitted disease (STD) must be considered despite the patient's age. Urethritis consists of inflammation of the urethra that occurs suddenly from acute infection or on a chronic basis. Urethral discharge is frequent in men but not usual in women.

A. History taking should include questions about
   • previous genitourinary problems or surgeries
   • previous STDs
   • current sexual behavior
   • onset of symptoms
   • precipitating factors
   • presence or absence of dysuria, including burning on urination, urgency, frequency, and nocturia
   • voiding history

B. Physical examination includes
   • vital signs
   • visualization of discharge when possible
   • external genitalia for redness, edema, and eversion of the meatus
   • inguinal lymph glands: tender and palpable?
   Laboratory evaluation is based on history and physical findings. Evaluative tests done may include
   • Gram's stain (Table 1) (diagnostic if positive in males; not diagnostic if positive in females)
   • Thayer-Martin culture or similar test for gonorrhea (see box below)
   • *Chlamydia* culture
   • syphilis serology
   If the Gram's stain is negative, it should be repeated in 24 hours. Instruct the patient not to urinate at least 4–8 hours before the examination. A second negative Gram's stain is followed by clean-catch midstream urine collection.

Obtaining a Urethral Swab

If no urethral discharge is present:
1. Obtain a urethral swab impregnated with calcium alginate
2. Insert the swab 2 cm into the anterior urethra
3. Roll the swab on a microscope slide
4. Z-track the swab on Thayer-Martin culture medium if a gonorrhea culture is desired

---

TABLE 1 Gram's Stain Result Analysis

Result	Findings
Gonococcus negative	No gram-negative diplococci (GND) found within polymorphonuclear leukocytes (PMNs) Many PMNs present 15 or more PMNs per high-power field indicates need for treatment for nongonococcal urethritis
Borderline	Gram-negative diplococci found, either atypical or extracellular
Gonococcus positive	Gram-negative diplococci found within PMNs

TABLE 2 Nongonococcal Urethritis (NGU)

Variable	Description
Types	*Chlamydia trachomatis* *Ureaplasma urealyticum*
Incubation	1–5 wk, peak 2 wk
Discharge:	
Appearance	Mucoid or watery in appearance
Presence	Less spontaneous 80% have discharge with stripping of urethra May be present only on arising in morning when bladder is full
Complications if not treated	Epididymitis (2%) Conjunctivitis Reiter's syndrome in genetically predisposed patients

C. If no STD is present, evaluate to determine a cause:
   • urethritis (Table 2)
   • cystitis
   • incontinence
   • prostatitis
   • epididymitis

D. If STD is diagnosed, sexual partners should be examined, treated, and instructed not to have intercourse until they return for a test of cure in 2 weeks. Report confirmed cases of STD to the state/local health department. Referral for drug therapy is indicated if not operating within protocols. Drug treatment depends on the organism found. *Neisseria gonorrhoeae* is treated with ceftriaxone and doxycycline according to CDC guidelines. NGU is treated with doxycycline, 100 mg twice daily for 2 weeks, unless the patient is allergic. Follow-up is needed only if symptoms persist or return after completion of treatment.

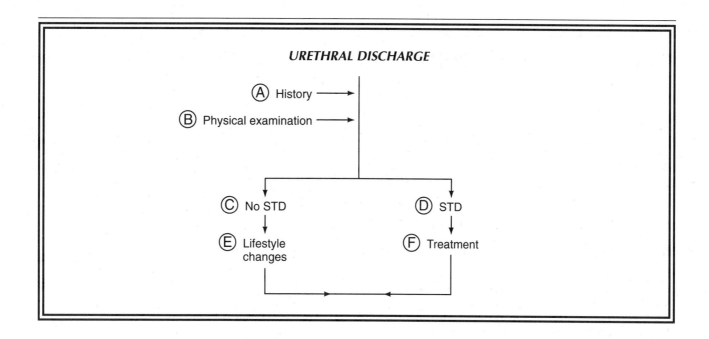

URETHRAL DISCHARGE

A. History

B. Physical examination

C. No STD → E. Lifestyle changes

D. STD → F. Treatment

E. Lifestyle changes to recommend include
- protected sex (condoms)
- use of a water-soluble lubricant during sex
- showers instead of baths
- avoidance of bubble baths, perfumed sprays, and feminine hygiene sprays
- avoidance of nylon undergarments, pantyhose, and constricting clothing
- proper hygiene (see box)

Proper Hygiene	
Men	*Women*
• Cleansing of glans penis • If not circumcised, retracting foreskin and cleansing thoroughly	• Wiping from urethra to anus (front to back) after toileting • Perineal cleansing after intercourse

F. Treatment focuses on the administration of systemic and/or topical antibiotics for positive test results and infection. Sitz baths and forcing fluids provide relief of symptoms of urethritis. Sexual intercourse should be avoided until treatment is completed. Lifestyle changes are advisable.

References

1989 Sexually transmitted diseases treatment guidelines. MMWR 1989; 38:5.

Bowie WR. Urethritis in males. In: Holmes KK, et al, eds. Sexually transmitted diseases. 2nd ed. New York: McGraw-Hill, 1990:638.

Holmes KK, et al, eds. Sexually transmitted diseases. 2nd ed. New York: McGraw-Hill, 1990.

Reilly B. Practical strategies in outpatient medicine. 2nd ed. Philadelphia: WB Saunders, 1991.

Stamm W, Kaetz S, Beirne M, Ashman J. The practitioner's handbook for the management of STD's. Seattle: Health Services Center for Educational Resources, 1988.

HOT FLASHES (VASOMOTOR INSTABILITY)

Carolyn M. Sutton

A physiologic response to estrogen deficiency present in over 50% of women after cessation of menstrual activity is vasomotor instability, commonly referred to as hot flashes. Hot flashes may continue for women in their seventies and eighties. Hot flashes are more common at night, lasting for seconds to minutes; are a feeling of heat within or on the body that spreads; and may be accompanied by flushing or change in skin color. Estrogen therapy is very effective in improving vasomotor symptoms. Concomitant progestin therapy is advised when the uterus is intact.

A. History-taking collects data about
- menstrual history including last normal menstrual period and menopause symptoms, such as
  - amenorrhea
  - vaginal dryness
  - dysuria, urgency, frequency
  - hot flashes
  - dyspareunia
- obstetric and gynecologic history: vaginal bleeding, breast, uterus
- family history: breast or endometrial cancer or coronary artery disease or hyperlipidemia
- personal history
  - cardiovascular disease
- thromboembolic disease
- liver disease
- gallbladder disease
- factors related to osteoporosis: sedentary lifestyle, calcium-poor diet, decrease in height

B. Physical examination assesses
- thyroid
- external and internal genitalia
- heart and lungs
- breasts
- abdomen
- uterus and adnexa
- rectum

Record height, weight, and blood pressure. Obtain mammogram, and investigate any abnormal findings before treatment. Obtain the following laboratory data
- complete blood count
- thyroid function studies
- fasting blood sugar
- liver profile
- lipid profile
- Pap smear with maturation index

TABLE 1   Hormone Replacement Regimens

Regimen	Administration	Comments
Cyclic therapy	Conjugated estrogen (Premarin), 0.625 or 1.25 mg, given days 1 to 25 *with* medroxyprogesterone acetate (Provera), 5 to 10 mg given days 14 to 25 *or* Conjugated estrogen (Premarin), 0.625 or 1.25 mg, given every day *with* medroxyprogesterone acetate (Provera), 5 to 10 mg, given days 1 to 10	Use lowest dose that relieves symptoms Based on calendar month Most commonly prescribed regimen in United States Progestin therapy needs to be at least 10 days, preferably 12 to 14 days, to prevent endometrial hyperplasia Cyclic withdrawal bleeding may lead to noncompliance with regimen Bleeding other than upon withdrawal requires an endometrial biopsy
Combined continuous low-dose therapy	Conjugated estrogen (Premarin), 0.625 mg daily, *with* medroxyprogesterone acetate (Provera), 2.5 mg or 5 mg daily	High prevalence of endometrial atrophy Promotes amenorrhea
Posthysterectomy	Conjugated estrogen (Premarin), 0.625 mg daily	No need for cycling No clear indication for progestin
Transdermal estradiol	Estraderm, 0.05 mg/24 hours, changed twice a week (every 3.5 days) (0.05 mg patch = 0.625 mg Premarin)	Rotate skin sites No metabolic effects of oral estrogen, including beneficial lipid effects Add oral progestin for 10 to 12 days per month if uterus is intact
Progestins	Medroxyprogesterone acetate (Provera), 20 mg orally daily *or* Medroxyprogesterone acetate injectable (Depo-Provera), 150 mg IM every 3 months	Use when estrogen therapy is contraindicated No beneficial effects on vagina and uterus

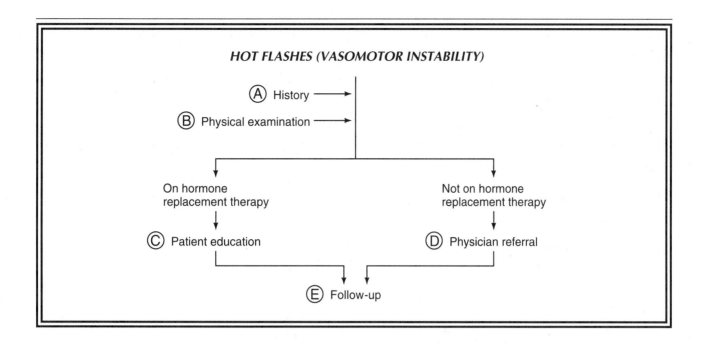

HOT FLASHES (VASOMOTOR INSTABILITY)

Ⓐ History

Ⓑ Physical examination

On hormone replacement therapy

Not on hormone replacement therapy

Ⓒ Patient education

Ⓓ Physician referral

Ⓔ Follow-up

C. Instruct patients concerning medication administration—purpose, dosage regimen, side effects. Patients should report problems, such as
- headaches
- hot flashes despite taking hormone replacement prescribed
- vaginal bleeding other than predictable withdrawal bleeding

D. If not functioning under a protocol, refer the patient to a physician for institution of hormone replacement therapy (Table 1). Referral for endometrial biopsy may also be in order to rule out developing hyperplasia or endometrial carcinoma before initiation of hormone replacement. Women who have a contraindication to estrogen therapy should be referred to a primary care physician or gynecologist.

E. Once exogenous hormones are initiated, periodic follow-up is necessary to evaluate the effectiveness of therapy and development of adverse side effects. Women receiving hormone replacement therapy should be examined and evaluated 3 months after initiation and at least annually thereafter. A breast and pelvic examination should be performed at these visits as well as monitoring of blood pressure, height, and weight.

References

Kjervik D, Martinson IM. Women in health and illness: Life experiences and crisis. Philadelphia: WB Saunders, 1986.

Ladewig P. Protocol for estrogen replacement therapy in menopausal women. Nurs Pract 1985; 10:44.

Nachtigall LE, Nachtigall RD. Evaluating the newly menopausal woman. Contemporary OB/Gyn 1985; 25:68.

Voda AM. Coping with the menopausal hot flash. Patient Counseling and Health Education 1982; 4:81.

VAGINAL DISCHARGE/BLEEDING

Carolyn M. Sutton

Vaginal discharge or bleeding may signal a benign, self-limiting, or life-threatening condition at any age. Be careful not to discount complaints of vaginal discharge or bleeding from postmenopausal women.

A. To compile an accurate database, ask about
   - chronic medical problems
   - current medications, prescription and over the counter
   - gynecologic history
     - menstrual problems
     - gynecologic surgeries, hysterectomy
     - menopause history
     - incidence of vaginitis, sexually transmitted diseases, or pelvic inflammatory disease
   - history of bleeding or discharge
     - onset
     - precipitating factors
     - duration
     - treatments used
     - other symptoms present
   - history of genital cancer
   - family history of genital cancer

B. Physical examination includes
   - blood pressure measurement
   - evaluation for volume deficit
   - breast examination
   - inspection of the vulva, vagina, and cervix for
     - hygiene
     - size
     - color
     - symmetry
     - lesions/polyps
     - vaginal discharge
       - color
       - amount
       - consistency
       - odor
     - inflammation
   - palpation of uterus and adnexal structures
     - size
     - tenderness
     - masses
   Laboratory evaluation may include
   - CBC
   - wet mount of vaginal secretions using saline and/or potassium hydroxide (KOH) to determine the involved organism
   - determination of vaginal pH
   - Papanicolaou smear with maturation index

C. Vaginal discharge may signal inflammation or infection of the vagina, cervix, or uterus because of
   - mechanical injury
   - pathogens causing vaginitis/cervicitis/endometritis (Table 1)
   Vaginal discharge may also occur as a normal physiologic response to changes in estrogen levels. When no pathologic organism is found in a postmenopausal woman, consider atrophic vaginitis (see Vaginal Dryness/Itching [Atrophic Vaginitis], p. 246).

D. Vaginal bleeding may be caused by
   - mechanical injury
   - irritation
   - malignancy
   Use vaginal examination to rule out mechanical injury or irritation due to atrophic vaginitis (see Vaginal Dryness/Itching [Atrophic Vaginitis], p. 246). If the cause of bleeding is not apparent, refer the patient for medical evaluation. The extent of vaginal bleeding may be difficult to determine by history or a single examination. Evaluation of CBC, especially hemoglobin and hematocrit, may be needed.

TABLE 1 Vaginal Discharge Identification

Problem	Characteristics of Discharge
Trichomonas vaginalis vaginitis	Heavy greenish-white or yellow Frothy Slightly malodorous
Candida albicans vaginitis	Thick white or yellow Curdlike Moderate amount
Bacterial vaginosis	Gray Malodorous Profuse
Mucopurulent cervicitis (often caused by *Chlamydia trachomatis*)	Thick, mucoid Purulent Blood-tinged
Gonorrhea	Purulent, yellow Small amount

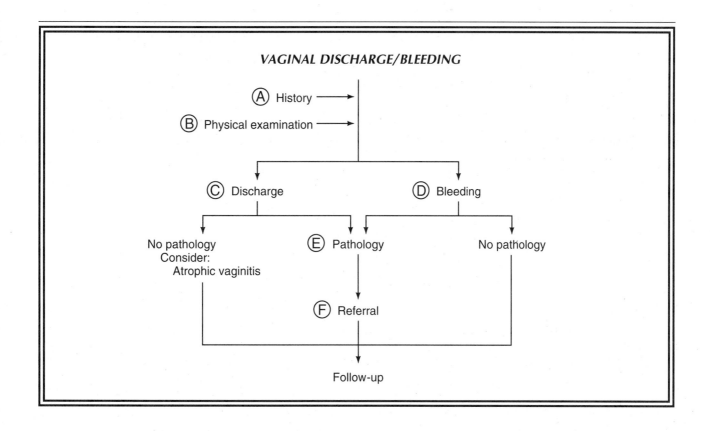

VAGINAL DISCHARGE/BLEEDING

E. When a pathologic cause of vaginal discharge or bleeding is found, referral should be made for medical treatment (see box below). Surgical intervention should be based on cytology of biopsy or Papanicolaou smear and clinical findings.

F. A referral to the primary care physician or gynecologist is indicated for pathologic clinical findings or medication. If functioning under protocols, treat accordingly for specific diagnostic findings.

Possible Medical Treatment	
Problem	*Treatment*
Vaginal discharge	Local or systemic antibiotics Treatment of sexual partner
Vaginal bleeding	Replacement of blood as needed Hormonal therapy (see Hot Flashes, p. 242) Surgical intervention

References

ACOG Technical Bulletin. Estrogen replacement therapy. April 1986; 93.

Kistner RW. Gynecology: Principles and practice. Chicago: Year Book, 1986.

Mishell DR, Brenner PF. Management of common problems in obstetrics and gynecology. Oradell, NJ: Medical Economics Books, 1983.

Speroff L, Glass R, Kase N. Clinical gynecologic endocrinology and infertility. Baltimore: Williams & Wilkins, 1983.

VAGINAL DRYNESS OR ITCHING (ATROPHIC VAGINITIS)

Carolyn M. Sutton

Dramatic changes occur in estrogen-dependent target tissues such as the vaginal epithelium at menopause (see box below). In some cases, atrophic vaginitis may develop with bleeding, itching, burning, and dyspareunia. Atrophic vaginitis can cause symptoms similar to a urinary tract infection, including frequency, urgency, and urge incontinence. These symptoms are not uncommon in women in their late 50s, 60s, and 70s.

A. History taking focuses on
   - menstrual history
   - current symptoms
   - change in soaps or detergents
   - use of feminine hygiene sprays or douches
   - medications, including estrogens
   - endometrial biopsy data
   - medical conditions, especially contraindications to systemic estrogen therapy
     - impaired liver function
     - vascular thrombolytic disease
     - undiagnosed vaginal bleeding
     - estrogen-dependent neoplasia of the
       - breast
       - uterus
       - vagina
     - family history of breast cancer
     - familial hyperlipidemia
     - seizure disorder
     - migraine
     - moderate to severe hypertension

B. In pelvic examination, inspect the vulva, vagina, and cervix for
   - hygiene
   - size
   - color
   - skin texture
   - symmetry
   - lesions
   - lumps or nodules
   - vaginal discharge if present
     - color
     - amount
     - consistency
     - odor
   - bleeding
   - vulvar inflammation

A foul-smelling discharge may suggest necrotic tissue or poor hygiene. If the vulva is inflamed, consider the possibility of an allergic reaction. Helpful laboratory tests to differentiate the cause of vaginal discharge include
   - wet mount evaluation of vaginal secretions using normal saline and/or potassium hydroxide (KOH)
   - determination of vaginal pH
   - Papanicolaou smear with maturation index

Normal vaginal pH is 3.5–4.0. A maturation index showing primarily parabasal cells is consistent with minimal or absent estrogen effect. Bacteriuria and pyuria can occur with urethritis in the presence of atrophic vaginitis. Vaginal secretions may reveal RBCs, many WBCs, and no other pathogens. Clinical findings with atrophic vaginitis may include
   - sterile urine
   - vulva
     - no visible lesions
     - tissue surrounding the introitus may appear atrophic and dry
   - vaginal canal
     - pale
     - smooth
     - thin and friable mucosa
   - discharge
     - scant
     - thin
     - yellowish
     - blood-tinged
   - vaginal pH of 6.5–7.5
   - KOH wet mount: no budding hyphae and a negative whiff

C. When there are pathologic findings, medical evaluation is indicated to rule out and treat benign gynecologic conditions or malignancy.

D. The most effective treatment for postmenopausal atrophic vaginitis is local or systemic estrogen supplementation. Advantages to systemic administration are that the absorption rate of the medication is predictable and concomitant treatment of vaginitis can occur. Topical estrogen in the form of vaginal cream is useful when oral estrogen is contraindicated or when only local symptom relief is sought. The aim of therapy is to restore vaginal moisture and thicken vaginal epithelium.

Postmenopausal Vaginal Changes

Physiologic Change	Observable Change
Decreased glycogen within epithelial cells	Smooth, shiny vaginal epithelium
Increased pH	Increased susceptibility to infection and trauma
Reduced thickness of epithelium	Smooth, shiny surface

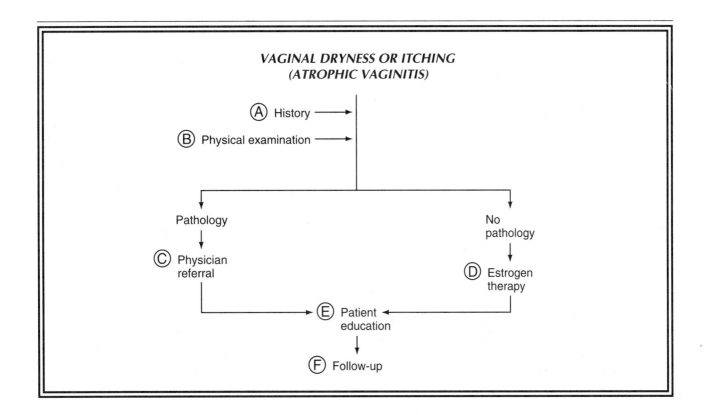

**VAGINAL DRYNESS OR ITCHING
(ATROPHIC VAGINITIS)**

Ⓐ History

Ⓑ Physical examination

Pathology

Ⓒ Physician referral

No pathology

Ⓓ Estrogen therapy

Ⓔ Patient education

Ⓕ Follow-up

E. Patient instructions should include
- medication/estrogen therapy (see Table 1 in Hot Flashes, p. 242)
  - purpose
  - dosage regimen
  - possible side effects
- reporting
  - breakthrough bleeding
  - excessive weight gain
  - tender or enlarged breasts
  - increased vaginal discharge
- use of water-soluble lubricant during sex
- maintenance of vaginal tone with regular sexual activity
- routine performance of Kegel or pelvic muscle exercises (see the tool *Modified Kegel Exercises* [*Pelvic Muscle Exercises for the Incontinent*], p. 216)

F. Postmenopausal women receiving exogenous estrogens should be examined 3 months after the therapy is initiated, and annually thereafter. Follow-up should include examination of
- blood pressure
- weight
- height
- pelvic organs
- breasts

References

Kistner RW. Gynecology: Principles and practice. Chicago: Mosby—Year Book, Inc., 1986.

Mishell DR, Brenner PF. Management of common problems in obstetrics and gynecology. Oradell, NJ: Medical Economics Books, 1983.

Speroff L, Glass R, Kase N. Clinical gynecologic endocrinology and infertility. Baltimore: Williams & Wilkins, 1983.

Psychosocial

COGNITION/PERCEPTION

AGGRESSIVE BEHAVIOR

Deborah Antai-Otong

Impaired cognition and feelings of losing control increase the risk of aggressive behaviors in the elderly. Aggression frequently results from sensory impairments that increase feelings of anxiety, suspiciousness, and paranoia. Patients with sensory loss or immobility often experience a loss of control over their environment and lack social support, which results in increased anxiety and aggressive behaviors such as physical and verbal abuse.

A. History taking should include
  • the time of day of aggressive behavior
  • precipitating factors or situations such as activities of daily living (ADL)
  • actions or environmental manipulations that alleviate behavior
  • memory deficits
  • ability to participate in ADL
  • medications
  • previous response to psychotropic agents
  When possible, determine from caregivers how the patient responds to touch.

B. A complete physical examination is indicated to rule out sources of pain, discomfort, or acute illness. In addition, specific assessment should target
  • thorough mental status evaluation (see Confusion/Cognitive Changes/Dementia, p. 254)
  • orientation
  • observed level of functioning
  Note interactions between caregivers and patient. Observe general appearance, gait, eye contact, and response to physical stimuli.

C. Physiologic changes that may precipitate aggressive behavior include
  • sleep disturbances (see Sleep Pattern Disturbances, p. 82)
  • impaired ADL (see Inability to Perform Activities of Daily Living, p. 6)
  • decreased sensation (see Decreased Sensation, p. 138)
  • decreased vision (see Decreased Vision, p. 118)
  • hearing loss (see Hearing Loss, p. 122)
  These physiologic changes may result in feelings of loss of control or helplessness that may trigger aggressive behavior in an attempt to gain control in some form.

D. Cognitive changes (see Confusion/Cognitive Changes/Dementia, p. 254) may produce aggressive behavior to combat fear, anxiety, or suspiciousness. Reactions to psychoactive drugs may be manifest in this way and should be eliminated as the cause of such behavior.

E. Life needs to be predictable. Common precipitating situations for aggressive behaviors include
  • changes in caregivers or unfamiliar visitors
  • disruptions in schedule or routine
  • ADL such as bathing
  • the onset of evening or dusk
  Disorientation or confusion at dusk, which may or may not be associated with aggression, is known as "sundowner" syndrome (see Confusion/Cognitive Changes/Dementia, p. 254).

F. Daily exercise, recreational or occupational therapy, must be included to allow and encourage independent functioning. Active and inactive range of motion exercises or daily walks improve the cardiovascular system and enhance self-esteem and social interaction. Such activity provides a physical outlet for the tension and frustration that often result from immobility and helplessness. Patients should be allowed to make decisions about daily activities and treatment schedules whenever possible. Choices as simple as menu items provide the capable patient with a sense of control or autonomy.

G. Ongoing reality orientation to surroundings and caregivers may decrease confusion and aggressive behaviors. Therapeutic communication skills include
  • a calm, soft voice
  • introducing oneself to the patient
  • a caring, firm manner
  • simple statements or explanations

H. Environmental control measures can encompass
  • adherence to a routine: same time, same place, same thing
  • maintenance of familiar caregivers
  • use of appropriate lighting (see Confusion/Cognitive Changes/Dementia, p. 254)
  If resistance to ADL and preliminary signs of aggressive behavior are evident, the following techniques may prove useful:
  • defer activity until later; do not insist upon or confront the patient with it
  • pair an unwelcome procedure (e.g., bathing) with a patient preference (e.g., eating ice cream, drinking a beverage)
  • sing or accompany activities with music
  • use a bubble bath

I. Touch may provide a calming effect, but be aware that some patients respond negatively to touch. They also can generally sense staff or caregiver anxiety, anger, or other emotions. Restraints should be considered as

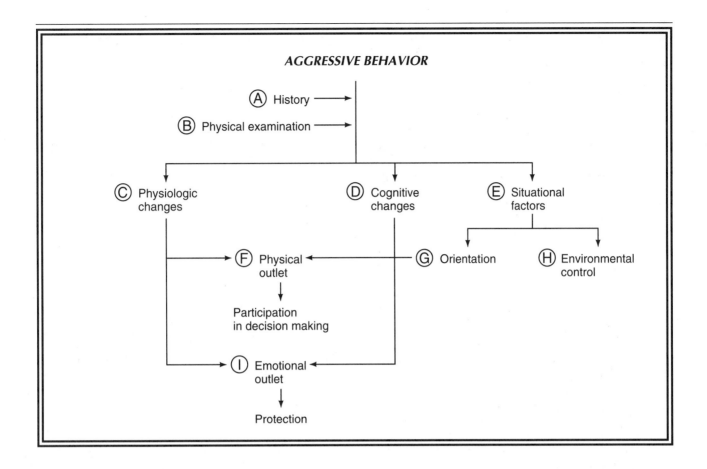

AGGRESSIVE BEHAVIOR

(A) History

(B) Physical examination

(C) Physiologic changes

(D) Cognitive changes

(E) Situational factors

(F) Physical outlet

(G) Orientation

(H) Environmental control

Participation in decision making

(I) Emotional outlet

Protection

a last resort to help patients gain control. The least restrictive choice of restraint is always most prudent. Begin with side rails or a Posey belt before using restraints on extremities. A low-dose neuroleptic or anxiolytic medication may be used to alleviate extreme anxiety, agitation, or fears. Observe for side effects, including
- sedation
- hypotension
- postural hypotension
- extrapyramidal symptoms such as drooling, dystonia, or tremors

Monitor vital signs before and after drugs are administered.

References

Antai-Otong DJ. Psychopharmacology. In: Johnson BS, ed. Psychiatric mental health nursing: Adaptation and growth. 2nd ed. Philadelphia: JB Lippincott, 1989:268.

Burgess AW. Psychiatric nursing in the hospital and the community. 4th ed. Englewood Cliffs, NJ: Prentice-Hall, 1985.

Mentes JC, Ferrario J. Calming aggressive reactions: A preventive program. J Gerontol Nurs 1989; 15:22, 35.

Winger J, Schirm V, Stewart D. Aggressive behavior in long term care. J Psychosoc Nurs Ment Health Serv 1987; 25:28, 38.

AGITATION

Catherine A. Hill

Excessive motor activity, short attention span, difficulty in completing a task, and destructive tendencies signal agitation in the elderly. Agitation may be a symptom of anxiety, suspiciousness, or aggression (see pp. 250, 264, and 278); a side effect of drug therapy; or an indication of a physiologic problem that the patient cannot articulate.

A. Gather information about
    • agitation
      • onset
      • duration
      • precipitating factors
      • alleviating factors
      • exacerbating factors
      • patterns of hyperactivity
      • alteration in attention span
      • difficulty in completing tasks
      • destructive activities
    • response to stimuli: environmental, psychosocial, physical
    • sleep and activity habits
    • ability to perform activities of daily living
    • nutrition and hydration
    • medical history: chronic illnesses, injuries, psychiatric history
    • medication history: current prescription and over-the-counter drugs, alcohol or recreational drug use, caffeine intake
    • psychosocial factors: coping skills, past use of violence, attention-seeking behaviors, support systems
    • fatigue (see p. 14)
    • toileting patterns

B. Physical examination evaluates
    • general appearance
      • restlessness
      • extraneous movements
      • hypersensitivity to noise or light
      • skin color and temperature
      • respiratory effort
    • mental status (see tools in Cognition/Perception Section), including
      • cognition
      • crying or angry behavior
      • violence or catastrophic reactions
      • mood and affect
      • aggressive behavior
    • neurologic status: sensory impairment, communication, reflexes, muscle tension
    • elimination: abdominal distention, constipation or impaction, urinary retention
    Laboratory tests to obtain include
    • complete blood count with differential
    • electrolytes and glucose
    • sedimentation rate
    • therapeutic drug levels
    • urinalysis
    • urine culture and sensitivity
    • oxygen saturation

C. Management and education to assist patient and caregivers with behavior control require a plan to
    • structure activities
    • remove patient from upsetting situations
    • alter the environment to decrease number and amount of stimuli by using soft music and soothing colors or removing abstract or confusing paintings or wall coverings
    • distract or redirect activities rather than criticize
    • communicate a calm, open manner verbally and nonverbally
      • approach with a relaxed, friendly expression
      • identify yourself
      • get patient's attention
      • use simple words
      • ask only one question at a time
      • orient the patient in a reassuring manner
    • assess for signs of pain, discomfort, need to toilet: grimacing, restlessness, or sudden onset of agitation
    • provide physical activity
    • schedule consistent caregivers
    • provide for physical safety by
      • removing contraband, sharps, or items that may cause harm
      • placing bed in low position
      • using siderails open at the end, if needed
      • avoiding restraints

D. Referrals may prove necessary for treatment of physical or psychological disorders. Intervention with psychoactive agents should follow correction or treatment of physical problems. Physical problems that may require medical treatment include
    • oxygen desaturation
    • electrolyte imbalances
    • urinary retention
    • drug levels not in therapeutic range
    • uncontrolled diabetes
    • adverse drug reactions
    • urinary tract infection
    Psychoactive drug therapy, when appropriate, includes low-dose major tranquilizers: haloperidol or thioridazine, or tricyclic antidepressants in the presence of depression. Pharmacologic agents are prescribed to alleviate uncomfortable symptoms for patients. Medications should be used not to act as a chemical restraint but rather to promote socially acceptable behaviors.

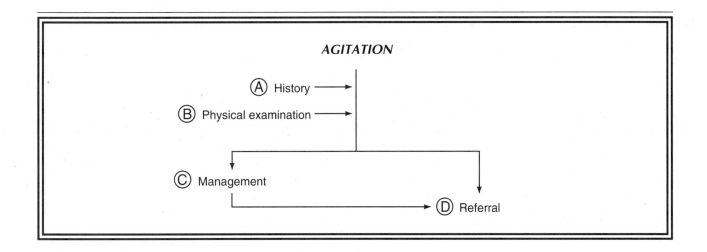

References

Burnside I. Nursing and the aged. 4th ed. New York: McGraw-Hill, 1988:55.

Maas M, Buckwalter KC, Hardy M. Nursing diagnoses and interventions for the elderly. Redwood City, CA: Addison Wesley, 1991:460.

Verwoerdt A. Clinical geropsychiatry. 2nd ed. Baltimore: Williams & Wilkins, 1981:72.

CONFUSION/COGNITIVE CHANGES/DEMENTIA

Deborah Antai-Otong

Confusion is a common description of many unspecified behaviors. For clinical purposes, confusion is defined as impairment of the following that results in functional limitations:
- cognition
- short- and long-term memory
- judgment
- orientation
- abstract thinking
- decision making

Dementia is another term used to describe the loss of brain function, the degenerative changes, and the accompanying clinical presentation. A clear distinction among dementia, delirium, and depression is essential (see Depression, p. 282). Dementias that arise from degenerative changes usually have an insidious course with lasting symptoms. Delirium, or an acute confusional state, may arise from infection, medications, or acute illness and may have a rapid onset and short duration. Delirium is life threatening. Symptoms include memory loss with the need to make frequent lists and notes. Patients often rationalize the forgetfulness. Confused patients often have labile moods and personality changes and may be apathetic. There is diminished concern for physical appearance and personal hygiene. The latter phase may be marked by extreme apathy and impairment in mental, sensory, and motor function. At this stage, patients may be bedridden and incontinent of stool and urine.

A. Ideally, the history should be obtained from the patient with collaboration from the family or significant others. Information to be gathered concerns
- onset and duration of confusion and cognitive impairment
- arteriosclerotic complications (cerebrovascular accidents, myocardial infarctions)
- hypertension
- psychiatric treatment, including previous treatment for depression
- prescribed and over-the-counter medications
- medication compliance
- alcohol use
- auditory or visual hallucinations
- recent losses
- head trauma or injury
- venereal disease

B. Make initial observations on general appearance, gait, and eye contact. Note interactions between caregivers and patients. Perform a neurologic examination to discover focal neurologic lesions. Specific mental status evaluation assesses
- affect
- cognitive functioning
- judgment
- orientation
- memory

Specific tools used to perform this evaluation are the Folstein Mini Mental State or short portable mental status examination and the tool *Geriatric Depression Scale* (see p. 268). Neuropsychological tests that assess cognitive functioning can help describe deficits and strengths more fully. Vision and hearing screening will identify sensory deprivation. Impaired sensory input may cause or contribute to confusion (see Hearing Loss, p. 122, and Decreased Vision, p. 118). Laboratory work-up aims at ruling out physical or chemical causes of confusion. Recommended routine testing includes
- chemistry panel
- CBC with differential
- sedimentation rate
- VDRL/RPR
- vitamin B_{12} and folate

Therapeutic blood levels of drugs the patient is taking may also be required. CT scan of the head is used to rule out normal-pressure hydrocephalus, intracranial lesions, or infarcts, particularly if gait changes occur. MRI may replace or be adjunctive to CT.

C. A safe, consistent environment may reorient the patient and assist in decreasing confusion and the agitation or delusions that may result. Caregivers should announce their presence and explain all procedures before beginning. Safety measures include
- clocks, calendars, and other visual clues to time and place
- activity schedule boards or lists
- well-lighted rooms
- noise control

Additional interventions may be necessary to ensure the safety of patients who experience "sun-downing" (increasing confusion at dusk). Strategies to distract patients during twilight include
- covering windows and turning on lights before dusk
- planning specific diversion or activity
- scheduling bedtime before sun-down

No single system has been universally successful in reducing the effects of sun-downing, and the phenomenon is still not clearly understood.

D. Therapeutic interventions may require referral to other health care professionals. Nursing interventions aim to protect patients from harm, increase patient orientation, and support caregivers. Medications used to treat confusion may include low-dose neuroleptics or anxiolytics (see Anger, p. 276). Ensure that these are taken regularly to maintain clinical efficiency. Physical restraint for aggressive or violent behavior should be used as a last resort after medications and reorientation measures have failed to ensure safety for the patient, other patients and staff. Nutrition assessment and referral is indicated when malnutrition is sus-

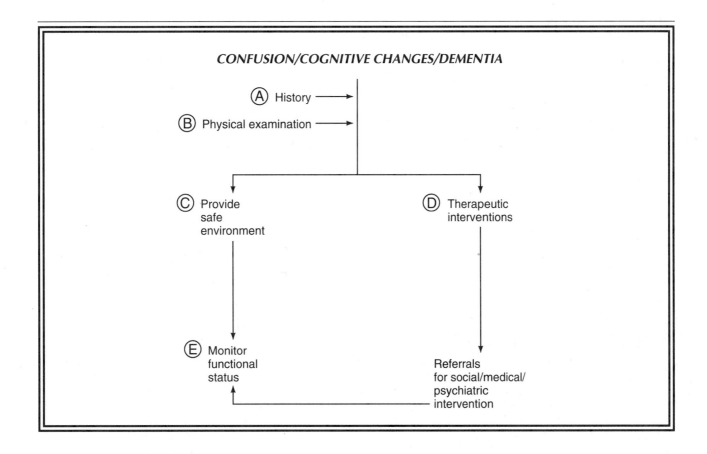

CONFUSION/COGNITIVE CHANGES/DEMENTIA

pected on the basis of findings from the history and physical examination. Nutritional support becomes critical when confusion results in functional decline.

E. With progressive decline in functional abilities, support and services are indicated. Ongoing monitoring is necessary to facilitate referrals to community and health care resources.

References

American Psychiatric Association. Diagnostic and statistical manual of mental disorders. 3rd ed, revised. Washington, DC: American Psychiatric Association, 1987:103.

Antai-Otong DJ. Psychopharmacology. In: Johnson BS, ed. Psychiatric mental health nursing. Philadelphia: JB Lippincott, 1989:268.

Berg R, Franzen M, Wedding D. Screening for brain impairment: A manual for mental health practice. New York: Springer, 1987.

For more information contact:
Alzheimer's Association
70 E. Lake St.
Chicago, IL 60601-5997
(1-800-621-0379)

INAPPROPRIATE SEXUAL BEHAVIOR

Kay Peterson

Sexual behavior deemed inappropriate includes display of body parts or functions or behaviors that are usually carried on in private or between consenting participants. Inappropriate sexual behavior may be manifest as a result of
- changes in cognitive function, progressive dementias
- decreased inhibition control secondary to cerebral tissue loss from a cerebrovascular accident (CVA) or transient ischemic attacks
- life-long difficulty dealing with sexuality
- anxiety
- impaired self-concept
- side effects of medications

A. Information to obtain in history taking includes
   - previous and current coping skills
   - medical history, especially CVA and psychological disorders and medications
   - recent injury, particularly head injury
   Ask specific questions about
   - the meaning of sexual behavior to the patient
   - fears, including loss of identity
   - the need for closeness
   - the level of anxiety during sexual behavior
   - the time, frequency, and setting in which behaviors occur (e.g., in relation to a need to toilet)
   - satisfaction with sexuality
   - beliefs regarding sexual function
   - the consequences for the patient and others of performing behaviors

B. Physical examination evaluates
   - cognitive function (see Confusion/Cognitive Changes/Dementia, p. 254)
   - neuromuscular control, particularly spastic limb movements or loss of gross motor coordination
   - dementia laboratory screen, including serum electrolytes; renal, liver, and thyroid function tests; and vitamin B_{12} and folate levels
   Observe for aggressive behavior (see Aggressive Behavior, p. 250). Ask the patient to bring all medication bottles (prescription and over the counter) to be reviewed.

C. Inappropriate sexual behavior may result from hormonal or neurologic changes. Substances that may affect sexual functioning or behavior include sedatives, narcotics, psychotropics, antidepressants, antihypertensives, antispasmodics, and alcohol. If changes in behavior coincide with the initiation of a minor tranquilizer, steroid, or antihypertensive, the medication should be suspected as the cause. With progressive loss of cerebral tissue, patients become increasingly disoriented. Consequently, sexual behavior may be inappropriate because of the time and place rather than the nature of the behavior itself.

D. Medical evaluation or intervention may be necessary if the cause of inappropriate sexual behavior is determined to be physiologic. Some physiologic causes are irreversible. Medication regimens should be reviewed to rule out iatrogenic effects; changes may be warranted. Monitor response to medication changes closely. Patients may require additional education regarding drug or food interactions.

E. Patient/caregiver education should emphasize the broader aspects of human sexuality (e.g., closeness, touch, sensuality). The environment can be changed to allow privacy and encourage others to respect the privacy and sexual needs of the patient. Removing the patient from a provocative setting should be recommended. Behavior can be targeted for stimulus control by identifying the
   - setting in which the behavior occurs
   - nature of the behavior
   - time of day
   - patient's level of awareness/orientation
   - precipitating factors, if any
   - immediate consequences for the patient and others
   A positive reinforcement system can be implemented to encourage sexual behaviors only in appropriate settings. Some patients respond to behavioral modification on the basis of reward. Patients who have greater insight and cognitive functioning may be capable of learning appropriate sexual behavior because of their higher functioning. The goals of health education should be to help patients regain control over sexual impulses and behavior, to identify appropriate ways in which sexual needs can be met, and to assist in maintaining sexual identity.

F. The decline of sexual functioning may produce anxiety that disrupts intimate relationships. In order to restore self-esteem, denial, projection, regression, or withdrawal may occur. Identifiable behaviors include
   - appearance of hypersexuality
   - becoming possessive
   - scapegoating a spouse or lover
   - hypochondriasis
   - social isolation

G. Sexuality counseling may be initiated when the patient's behavior results from psychological losses. Nurses should examine their personal beliefs, values, and attitudes to determine any factors that might inhibit their acting as an effective counselor. A relaxed, private atmosphere should be available for discussion of sexual concerns. Be alert for nonverbal cues to patient anxiety or reluctance to continue the discussion. A knowledge of normal sexual changes that accompany aging is imperative. Counseling may

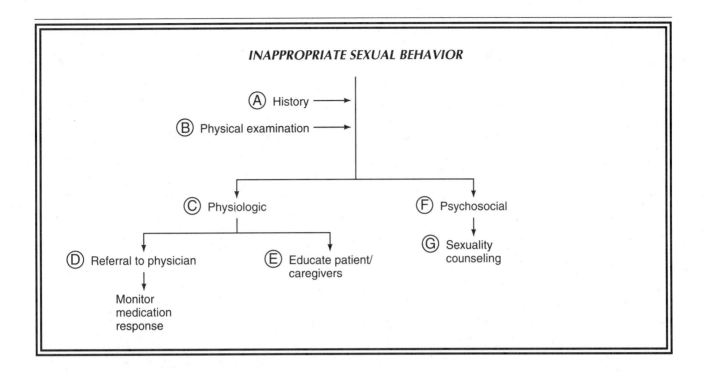

INAPPROPRIATE SEXUAL BEHAVIOR

(A) History

(B) Physical examination

(C) Physiologic

(D) Referral to physician

Monitor
medication
response

(E) Educate patient/
caregivers

(F) Psychosocial

(G) Sexuality
counseling

involve a review of sexual physiology: an assessment of the patient's sexual knowledge and concerns and level of anxiety associated with the presenting sexual problem. If appropriate, instruction may be indicated in sexual techniques that may serve as substitutes for usual approaches to sexual expression, which may now be limited. Be prepared to counsel those of differing sexual preferences or to refer patients to a therapist who can effectively and nonjudgmentally provide counseling services.

References

Adams C, Macione A. Handbook of psychiatric mental health nursing. New York: John Wiley, 1983:177.

Hussian R, Davis R. Responsive care: Behavioral interventions with elderly persons. Champaign, IL: Research Press, 1985:143, 177.

Steffl B. Handbook of gerontological nursing. New York: Van Nostrand Reinhold, 1984:461.

Verwoerdt, A. Clinical geropsychiatry. Baltimore: Williams & Wilkins, 1976:262.

MEMORY CHANGES

Nina A. Klebanoff

Memory is divided into three areas: immediate, recent, and remote (or long-term). It is a three-phased information-processing activity: (1) receipt, (2) storage or retention, and (3) retrieval, which remains relatively stable as individuals age. Marked variation in a person's memory ability, whether sudden or progressive, suggests a physical or mental disorder, or both. Memory changes without impairment of activities of daily living (ADL) or pathologic etiology may be termed "benign forgetfulness." Normal memory changes are associated with minimal progression, variability over time, and an inability to recall unimportant facts or parts of an experience, but not the experience itself. Normal older adults tend to need more time to learn and recall new information. They have little difficulty with immediate and remote memory, but often do worse on tests of recent memory in comparison with normal younger adults. Anxiety, changes in social milieu, and loneliness can contribute to changes in recent memory. Remote memory usually remains intact as a person ages.

A. Elicit any history of
- onset and course of memory changes
- signs and symptoms of depression
- cardiovascular complications
- venereal disease
- psychiatric care
- falls and injuries
- medications
- allergies
- alcohol use
- pain
- bowel and bladder continence
- stressful life events, including recent losses or changes
- coping and personal habits
- level and frequency of socialization
- patterns of exercise and rest
- accidents such as burning of pots and pans
- financial management problems
- patient and family perception of, and response to, memory changes

Also, seek collaborative data from the family or significant others.

B. Observe mobility, general appearance, and ability to respond to specific questions. Obtain vital signs. Perform neurologic assessment and pay particular attention to sensory deficits (see Hearing Loss, p. 122, and Decreased Vision, p. 118). Assess ability to perform ADL. Patients with memory changes may not be able to sequence self-care activities appropriately. Mental status evaluation should assess
- affect
- cognitive functioning
- judgment
- orientation
- memory

Test immediate memory by asking patients to remember a color and a name, and requesting them to recall it 3–5 minutes later. More specific tools used to perform a mental status evaluation are the Folstein Mini-Mental State or short portable mental status examination and the Geriatric Depression scale (see p. 268). Direct specific questions about times, the sequence of events for the past 2 days, or current news events to test recent memory. A recent memory problem is suggested if patients cannot give a coherent presentation of the past few days or current events. Remote memory is assessed by asking patients specific questions about meaningful events in their past, such as date of birth and life milestones. Laboratory studies are similar to those for confused patients (see Confusion, p. 254). The purpose is to rule out physical or chemical abnormalities (neurosyphilis, vitamin deficiency, uncontrolled hypertension or diabetes mellitus, pernicious anemia, electrolyte and endocrine disorders, infection) as the cause of memory loss.

C. Services are available in many communities to support patients with memory loss so that they may remain at home. In-home services for patient and family include
- meal service
- custodial care
- housekeeping services
- respite

Adult day care and senior centers may also provide supervision, nutrition, socialization, and a structured environment.

D. Even when someone has a considerable degree of memory loss due to dementia, it is known that learning by action and rehearsal can take place. An individualized program of behavioral techniques (shaping, prompting, reinforcement) can permit older adults with dementia to maintain higher levels of self-care and independence. Rehearsal and repetition strategies, categorization, organization and cueing (both visual and verbal) techniques, visual imagery, reminders, mild exercise, reassurance and integrative therapies, mnemonics, and environmental manipulation (for the purpose of constancy and predictability) are all indicated to enhance memory performance in older adults with normal, age-related memory changes. Various adaptive devices and new technologies such as medication dispensers, are available to help people remember via alarms or buzzers. Older adults who have normal cognitive function and wish to improve their memory performance can be referred to various memory training programs and resources, if available in the community. Anxiety reduction techniques such as relaxation training can assist with improved recall, as can the treatment of depression (see Depression, p. 282).

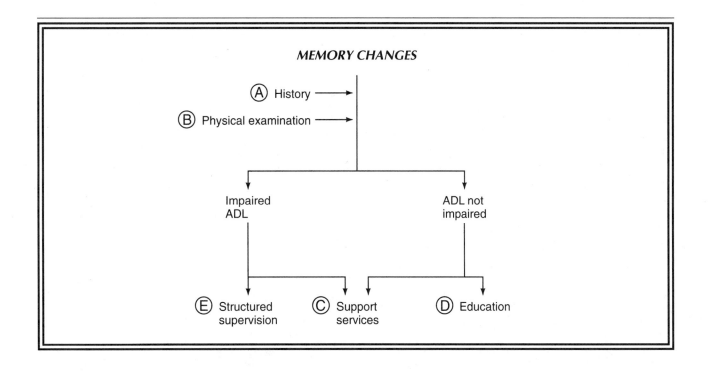

MEMORY CHANGES

(A) History →

(B) Physical examination →

Impaired ADL

ADL not impaired

(E) Structured supervision

(C) Support services

(D) Education

E. When impairment in ADL becomes so severe that periodic support or supervision no longer ensures patient safety, a change of environment becomes necessary. Around-the-clock supervision is now possible in some retirement communities, nursing homes, and convalescent centers. The decision to obtain 24-hour supervision is a difficult and emotional one for many families. A referral to Social Services to provide information concerning local options is helpful. The ongoing relationship between patient/family and nurse requires that the nurse become involved in the decision to keep the patient at home. Compassion and knowledge of the family's strengths and weaknesses are necessary to facilitate the decision-making process.

References

Ciocon JO, Potter JF. Age-related changes in human memory: Normal and abnormal. Geriatrics 1988; 43:43.

Clites J. Maximizing memory retention in the aged. J Gerontol Nurs 1984; 10:34.

Gillies DA. Patients suffering from memory loss can be taught self-care. Geriatr Nurs 1986; 7:257.

LaRue A. Memory loss and aging distinguishing dementia from benign senescent forgetfulness and depressive pseudodementia. Psychiatr Clin North Am 1982; 5:89.

Poon LW. Handbook for clinical memory assessment of older adults. Washington, DC: American Psychiatric Association, 1986.

PERCEPTUAL DISTURBANCES

Karen R. Perkins

Perception is the interpretation of or assignment of meaning to stimuli rather than just an awareness of the sensation. The elderly are susceptible to perceptual disturbances due to
- decreased vision
- auditory acuity loss
- multiple physical and medical disorders
- decline in physical or mental function

Two types of perceptual disturbances that can occur are illusions (distortions or false perceptions of actual sensorial stimulation, usually short-lived and disappearing with proper identification) and hallucinations (sense perceptions to which there are no external stimuli; more chronic in nature) (Table 1).

Perceptual disturbances may not be readily disclosed for fear of rejection and being thought "crazy" and at risk for hospitalization. It should never be assumed that there is a psychiatric dysfunction only.

A. Ask questions about
- onset and duration of perceptual disturbances
- sensory problems
  - hearing loss (see p. 122)
  - decreased vision (see p. 118)
  - decreased sensation (see p. 138)
  - taste changes (see p. 136)
  - decreased smell (see p. 126)
- medical history
  - cardiovascular disease
  - other chronic illnesses
  - psychiatric history
  - allergy history
- medication history
  - prescription and over-the-counter drugs
  - recent medication changes
  - home remedies
  - recreational drug use
  - alcohol use
- psychosocial factors
  - recent stressors
  - changes in social situation
  - support systems
- behavior
  - violence
  - suicidal ideation

A directed but supportive, unhurried approach during history taking creates an atmosphere in which specific questions can be asked, such as
- Have you experienced any strange happenings?
- Have you seen, heard, or felt something odd that has you concerned or worried?

B. Physical assessment should focus on
- sensory factors
  - hearing screen (see Hearing Loss, p. 122)
  - repair, fit, and operation of hearing amplification devices
  - visual acuity and fields (see Decreased Vision, p. 118)
    - without correction
    - with correction
  - repair, appropriateness, cleanliness and fit of glasses
- mental status (see tools on pp. 268–272)
  - cognitive functioning
    - judgment
    - memory
    - orientation
    - affect and mood
  - cardiovascular
    - peripheral pulses
    - capillary refill
    - bruits

Laboratory tests to rule out systemic or chemical problems include
- CBC with differential
- electrolytes
- glucose
- vitamin B_{12} level
- folate
- heavy metals
- therapeutic drug levels
- thyroid profile/thyroid stimulating hormone
- VDRL/RPR
- oxygen saturation

C. Reorientation of patients experiencing illusions requires that vision and hearing be corrected or improved as much as possible, since visual and hearing problems account for most instances of illusion. Disruption in the physical environment or a move to a new facility may precipitate illusions that contribute to confusion (see Confusion/Cognitive Changes/Dementia, p. 254) and resultant agitated behavior (see Agitation, p. 252). Listen carefully and position yourself to better see and hear what is in the patient's field of vision, to help identify objects or sounds that may be easily misconceived by a sensory-impaired patient. An accepting, supportive attitude may yield disclosures of perceptual disturbances from the most reluctant patient. Explain that decreasing eyesight or hearing, medications, depression, or even loneliness may often contribute to perceptual disturbances.

Text continued on page 262.

PERCEPTUAL DISTURBANCES

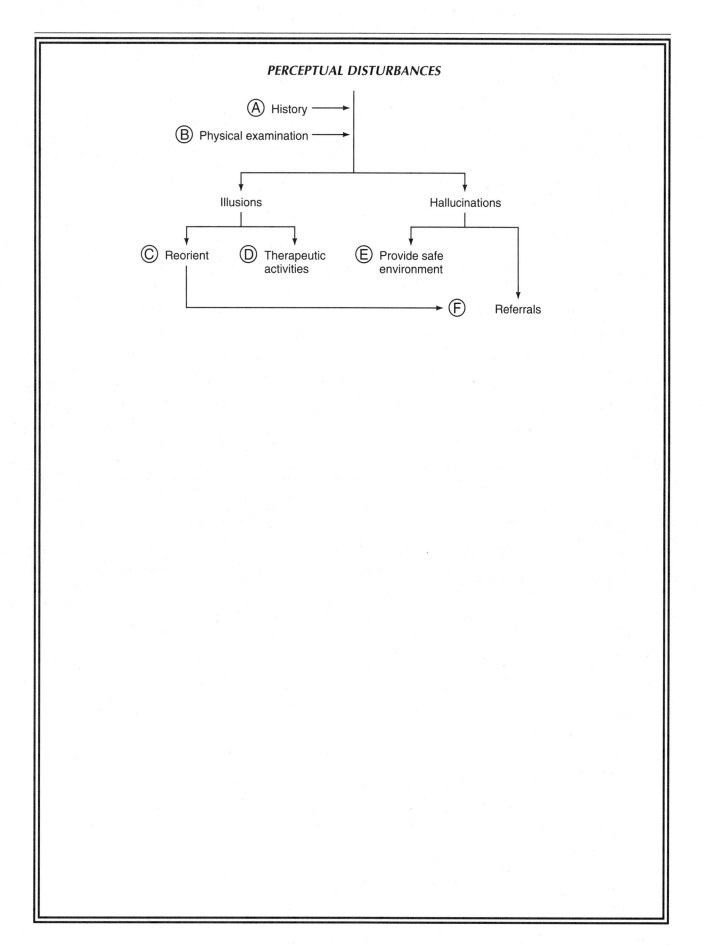

D. Therapeutic activities might be summarized and remembered as SENSE.
- *Support*
  - patients and caregivers in obtaining
    - consultations
      - ophthalmology
      - audiology
      - psychiatry
    - community services
      - home-delivered meals
      - transportation
      - socialization
    - health care services
      - home health care
      - mental health follow-up
- *Education*
  - teach normal sensory changes of aging
  - help caregivers identify situations in which patient frequently experiences sensory disturbances
    - twilight
    - mealtimes
    - change of shift or caregiver
- *Nutrition*
  - maintain adequate fluid and nutritional intake
  - avoid laxatives and use high-fiber diets
- *Schedule*
  - establish a schedule of activities and care
  - orient some patients several times a day
    - provide large numeral calendars and clocks
    - label items
- *Equipment*
  - obtain assistive devices and equipment such as
    - corrective lenses
    - magnifiers
    - hearing amplification or listening devices

TABLE 1 Clinical Groupings of Hallucinations

Type	Description	Nursing Actions
Psychiatric disorder	May be seen in manic states schizophrenia major depression	1. Observe for staring and talking into space
	Command hallucinations in which "voices" say to harm self or others	2. Watch for violent or suicidal behavior
Medication induced	May be related to drug interaction drug absorption, distribution, metabolism and excretion	1. Obtain complete medication history
	Common medications that precipitate visual hallucinations: digoxin antidepressants beta blockers atropine cholinergics corticosteroids antibiotics	2. Watch for signs of medication side effects or interactions
Delirium tremens (DTs)	Caused by abrupt alcohol withdrawal Usually accompanied by vivid visual hallucinations May be accompanied by intense fear and restlessness	1. Obtain a history of alcohol use 2. Watch for signs of DTs 3. Report onset to physician
Delirium	May be caused by unsuspected infection endocrine abnormalities vitamin deficiences heavy metal poisoning mercury lead	1. Obtain laboratory indices appropriate to history 2. Report onset to physician

E. Environmental safety can be promoted by
- removal of contraband, sharps, or items that may cause harm
- provision of adequate supervision
- maintenance of a schedule for sleep, meals, rest, and activities
- correction of vision or hearing impairments when possible
- avoidance of restraints
- provision of a room easily observed
- use of side rails, open at the end, if necessary

F. Referral to a physician or biologically oriented psychiatrist is appropriate when evaluation and medical work-up is indicated. Other referrals may be for
- eye examination
- hearing testing
- community services
- respite services, either in the home or institution
- family/caregiver counseling
- long-term care planning
- legal resources

References

Assad G, Shapiro B. Hallucinations: Theoretical and clinical overview. Am J Psychiatry 1986; 143:1088.

Burnside I, ed. Nursing and aged—a self-care approach. New York: McGraw-Hill, 1988.

SUSPICIOUSNESS

Catherine A. Hill

Suspiciousness may be defined as an extreme distrust of others. This distrust is frequently manifested by
- living alone
- a tendency toward inflexible or rigid thinking
- misinterpreting the acts of others
- fearing loss of control
- exhibiting behaviors that increase isolation from others

A. Ask about
- psychosocial factors
  - contact with significant others
  - areas in which the patient accepts help
  - hallucinations (see Perceptual Disturbances, p. 260)
  - delusions
  - aggressive behavior
  - coping skills
- activities of daily living (ADL)
  - ability to perform ADL
  - avoidance or neglect of ADL
  - hydration
  - nutrition
  - sleep and activity patterns
- medical history
  - chronic illness
  - injuries
  - psychiatric history
- medication history
  - prescription and over-the-counter drugs
  - alcohol use
  - recreational drug use

B. Assess
- general appearance
  - hygiene
  - appropriateness of clothing
  - restlessness
  - poor eye contact
  - wariness/hypervigilance
  - avoidance of touch/contact with others
- nutritional state
  - hydration
  - muscle wasting
  - skin appearance/lesions
- mental status
  - cognition (see tools on pp. 268–272)
  - mood and affect (see tool on p. 268)
  - delusions
  - hallucinations (see Perceptual Disturbances, p. 260)
- neurologic status
  - muscle tension
  - guarding
  - communication
- sensory factors
  - hearing (see Hearing Loss, p. 122)
  - vision (see Decreased Vision, p. 118)

C. Effective interventions for patients who are not hallucinating include
- avoiding whispering
- talking *to* patients, not *about* them
- informing patients about and seeking consent for scheduling all tests and treatments
- providing information
- providing simple, brief explanations for procedures or examination steps
- giving concrete tasks to increase reality orientation
- adapting the environment
- use of consistent staff and caregivers
- following a predictable schedule
- encouraging development of a confidante relationship
- not rushing patients
- use of educational materials at proper reading level
- use of hearing amplification devices or magnification if necessary to enhance communication
- treating patients with respect and like adults, *not* children
- avoiding the assumption that the elderly cannot learn

D. Referral to a primary care physician or consultation of a psychiatrist is warranted if hallucinations are present. Careful review and discontinuation of causative agents, including medications or alcohol, may be required. Treatment for suspiciousness with hallucinations may necessitate hospitalization, psychotropic drug therapy, or supportive psychosocial counseling. Psychotropic drugs of choice are generally the antipsychotic agents
- haloperidol (Haldol)
- thiothixene (Navane)
- chlorpromazine (Thorazine)
- thioridazine (Mellaril)

The most common side effects with antipsychotic drugs are extrapyramidal. Careful prescribing at low doses with gradual increase, and monitoring of tolerance and efficacy, are indicated. Long-term psychological treatment and monitoring of drug effects may be provided in a community setting. Referral to community mental health services or groups is appropriate.

References

Ebersole P, Hess P. Toward healthy aging. 2nd ed. St. Louis: Mosby–Year Book, 1990.

Miller CA. Nursing care of older adults: Theory and practice. Glenview, IL: Scott Foresman/Little, Brown Higher Education, a division of Scott Foresman Company, 1990.

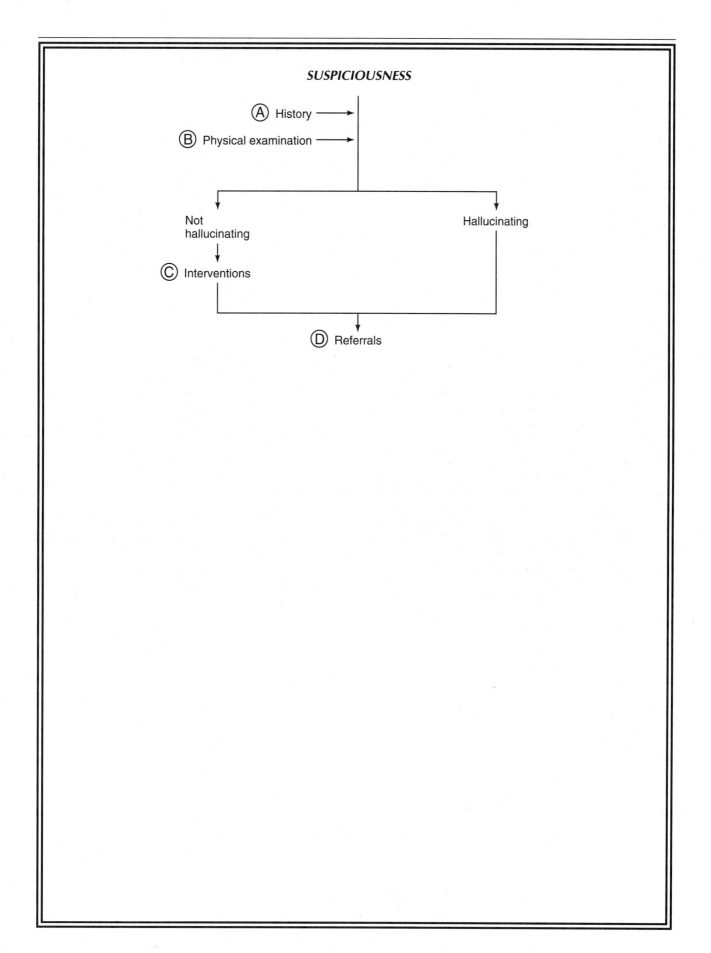

SUSPICIOUSNESS

Ⓐ History ⟶

Ⓑ Physical examination ⟶

Not hallucinating

Hallucinating

Ⓒ Interventions

Ⓓ Referrals

WANDERING

Nina A. Klebanoff

Wandering behavior is defined as time spent in motion and different purposeful and nonpurposeful behaviors. Wandering may signal unmet physical needs such as hunger, pain, temperature regulation, and toileting or response to psychosocial factors such as
• boredom
• anxiety
• isolation
• tension
• depression
• loneliness
• neurotic or affective disorders
• impaired cognition
• separation

Persons who exhibit wandering behavior tend to have deficits in judgment and memory, have had more stressful life experiences, and respond to stress with psychomotor reactions. They are more likely to have engaged in physically active leisure and social activities than those who do not display wandering behavior. Unfamiliarity with the environment does not seem to be a strong factor in promoting wandering behavior, but weather and seasonal changes do play a part. Three types of wandering behavior have been identified and defined (see the box below). Akathisiac wandering is paradoxic agitation or hyperactivity in response to psychoactive medications and does not constitute true wandering. When identifiable, the cause of wandering should be reduced or eliminated.

A. Sources for history may be either patients or caregivers. General questions to ask are
   • onset and precipitating factors
   • family mental health
   • somatic complaints
   • socialization
   • past and current medications
   • interests and hobbies

Types of Wandering

Type	Definition
Exit-seeking	Overtly goal-directed or searching behavior to get away
Modeling	Following someone else who is ambulating with no goal
Self-stimulating	Goal-directed, industrious behavior to produce auditory or tactile stimulation

TABLE 1 Approaches by Type of Wandering

Type	Environmental Intervention	Psychosocial Intervention
Exit-seeking	Use keypad locks for exit doors Provide personal alarm system Use personal identification or photographs	Observe closely
Modeling	Instruct staff and caregivers NOT to go through doorways with patient behind or near them	Pair patient with "safe" model
Self-stimulating	Provide items that can be touched, squeezed, listened to, and so on Allow movements to continue while patient is sitting or sleeping Camouflage doorways Place chairs near high-activity areas	Institute a behavior modification program

• coping patterns
• responses to touch
• stressful life events
• perceptions of heat and cold in the environment
• recent losses or changes

Personal health history should elicit
• injuries, falls, or trauma
• dizziness or orthostatic hypotension
• bowel and bladder continence
• cardiovascular and cerebrovascular disease
• presence of pain
• allergies
• exercise and rest patterns
• toileting habits

Mapping wandering behavior can determine
• incidence
• location
• associated behaviors
• environmental stressors
• response of caregiver

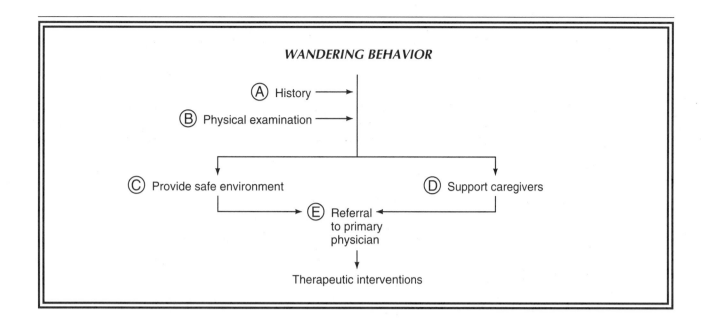

WANDERING BEHAVIOR

- (A) History
- (B) Physical examination
- (C) Provide safe environment
- (D) Support caregivers
- (E) Referral to primary physician
- Therapeutic interventions

B. Take a photograph as part of the physical examination as well as take vital signs; evaluate functional ability: gait, use of assistive devices, bowel and bladder function; evaluate vision, hearing, smell, taste, and rate of speech; and perform laboratory evaluation (see Confusion/Cognitive Changes/Dementia, p. 254). Temporary close observation promotes a thorough mental status assessment
- orientation
- judgment
- memory
- cognitive abilities
- mood
- affect

Use tools available in the section Cognition/Perception, pp. 268–272, for this purpose. Consider medical evaluation of possibly reversible etiologies.

C. Providing a safe environment can eliminate the need for physical and chemical restraints; promote dignity, freedom, and independence; stimulate circulation and oxygenation; promote physical activity that reduces stress; and reduce contractures and skin changes. Environmental interventions may include
- reducing background noise
- installing door buzzers or alarms
- providing visual cues or signs
- color coding belongings
- monitoring activities
- using nonglare glass, shadowless lighting
- covering stove burners, plugs, thermostats
- providing safe area with tactile stimuli
- scheduling activity and rest periods
- applying reflective tape to clothing

Caution caregivers that environmental adaptations may provide a false sense of security. Psychosocial interventions are to
- not confront or argue with wanderer
- instill trust through one-to-one interactions

- secure identifying information on patient
- develop a plan to follow if the patient is reported missing

D. Acknowledge the efforts of caregivers dealing with wandering. Observe caregivers for physical and mental decompensation. Make referrals to social service agencies. Support groups can provide creative ideas to control wandering behavior from other caregivers' experiences. Other sources of support to caregivers are respite care, home health aides or homemakers, institutional care, legal advice, family counseling, and day care.

E. Therapeutic interventions aim to protect the patient from injury and provide appropriate physical stimulation. Confusion will influence the choice of interventions specific to the type of wandering (Table 1). General approaches that benefit any type of wanderer are
- assisting the patient to express emotion
- identifying and assisting with patient's physical needs
- providing a routine exercise program to promote sleep

Physical and/or pharmacologic restraints should be a last resort.

References

Fopma-Loy J. Wandering: Causes, consequences, and care. J Psychosoc Nurs Ment Health Serv 1988; 26:8.

Heim KM. Wandering behavior. J Gerontol Nurs 1986; 12:4.

Hussian RA, Davis RL. Responsive care behavioral interventions with elderly persons. Champaign, IL: Research Press, 1985.

Steffl BM. Handbook of gerontological nursing. New York: Van Nostrand Reinhold, 1984:127.

Geriatric Depression Scale OR Mood Assessment Scale

Choose the best answer for how you felt over the past week.

Are you basically satisfied with your life?	(0)	Yes	No	(1)
Have you dropped many of your activities and interests?	(1)	Yes	No	(0)
Do you feel that your life is empty?	(1)	Yes	No	(0)
Do you often get bored?	(1)	Yes	No	(0)
Are you hopeful about the future?	(0)	Yes	No	(1)
Are you bothered by thoughts you can't get out of your head?	(1)	Yes	No	(0)
Are you in good spirits most of the time?	(0)	Yes	No	(1)
Are you afraid that something bad is going to happen to you?	(1)	Yes	No	(0)
Do you feel happy most of the time?	(0)	Yes	No	(1)
Do you feel helpless?	(1)	Yes	No	(0)
Do you often get restless and fidgety?	(1)	Yes	No	(0)
Do you prefer to stay at home rather than going out and doing new things?	(1)	Yes	No	(0)
Do you frequently worry about the future?	(1)	Yes	No	(0)
Do you feel you have more problems with memory than most?	(1)	Yes	No	(0)
Do you think it is wonderful to be alive now?	(0)	Yes	No	(1)
Do you feel downhearted and blue?	(1)	Yes	No	(0)
Do you feel pretty worthless the way you are now?	(1)	Yes	No	(0)
Do you worry a lot about the past?	(1)	Yes	No	(0)
Do you find life very exciting?	(0)	Yes	No	(1)
Is it hard for you to get started on new projects?	(1)	Yes	No	(0)
Do you feel full of energy?	(0)	Yes	No	(1)
Do you feel that your situation is hopeless?	(1)	Yes	No	(0)
Do you think that most people are better off than you are?	(1)	Yes	No	(0)
Do you frequently get upset over little things?	(1)	Yes	No	(0)
Do you frequently feel like crying?	(1)	Yes	No	(0)
Do you have trouble concentrating?	(1)	Yes	No	(0)
Do you enjoy getting up in the morning?	(0)	Yes	No	(1)
Do you prefer to avoid social gatherings?	(1)	Yes	No	(0)
Is it easy for you to make decisions?	(0)	Yes	No	(1)
Is your mind as clear as it used to be?	(0)	Yes	No	(1)

TOTAL SCORE: Add together the numbers that are circled and place that number on the total score line.

TOTAL SCORE: _____

Useful for depression screening and to determine level of depression e.g., normal, mildly or severely depressed. A score of 10 or more warrants further evaluation.

From Yesavage J, Brink T, Rose T, et al. Development and validation of a geriatric screening scale: A preliminary report. J Psychiatr Res 1983; 17:37; with permission.

Mini–Mental State Examination

Patient's Name: _____   Patient No.: _____

Examiner's Name: _____   Date: _____

Patient Score	Maximum Score	
		Orientation
_____	5	What is the (year) (season) (date) (day) (month)?
_____	5	Where are we (country) (state) (county) (city) (clinic)?
		Registration
_____	3	Name three objects, allotting one second to say each one. Then ask the patient to name three objects after you have said them. Give one point for each correct answer. Repeat this until he hears all three. Count trials and record number.
		APPLE . . . BOOK . . . COAT Number of trials _____
		Attention and Calculation
_____	5	Begin with 100 and count backward by 7 (stop after five answers): 93, 86, 79, 72, 65. Score one point for each correct answer. If the patient will not perform this task, ask the patient to spell "WORLD" backwards (DLROW). Record the patient's spelling: _____. Score one point for each correctly placed letter.
		Recall
_____	3	Ask the patient to repeat the objects above (see Registration). Give one point for each correct answer.
		Language
_____	2	Naming: Show a pencil and a watch, and ask the patient to name them.
_____	1	Repetition: Repeat the following: "No ifs, ands, or buts."
_____	3	Three-stage command: Follow the three-stage command, "Take a paper in your right hand; fold it in half; and put it on the table."
_____	1	Reading: Read and obey the following: "Close your eyes" (show the patient the item written on the illustration on the following page).
_____	1	Writing: "Write a sentence" (see the illustration on the following page).
_____	1	Copying: "Copy the design of the intersecting pentagons" (on the following page).
_____	30	Total Score Possible

Interpretation and scoring: Score of 25 or greater is normal; 15 to 24 indicates cognitive impairment and warrants further evaluation; less than 15 has high correlation with dementia. Low score is possible in presence of physical illness, low intelligence, and affective disorder.

Helpful hint: Write patient responses on form for later reference and interpretation of findings.
Adapted from Folstein MF, Folstein S, McHugh PR. Mini-mental state: A practical method for grading the cognitive state of patients for the clinician. J Psychiatr Res 1975; 12:189; with permission.

CLOSE   YOUR   EYES

_____

WRITE   A   SENTENCE

_____

_____

COPY   DESIGN

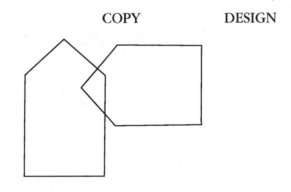

Short Portable Mental Status Questionnaire

Instructions: Ask questions 1 through 10 in this list and record all answers. Ask question 4A only if patient does not have a telephone. Record total number of errors based on ten questions.

1. What is the date today? _____
   Month   Day   Year
2. What day of the week is it? _____
3. What is the name of this place? _____
4. What is your telephone number? _____
4A. What is your street address? _____
    (Ask only if patient does not have a telephone.)
5. How old are you? _____
6. When were you born? _____
7. Who is the president of the
   United States now? _____
8. Who was president just before him? _____
9. What was your mother's maiden name? _____
10. Subtract 3 from 20 and keep subtracting 3 from
    each new number, all the way down.

_____   Total Number of Errors

Scoring: 0–2 errors = intact mental function
         3–4 errors = mild intellectual impairment
         5–7 errors = moderate intellectual impairment
         8–10 errors = severe intellectual impairment
         Allow one more error if subject had only grade school education.
         Allow one fewer error if subject has had education beyond high school.

From Pfeiffer E. A short portable mental status questionnaire for the assessment of organic brain deficit in elderly patients. J Am Geriatr Soc 1975; 23:433; with permission.

The Set Test

Patient's Name _____ Date _____

- A simple procedure for cognitive screening of patients over 60 years of age
- Easily administered during a routine visit

General Instructions
- After asking the patient how his or her memory is, say that you would like to ask a few routine questions.
- Ask the patient to tell you all the colors he or she can think of.
- Keep count of the colors mentioned, to a maximum of 10.
- Use the same procedure and ask the patient to name all the animals he or she can think of, then fruits, and finally towns.

SCORE
(number named)
(maximum 10)

1. COLORS   ☐

2. ANIMALS   ☐

3. FRUITS   ☐

4. TOWNS   ☐

TOTAL (maximum 40) _____

Evaluation of Score

25–40: no cognitive impairment
15–24: significant impairment of
       cognitive function
5–14: severe cognitive impairment
0–5: severely demented or poorly
     motivated to perform test

Further Considerations
- The Set Test cannot be used in patients who have a severe hearing impairment, are dysphasic, or have a language barrier.
- The test should not be given to patients who are physically ill, in pain, or under the influence of drugs.
- The test should not be performed in the presence of relatives, who may not be able to resist the temptation to "help."
- In administering the test, do not ask, "Can you think of any more?" or in any other way influence the patient's response.
- A diagnosis of cognitive impairment should never be based solely on a low score on the Set Test. This score is just one factor to be considered in evaluating the total clinical picture.

Adapted from Isaacs B. A simple screening test for dementia in the elderly. Geriatr Med Today 1985; 4:49; with permission.

Blessed Dementia Rating Scale

1. Memory and performance of everyday activities
   Loss of ability

None	Some	Severe	
0	0.5	1	A. Ability to perform household tasks
0	0.5	1	B. Ability to cope with small sums of money
0	0.5	1	C. Ability to remember a short list of items (e.g., shopping list)
0	0.5	1	D. Ability to find way about indoors (patient's home or other familiar locations)
0	0.5	1	E. Ability to find way around familiar streets
0	0.5	1	F. Ability to grasp situations or explanations
0	0.5	1	G. Ability to recall recent events
0	0.5	1	H. Tendency to dwell in the past

   (Score: 0 = none; 0.5 = sometimes; 1 = frequently)

2. Habits
   A. Eating
      0 = Feeds self without assistance
      1 = Feeds self with minor assistance
      2 = Feeds self with much assistance
      3 = Has to be fed

   B. Dressing
      0 = Unaided
      1 = Occasionally misplaces buttons; requires minor help
      2 = Wrong sequence, forgets items, requires much assistance
      3 = Unable to dress

   C. Toilet
      0 = Clean; cares for self at toilet
      1 = Occasional incontinence or needs to be reminded
      2 = Frequent incontinence or needs much assistance
      3 = No control

3. Total score of all items
   (maximum score 17) _____

From Blessed G, Tomlinson BE, Roth M: The association between quantitative measures of dementia and of senile change in the cerebral gray matter of elderly subjects. Br J Psychiatry 1968; 114:797; with permission.

SELF-IMAGE

UNDIAGNOSED ALCOHOL ABUSE

Karen R. Perkins

Many health problems of the elderly such as falls, confusional states, dementia, mood fluctuations, poor nutrition, and gastritis may be dismissed as secondary to aging rather than identified as undiagnosed alcohol abuse. The criteria for diagnosing alcohol abuse are
- quantity of alcohol consumption
- frequency of alcohol consumption
- tolerance
- withdrawal symptoms

These may not be distinguishable because of confounding factors such as medication interactions, alcohol and medication interactions, and the presence of chronic illness. Alcohol abuse if left untreated can be fatal. Any time alcohol abuse is suspected in a medically compromised patient, a referral to professionals knowledgeable about detecting and treating alcohol abuse is essential. The elderly alcohol abuser is at higher risk for suicide than the general population. Major stressors that contribute to suicide risk include
- social isolation
- multiple losses
- loneliness
- major depression

A. History taking is best accomplished when rapport has been established to reduce the patient's stress level. Start with nonthreatening subjects such as past medical history, family medical history, and medication review, including over-the-counter drugs.
   Eliciting history of family psychiatric profile, alcohol use, and drug use may introduce these topics for later exploration of the patient's drug or alcohol history and current use. Obtain information about
   - current symptoms—onset, duration, factors that alleviate, and factors that exacerbate
   - self-medication

- recent major life changes
- stressors, especially significant losses
- past and present coping mechanisms
- ability to perform activities of daily living
- nutritional intake, including beverages

The dietary history can serve as an excellent and nonthreatening approach to elicit alcohol use. Listen for oblique references to use of alcohol or drugs and expressions of suicidal thoughts. Use of tools such as the *Michigan Alcoholism Screening Test* (MAST) (see p. 288) or CAGE (see the box "CAGE Questionnaire") may be useful.

B. Physical examination should assess body systems that demonstrate alcohol-related complications such as liver size, peripheral neuropathies, and body weight change. Use a mental status questionnaire (see tools on pages 268–272) to evaluate cognitive status. Administer the depression scale (see tool on page 268). Perform tests to rule out other physiologic causes
   - electrolytes
   - thyroid function
   - electrocardiogram
   - blood glucose level
   - B_{12} level, serum protein, albumin
   - liver enzymes
   - serum alcohol level

C. Primary or early-onset alcoholism is thought to have a genetic predisposition. This form of alcoholism usually develops at an early age and follows a fairly predictable course. Patients with this form of alcoholism are more readily identified as problem drinkers because their history is strongly indicative of classic alcohol abuse, including
   - tolerance
   - withdrawal symptoms
   - medical problems associated with chronic alcohol abuse
   - social and work problems due to drinking
   - trouble with the law such as driving while intoxicated (DWI)

CAGE Questionnaire

- Have you ever felt you ought to **C**ut down on your drinking?
- Have people **A**nnoyed you by criticizing your drinking?
- Have you ever felt bad or **G**uilty about your drinking?
- Have you ever had a drink first thing in the morning to steady your nerves or get rid of a hangover (**E**ye-opener)?

Purpose: For screening and detection of alcoholism
Rating: Two or three positive responses = high suspicion of alcoholism
Four positive responses = pathognomonic for alcoholism

From Ewing JA. Detecting alcoholism: The CAGE questionnaire. JAMA 1984; 252:1905; with permission.

Chlordiazepoxide Treatment Regimen

Day	Dosage
1	25–50 mg QID
2	20–40 mg QID
3	15–30 mg QID
4	10–20 mg QID
5	5–10 mg QID

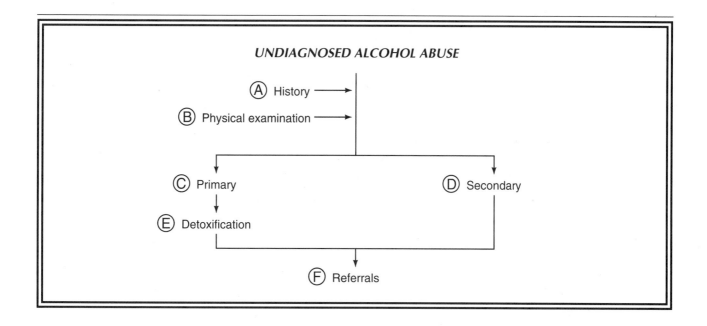

D. Secondary or late-life-onset alcoholism may develop as a result of a psychiatric disorder such as major depression or an anxiety disorder. Patients with a painful chronic disease such as arthritis may start drinking to decrease the discomfort. The sociologic changes associated with aging—loss of status, loss of income, loss of loved ones, loss of meaningful work, and illness—may also contribute to the development of secondary alcoholism. For many overwhelmed elderly persons, alcohol temporarily helps to decrease the sense of anxiety and psychic pain.

E. Detoxification is essential. Almost all active primary alcohol abusers will experience some degree of alcohol withdrawal syndrome upon cessation of alcohol intake. For patients with major medical illnesses such as pneumonia, cirrhosis, or uncontrolled diabetes, untreated withdrawal symptoms can be life-threatening. The decision of whether hospitalization is required to manage withdrawal is made by the physician based on
  • severity of symptoms
  • use or misuse of other drugs
  • social support systems
  • patient cooperation
  • medical complications
  • ability to follow directions
  • past history
Outpatient detoxification includes a standard treatment regimen of chlordiazepoxide (see the box "Chlordiazepoxide Treatment Regimen"). Use of an outpatient chlordiazepoxide protocol requires a motivated patient in good health with support systems and mild withdrawal symptoms. The patient should be monitored daily and encouraged to actively participate in Alcoholics Anonymous to reinforce the resolve to abstain.

F. Determining and appropriately treating the precipitating medical or psychosocial contributing cause of secondary alcoholism is a starting point. Treatment may be both physical and emotional to deal with the dynamics that lead the patient to rely on alcohol as a means of coping with problems. Referral must always be made for alcohol cessation treatment. Other referrals may include
  • pain management programs
  • socialization activities such as senior citizen programs
  • psychosocial counseling
  • home visitation and community outreach

References

Blazer DG, Pennybacker MR. Epidemiology of alcoholism in the elderly. In: Hartford J, Samorajki T, eds. Alcoholism in the elderly. New York: Raven Press, 1984:25.

Dunlop J. The older client who is alcoholic. In: Jack L, ed. Nursing care planning with the addicted client. Skokie, IL: National Nurses Society on Addictions, 1989:41.

Ketcham M. The client with physical complications from chronic alcoholism. In: Jack L, ed. Nursing care planning with the addicted client. Skokie, IL: National Nurses Society on Addictions, 1989:25.

Krach P. Discovering the secret: Nursing assessment of elderly alcoholics in the home. J Gerontol Nurs 1990; 16:32.

ANGER

Deborah Antai-Otong

Anger may stem from feelings of helplessness, powerlessness, loss of control, or dependency. The elderly experience social and physical changes (loss of a spouse, home, or financial security; hospitalization) that can precipitate feelings of anger. Anger, like depression, may be manifested by either physical or psychological symptoms. Expressions of anger that are not socially acceptable signal the loss of impulse control.

A. Ask questions to identify
    • onset and duration of symptoms
    • previous coping patterns
    • available resources
    • number and significance of recent stressors
    • sleep patterns
    • nutrition
    • previous psychiatric treatment
    • suicide ideations or attempts
    • participation in and enjoyment of activities
    Elicit triggers for anger by asking when irritability or agitation increases. Loud noise or overstimulation may precipitate angry outbursts. Determine specific symptoms or behaviors that demonstrate anger, such as
    • physical aggression
    • verbal abuse and screaming (see Aggressive Behavior, p. 250)
    • communication patterns with significant others
    Ascertain methods that have worked to diffuse the anger or stop the behavior.

B. Initial assessment should rule out any organic or physical cause of complaints and symptoms. Also obtain information about
    • cognition (see Confusion/Cognitive Changes/Dementia, p. 254)
    • level of functioning
    • mood and affect: specifically, depression, anxiety, irritability, or agitation
    • physical or verbal aggressive behavior
    Observe interactions between the patient and significant others or caregivers.

C. The nursing approach to angry patients should avoid
    • personalizing the expression of anger
    • treating patients as children
    • using endearments such as "honey," "dearie," or "granny"
    It is important to provide advocacy by protecting patients' desire for modesty and a sense of control, especially in health care settings. Allow patients' legitimate need to express dissatisfaction and acknowledge their rights. Encourage patients to verbalize their feelings while actively listening and promoting emotional comfort. Other ways to minimize anger and feelings of helplessness include allowing active participation in treatment and decisions. These measures facilitate readjustment and reorganization in dealing with associated anger.

D. To redirect anger, patients must have some insight into the underlying feelings or irritational beliefs that contribute to the anger. Teach them to identify the source of provocation or how to recognize emotional and physical reactions that indicate anger. Once the patient recognizes situations that provoke anger, techniques can be used to change behavior or response. Both physical and emotional outlets for anger are possible (see Aggressive Behavior, p. 250).

E. Patients with personality disorders and other psychiatric illnesses often have poor impulse control, are easily angered, and may act out their feelings both verbally and physically. Relaxation techniques and imagery can help patients deal with situations that provoke anger and feelings of losing control. Appropriate behavior should be rewarded to cultivate its adoption. A common error that nurses make is to reward inappropriate behavior by spending more time with patients who display anger.

F. Effective coping patterns lead to socially acceptable expressions of anger. Patients need help in developing new behaviors or responses to situations that leave them feeling helpless, hopeless, or dependent. Practice problem-solving strategies with patients in a nonthreatening environment. The nurse can also assist patients to identify events that trigger justifiable anger. Since anger may stem from irrational beliefs, patients may benefit from homework assignments such as practicing daily positive self-statements.

G. Nurses may be required to administer anxiolytic or neuroleptic medications (e.g., Ativan, Haldol) to patients who are unable to control anger. Dosages of psychoactive drugs should reduce aggressive behavior without undue sedation. Watch for side effects such as extrapyramidal symptoms, hallucinations, agitation or anxiety, and anticholinergic effects (dry mouth, dysuria, confusion).

H. The application of physical restraints may be necessary as a last resort when patients do not respond to redirection, behavioral techniques, or medical management or become physically aggressive. Physiologic and psychological effects of restraint include increased anger and hostility or extreme passivity and regression. Regression can lead to incontinence and lack of motivation to deal with activities of daily living. Restraints can also lead to drastic mental status changes and confusion. Physiologic hazards include limitations in musculoskeletal movement and impaired circulation. Restraints must be constantly reevaluated and removed as quickly as possible to prevent debilitating effects. Follow institutional guide-

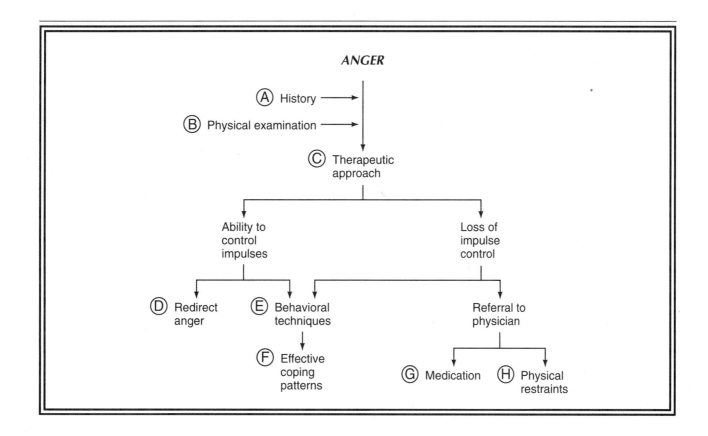

ANGER

- Ⓐ History
- Ⓑ Physical examination
- Ⓒ Therapeutic approach
  - Ability to control impulses
    - Ⓓ Redirect anger
    - Ⓔ Behavioral techniques
      - Ⓕ Effective coping patterns
  - Loss of impulse control
    - Referral to physician
      - Ⓖ Medication
      - Ⓗ Physical restraints

lines for restraints and use only when absolutely necessary. General guidelines for caring for patients in restraints include nonpunitive use, documenting reasons for their use, documenting release of restraints at frequent intervals, and treating patients with respect.

References

Burgess AW. Psychiatric nursing in the hospital and the community. 4th ed. Englewood Cliffs, NJ: Prentice-Hall, 1985.

Kolcaba L, Miller CA. Geropharmacology treatment. J Gerontol Nurs 1989; 15:29.

McHutchion E, Morse JM. Releasing restraints, a nursing dilemma. J Gerontol Nurs 1989; 15:16.

Meichenbaum D. Cognitive-behavior modification. 2nd ed. New York: Plenum Press, 1979.

ANXIETY

Catherine A. Hill

As the elderly cope with changes in body image, living situations, and physiologic function, they sometimes exhibit apprehension, tension, or uneasiness. Any loss of control over their lives can be perceived as a threat that triggers feelings of anxiety. Anxiety may be
- reactive—response to stressful situations
- phobic—intense fear
- panic—sudden occurrence of overwhelming fear
- free-floating—general persistent sensation unrelated to events

A. Elicit information about
- exacerbating and alleviating factors
- coping skills
- recent psychosocial changes, such as
  - death of loved one
  - marriage
  - retirement or financial status
  - perceived satisfaction with life
  - divorce or separation
  - recreation or church activities
  - birth of grandchildren
- medical history: chronic illnesses; recent falls, accidents, or injuries; past psychiatric history; sexual disorders such as impotence or orgasmic dysfunction
- medication history: current prescription and over-the-counter medications, alcohol and recreational drug use
- physiologic symptoms or changes, such as

Concerns About Antianxiety Medications

Minor Tranquilizers
Chlordiazepoxide and diazepam can cause confusion or gait disturbances.
Lorazepam and oxazepam, with shorter half-lives, are preferred.
Short-acting benzodiazepines should be tapered to avoid withdrawal symptoms; do not discontinue abruptly.

Major Tranquilizers
Use major tranquilizers such as trifluoperazine (Stelazine) or thioridazine (Mellaril) in small doses for severe anxiety.

General Considerations
Excessive lowering of anxiety may decrease motivation to solve problems.
Patients may develop paradoxic responses.
Significant side effects include
- *agitation or hallucinations
- *confusion or delirium
- *hypotension or cardiotoxicity
- *insomnia
- *drowsiness or oversedation
- *anticholinergic symptoms

- headache
- muscle tension
- fatigue (see p. 14)
- pain
- frequent urination
- nausea or vomiting
- diarrhea
- tachycardia, palpitations
- restlessness
- cold, clammy hands
- dry mouth
- dizziness (see p. 140)
- changes in elimination pattern
- profuse sweating
- poor concentration
- limited attention span
- sleep alterations
- nutrition history: 24-hour recall, fluid intake, appetite changes
- sociocultural influences: support systems, religious beliefs, ethnic mores, holiday celebrations

B. Physical factors to be assessed include
- vital signs, such as blood pressure for elevation or orthostatic hypotension, pulse for tachycardia, and respirations for rate, hyperventilation, or sighing
- general appearance
  - restlessness
  - wariness
  - dishevelment
  - trembling or hand tremors
  - quivering voice
  - extraneous movements
  - glancing about
  - hypersensitivity to noise or light
  - poor eye contact
  - wringing of hands or tapping of fingers
  - meaningless, rapid speech
  - facial tightness
- integument changes: profuse sweating, rashes or hives, hydration
- mental status (see Cognition/Perception Section tools), including
  - cognition
  - vegetative signs
  - crying or angry behavior
  - mood and affect
  - false cheerfulness
- musculoskeletal signs: tension, ability to perform activities of daily living
- neurologic signs: dilated pupils, hypersensitive reflexes
Laboratory tests may include measurement of electrolytes, thyroid profile, thyroid-stimulating hormone, and glucose.

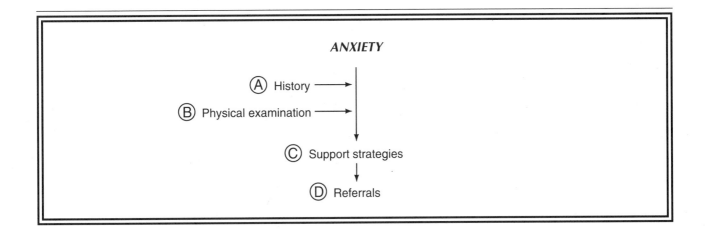

ANXIETY

- (A) History
- (B) Physical examination
- (C) Support strategies
- (D) Referrals

C. Anxiety may be a result of ineffective coping or provide a source of secondary gains. Strategies to help the patient deal with anxiety should include a support system for both the patient and caregiver. The nurse should
- evaluate current coping strategies
- facilitate changing behavior by
  - reducing tension
  - problem solving
  - clarifying cause of anxiety
  - developing course of action
- teach new coping strategies congruent with patient belief systems
- encourage caregivers to listen, reinforce positive coping activities, and report progress
- reassure patient that symptoms are not signs of physical deterioration
- develop a plan with patient and caregiver to meet patient needs, such as acknowledging and rewarding appropriate behavior and determining responsibilities for all parties
- maintain a safe, familiar environment, which includes
  - routine daily schedule
  - appropriate nutrition
  - adequate supervision and privacy
  - balanced rest and activity times

D. Referral for primary care, clinical psychology, or psychosocial counseling may be warranted. Antianxiety medications include
- minor tranquilizers: benzodiazepines or meprobamates
- major tranquilizers: phenothiazines or butyrophenones (see the box)

Patients and caregivers must be aware that antianxiety medications treat the symptoms, not the cause, which still requires attention. Other referrals to be explored for treatment include
- behavioral therapies: relaxation, biofeedback, sensitivity training
- psychotherapy to return the sense of control to the patient

References

Burgess AW. Psychiatric nursing in the hospital and the community. 4th ed. Englewood Cliffs, NJ: Prentice-Hall, 1985.

McConnell ES. Nursing diagnoses related to psychosocial alterations. In: Matteson MA, McConnell ES, eds. Gerontological nursing: Concepts and practice. Philadelphia: WB Saunders, 1988:530.

Schultz JM, Dark SL. Manual of psychiatric care plans. Boston: Little, Brown, 1982.

APATHY

Kay Peterson

Apathy is a condition of emotional exhaustion or profound emotional withdrawal. This detachment or dulled emotional tone may be a reaction to either long-term or acute illness. Apathy and the accompanying withdrawal are often interpreted as a depressive reaction when the cause may be an underlying organic or metabolic disorder. The observation of apathy does not justify a diagnosis of depression or schizophrenic withdrawal.

A. Elicit any history of
  • mental illness (psychosis, depression)
  • cognitive impairment
  • metabolic imbalance
  • recent illnesses
  • medications, prescribed and over the counter
  • significant losses
  • changes in environment or stimulation
  • appetite changes
  • sensory losses
  • sleep patterns or disturbances
  • loss of interest in activities
  • support systems
  • nutritional status
  • ability to perform activities of daily living (ADL)
  The patient may not be a reliable source of information, so caregiver or family input is essential.

B. Physical examination should evaluate
  • cognitive level
  • functional motor skills
  • presence of psychomotor retardation
  • skin condition
  • GI function
  • presence or absence of sensory impairment (see Hearing Loss, p. 122, and Decreased Vision, p. 118)
  • mood, restricted affect
  • neurologic assessment
  Laboratory studies are used to rule out organic disease. Helpful tests include CBC, erythrocyte sedimentation rate, electrolytes, renal function tests, serologic test for syphilis, and thyroid function; and nutritional variables such as albumin, vitamin B_{12}, thiamine, and folate levels.

C. Social isolation can be the result of
  • decreased gratification with roles and relationships
  • loss of ambition or interest
  • social withdrawal from environmental stimulation
  • lack of resources
  • loss of friends and support systems
  • feelings of powerlessness
  • stereotyping of the older adult
  The many losses that accompany the aging process can be severely disabling.

D. Apathy may be manifest as depression, regression, or schizophrenia. Observed behaviors include
  • withdrawal into delusional thinking in an effort to cope with anxiety in a confusing, threatening world
  • impairment of memory, abstract reasoning, and concentration (see Confusion/Cognitive Changes/Dementia, p. 254, and Depression, p. 282)
  Iatrogenic apathy may result from excessive tranquilization, overly aggressive medical procedures, and extended hospitalization.

E. Physiologic causes of apathy may be drugs, including tranquilizers; electrolyte or hormonal imbalance; vitamin deficiency; or anemia (Table 1). Organic brain disease, trauma or brain tumors of the frontal lobes or right hemisphere, hydrocephalus, Pick's disease, Huntington's chorea, and bilateral brain disease may cause apathetic behavior. In particular, injury or disease of the frontal lobe affects reason and ability to control emotions.

F. Counseling may be informal or intensive; the type required is determined by the extent to which the apathy interferes with ADL. For patients who have begun to isolate themselves, take steps to
  • mobilize support systems
  • correct sensory impairments to maximal level
  • identify areas of loss
  • facilitate the grief process
  • expand coping capabilities and sense of control
  • assist in setting realistic goals
  • support beyond the crisis

TABLE 1   Physiologic Manifestations of Apathy

Problem	Symptoms
Hyponatremia	Lethargy and mental sluggishness
Hyperglycemia	Hyperactivity
	Difficulty concentrating
Hypoglycemia	Confusion
	Personality changes
Vitamin deficiencies	Confusion
(folic acid, B_{12}, thiamine)	Appearance of emotional exhaustion
Anemia	Confusion
	Apathy
Hyperthyroidism	Depression
(apathetic thyrotoxicosis)	Withdrawal
Hypothyroidism	Irritability
	Psychomotor retardation
	Impaired cognition

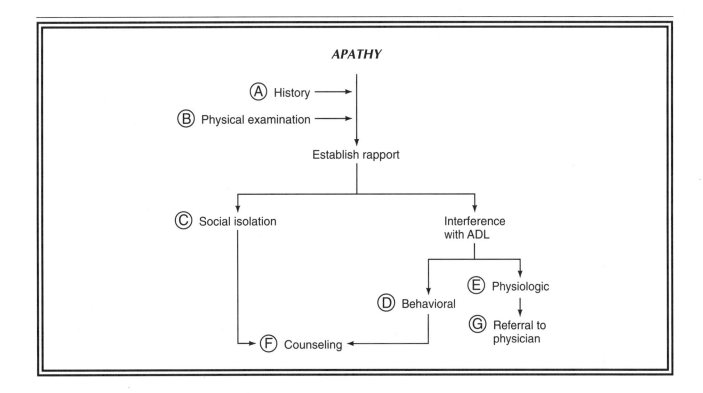

APATHY

(A) History

(B) Physical examination

Establish rapport

(C) Social isolation

Interference with ADL

(D) Behavioral

(E) Physiologic

(G) Referral to physician

(F) Counseling

Patients who are unable to perform ADL or maintain reality orientation may require extensive psychological intervention and support. Basic principles of care include
* continual orientation to time and the caregiver role, including how long interactions will be and when the caregiver will be accessible
* consistent caregiver and approach
* frequent, brief interactions
* planned, supervised activity periods
* avoidance or judicious use of touch
* role model and effective communication in a comfortable, nonthreatening manner
* development of a trusting relationship

G. The apathetic patient with impaired neurologic and physical function needs referral to a primary care physician. Assessment with head CT scan, MRI, or electroencephalography may be indicated for diagnostic evaluation. Once a differential diagnosis has been made, a medication regimen can be started. In cases of dementia or clinical depression, a psychiatric consultation and neuropsychological testing may be recommended (see Confusion/Cognitive Changes/Dementia, p. 254, and Depression, p. 282).

References

Birren J, Sloane R. Handbook of mental health and aging. Englewood Cliffs, NJ: Prentice-Hall, 1980:701.
Miller J. Inspiring hope. Am J Nurs 1985; 85:22.
Ravish T. Prevent social isolation before it starts. J Gerontol Nurs 1985; 11:10.
Verwoerdt A. Clinical geropsychiatry. Baltimore: Williams & Wilkins, 1976:169.

DEPRESSION

Karen R. Perkins

Depression is the most common psychiatric disorder in the elderly, unfortunately often unrecognized by both patient and health care provider. Undiagnosed and untreated depression results in unnecessary suffering, which may lead to death. Many medical illnesses, as well as medication and alcohol abuse, may precipitate or contribute to the development of depression in the elderly.

A. The first several minutes of a depressed patient's encounter with the nurse are crucial in setting the tone for successful intervention. A sensitive, patient, interested manner helps to establish rapport. Without a comfortable relationship, the depressed patient may refuse to cooperate or leave against advice before evaluation and treatment is complete. Allow additional time to gather information. Elders have more life history, and the questions asked may stimulate a need to engage in a life review that may be therapeutic. Many suicidal patients see a health care provider before attempting suicide. It is therefore imperative to establish rapport and determine the potential for suicide.

B. Concerns to address in history include
    • onset and duration of symptoms
    • weight or appetite change
    • recent major life changes and stressors
    • situations or actions that increase or decrease symptoms or comfort level
    • psychiatric history or treatment
    • family history of depression, dementia, mental illness, alcohol or drug problems
    • allergies
    • current medications, prescription and over the counter
    • support systems or changes in the support network
    • previous coping mechanisms
    • sense of feeling helpless and worthless
    • medical history
    • change in sleeping pattern or new onset of insomnia
    • recent change in level of functioning in several life areas
        • household management
        • personal care
        • recreational
        • social
    Observe how the patient interacts with caregivers, relatives, and health care workers. It is often difficult to identify a chief complaint in a depressed patient. The presentation of depression in the elderly is commonly nonspecific and atypical.

C. A complete physical examination may be necessary to rule out systemic illness based on nonspecific somatic complaints such as fatigue, weakness, diffuse pain, and anorexia. Basic laboratory evaluation may include
    • complete blood count
    • sedimentation rate
    • serum electrolytes
    • glucose
    • calcium
    • renal studies
    • liver battery
    • thyroid function tests
    Optional tests include
    • heavy metals screen
    • drug toxicology screen
    • therapeutic drug level
    The aim is to rule out anemia, electrolyte imbalances, acute illness, or drug and heavy metal poisoning. Sensory impairments may indicate a need for a hearing screen (see Hearing Loss, p. 122) and visual evaluation (see Decreased Vision, p. 118). Specific components in the assessment of depression include:
    • mental status examination (see tools on pp. 268–272)
    • a geriatric-specific depression screening instrument (see tool on p. 268)
    • affect/mood
        • apathy
        • withdrawal
        • restricted affect
    • presence of psychomotor retardation

D. Suicide risk is not always correlated with presence of risk factors (see the box "Suicide Risk Factors"). Asking about suicidal thoughts and intent will *not* give the idea of suicide to someone who has not already entertained the idea. Express concern and ask if the patient feels that life is not worth living and if suicide is being contemplated. Determine whether the patient experiences thoughts of suicide or self-harm and has a plan to accomplish it. A specific plan indicates a higher level of risk. Of even more concern is someone who already has a means to accomplish the plan, such as
    • a gun, bullets, and a plan
    • stockpiling medication with a history of suicide attempts
    • an alcohol user with a history of impulsive behavior
    Be especially alert for subtle signs of suicidal thought (e.g., suddenly giving away personal possessions or making a will). The elderly have the highest rate of suicide and are more likely to be successful.

Text continued on page 284.

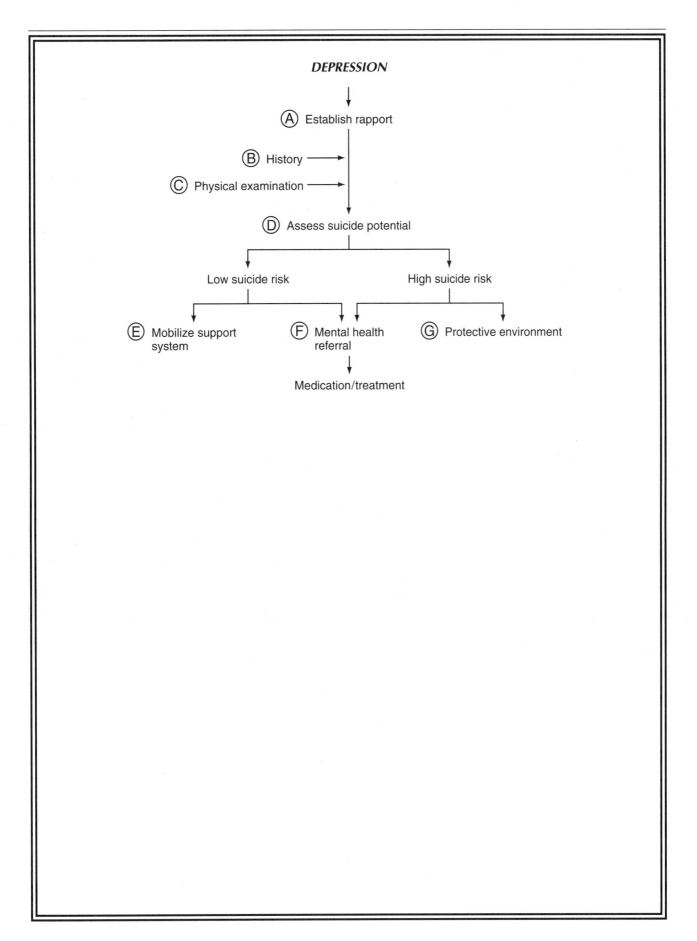

E. Support systems should be mobilized to
  - provide encouragement and information
  - increase interaction
  - decrease isolation
  - support treatment plans
  - increase activity, both mental and physical
  - promote past and present interests
  - diminish sensory deprivation
  - follow through with psychiatric evaluation
  - assist with treatment recommendations

  The goals of all interaction are to decrease feelings of worthlessness and loneliness, teach significant others about depression and suicide, and promote maintenance of the medication regimen and psychotherapy follow-up services.

F. Referral to a mental health professional is necessary to obtain pharmacologic treatment. Successful response to antidepressant therapy often confirms the diagnosis of depression. Obtaining the correct help for an actively suicidal patient can be time-consuming and requires the services of staff proficient in crisis intervention. Medications for depression management include antidepressants, monoamine oxidase (MAO) inhibitors, and occasionally stimulants. Antidepressants are the most common agents used in the elderly. Management usually involves a significantly lower dose initiation, about half or less of the usual adult dose, with documentation of target symptoms to follow and evaluation of the efficacy of drug treatment. Common side effects of antidepressants that may be annoying but manageable in younger patients may be debilitating or even lethal in susceptible elders. Postural hypotension may lead to falls and hip fractures (see Falls, p. 90). Anticholinergic side effects associated with antidepressants are of particular concern and may be misdiagnosed. See the box "Common Adverse Effects of Antidepressants." Short-acting anxiolytics may be prescribed for anxiety or agitation accompanying the depression, and antipsychotics for associated psychoses. Electroconvulsive therapy (ECT) may be the treatment of choice for acutely suicidal or medically compromised patients. In the depressed elderly, ECT is often a preferred therapy.

Suicide Risk Factors

Socioeconomic
- middle and upper class
- the myth of urban dwellers being more prone than rural dwellers has been discredited

Ethnicity
- white

Religion
- no statistical differences

Gender
- male:female ratio 3:1

Age
- 85 years of age or older

Life-style
- lives alone
- isolated
- recent relocation
- previous attempts, especially in males

Social support
- lacking

Marital status
- never married
- widower
  - high risk 6–12 months after loss (both sexes)
  - remains higher for males

Health status
- alcoholism
- poor health
- terminal illness
- chronic pain or disease
- mental illness
- depression

Psychological status
- helplessness
- hopelessness
- haplessness

Common Adverse Effects of Antidepressants

Anticholinergic
- dry mouth
- blurred vision
- constipation
- urinary retention
- tachycardia

Cardiovascular
- tachycardia
- postural hypotension

Neurologic
- tremors
- confusion
- sedation
- weakness

G. Removing the means to commit suicide is the first step needed to promote a protective environment. The overtly suicidal patient may be hospitalized to allow for safety and concentrated intervention. Once the threat to life has been eliminated, increasing social contacts with significant others and involving outpatient services provide continued protection from isolation. An organized plan of after-care in the home or in community/health care centers is essential.

References

Barbato L. Crisis intervention. In: Decision making in emergency nursing. Toronto: BC Decker, 1987:198.

Bernstein JG. Drug therapy in psychiatry. 2nd ed. PSG Publishing, 1988:459.

Burnside IM, ed. Nursing and the aged: A self-care approach. New York: McGraw-Hill, 1988:687.

HELPLESSNESS

Deborah Antai-Otong

Feelings of helplessness may be precipitated by uncontrollable events. The elderly often lose control over their lives when they are in extended care facilities or living with family members. Patients experiencing feelings of helplessness tend to overgeneralize negative life events, thereby reinforcing their feelings of losing control, powerlessness, and dependency. They may take a single shortcoming or failure as a sign of personal or social inadequacy.

A. Elicit information about
   • social withdrawal
   • apathy or fatigue
   • decreased motivation to participate in daily activities
   • increased dependency or passivity
   • recent stressors such as the loss of a loved one or a recent move
   • previous and current coping patterns
   • social and emotional support systems
   • previous psychiatric history
   • suicidal ideations or previous attempts
   • adherence to medical regimens
   • current medications used, prescription and over the counter
   • alcohol or drug use

B. Factors to be assessed include
   • cognition
   • mood and affect
   • use of negative self-statements
   • psychomotor agitation or retardation
   If alcohol or drug abuse is suspected, appropriate laboratory toxicity screens should be performed.

C. Continuously assess patients exhibiting symptoms of helplessness for suicide risk. Feelings of helplessness can lead to pessimism, powerlessness, and hopelessness. If uninterrupted, this spiral may end in a depression so severe that suicide seems the only answer.

D. Assist patients to work through a crisis and take control of their lives by
   • developing goals to deal with present stressors
   • encouraging independence
   • reassurance and inviting an expression of feelings
   • allowing them to participate in decision making
   • exploring through reminiscence the meaningfulness and purpose of their lives
   • changing or minimizing negative thought processes through realistic evaluation of situations
   • homework assignments that provide fulfilling activity and diminish poor self-concepts (Table 1)

E. Modifying behavior can result in more effective coping patterns and a decrease in feelings of helplessness. Specific strategies aim to develop attainable goals, decrease stressors, and promote independence/control (Table 1). Suicide is a serious consequence of unresolved feelings of helplessness. Clinical depression and a history of drug abuse are additional risk factors for suicide.

F. Because of the high rate of successful suicides in the elderly, efforts to prevent suicide should be directed at assessing the potential, means, and opportunity. Environmental modifications and removal of specific means such as firearms or hoarded medications are indicated.

G. Suicidal ideation dictates referral to a primary care physician and probable psychiatric consultation. For depression, antidepressants, electroconvulsive therapy, or other medical management may be necessary. Of course, helplessness associated with disease processes, pain, immobility, or other functional limitations deserves a second or fresh look to see whether further intervention may be beneficial.

H. Community activities may include structured day programs that provide activities geared to fit the patient's needs and ability to participate. Social outlets and activities that reinforce social support systems or volunteer work at local health facilities may be appropriate. Increased social interactions promote a sense of well-being and belonging while decreasing remorse and self-deprecation. The homebound elderly may benefit from home visitation or outreach programs. If the risk of suicide is suspected, referrals to State Departments of Human Resources/Adult Protective Services, mental health services, or suicide prevention and crisis centers should be initiated, depending on the community's recognized response network.

TABLE 1 Strategies to Decrease Helplessness

Strategy	Actions
Develop attainable goals	Give cues for performance
	Provide rewards for success
	Define options allowable
Decrease stressors	Teach relaxation techniques
	Have patient engage in physical activity
	Ensure social support
	Provide consistent, structured environment
Promote independence/ control	Allow decision making
	Introduce minimal change
	Reward attempts at independent activities
	Discourage negative self-talk

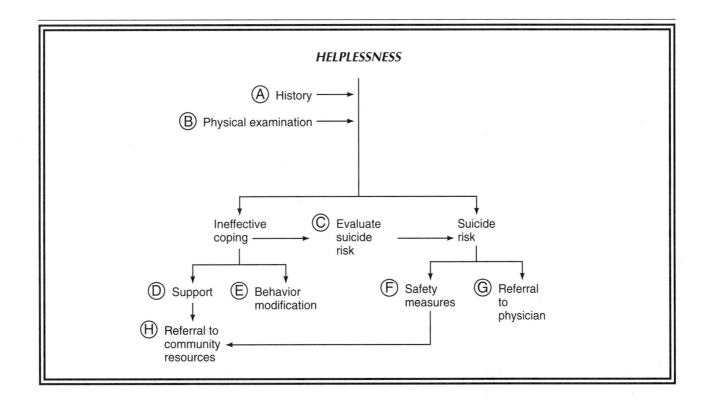

HELPLESSNESS

References

LeSage J, Slimmer LW, Lopez M, et al. Learned helplessness. J Gerontol Nurs 1989; 15:8, 42.

Meichenbaum D. Cognitive-behavioral modification. 2nd ed. New York: Plenum Press, 1979.

Seligman M. Helplessness: On depression, development, and death. San Francisco: WH Freeman, 1975.

Michigan Alcoholism Screening Test (MAST)

	Scoring Weights
1. Do you feel you are a normal drinker?	No (2)
2. Have you ever awakened the morning after some drinking the night before and found that you could not remember a part of the evening before?	Yes (2)
3. Does your wife/husband/companion ever worry or complain about your drinking?	Yes (1)
4. Can you stop drinking without a struggle after one or two drinks?	No (2)
5. Do you ever feel bad about your drinking?	Yes (1)
6. Do friends or relatives think you are a normal drinker?	No (2)
7. Are you always able to stop drinking when you want to?	No (2)
8. Have you ever attended a meeting of Alcoholics Anonymous (AA)?	Yes (5)
9. Have you gotten into fights when drinking?	Yes (1)
10. Has drinking ever created problems between you and your wife/husband?	Yes (2)
11. Has your wife/husband (or other family member) ever gone to anyone for help about your drinking?	Yes (2)
12. Have you ever lost friends or girlfriends or boyfriends because of drinking?	Yes (2)
13. Have you ever gotten into trouble at work because of drinking?	Yes (2)
14. Have you ever lost a job because of drinking?	Yes (2)
15. Have you ever neglected your obligations, your family, or your work for two or more days in a row because you were drinking?	Yes (2)
16. Do you ever drink before noon?	Yes (1)
17. Have you ever been told you have liver trouble? Cirrhosis?	Yes (2)
18. Have you ever had delirium tremens (DTs), severe shaking, heard voices or seen things that weren't there after heavy drinking?	Yes (2)
19. Have you ever gone to anyone for help about your drinking?	Yes (5)
20. Have you ever been in a hospital because of drinking?	Yes (5)
21. Have you ever been a patient in a psychiatric hospital or on a psychiatric ward of a general hospital where drinking was a part of the problem?	Yes (2)
22. Have you ever been seen at a psychiatric or mental health clinic or gone to a doctor, social worker or clergyman for help with an emotional problem in which drinking has played a part?	Yes (2)

Scoring: 3 − 4 indicates possible alcoholism
5 or greater correlates with definite alcoholism

Adapted from Selzer ML. The Michigan Alcoholism Screening Test (MAST): The quest for a new diagnostic instrument. Am J Psychiatry 1971; 127:1653; with permission.

ROLE RELATIONSHIPS

ABUSE

Barbara Harrison Nauss

Abuse is the deliberate and willful act of a caregiver in inflicting injury. The elder abuse victim is typically female, over age 75 years, living with a relative, and with physical or mental impairment. Abuse should be suspected when history taking reveals
- conflicting information from caregiver and patient
- a frightened, ambivalent, withdrawn, or untrusting patient
- repeated injuries or accidents

Abuser characteristics include
- most likely a family member providing care in the home
- substance abuse
- poor relationship with the patient in the past or at present
- poor impulse control
- mental illness
- ineffective coping skills with expression of significant stress or frustration (see Caregiver Stress, p. 292)
- unrealistic expectations
- dependency needs of his or her own
- a feeling of being forced to care for the patient

A. When abuse is suspected, interview the patient first and alone to build trust. Patients may fear displacement or reprisals from the caregiver. The patient must understand that the information is being obtained to promote health and welfare, and that all decisions will be made with their input.
    Important social history information includes
    - the relationship of the caregiver to the patient
    - living arrangements
    - monetary arrangements
    - previous and present nature of the relationship with the caregiver
    - events in a typical day
    - names of family and friends
    - the degree of dependence on the caregiver
    - the adequacy of medicine, supplies, and assistance
    - any history of family violence

    Health history taking elicits
    - chronic conditions
    - medications
    - treatments
    - recent illnesses or injuries
      - events surrounding injury
      - time interval between injury and seeking care
    - ability to perform activities of daily living
    - recent changes in health status
    - source of primary care
    - the number of physicians seen in the previous 6 months

    If possible, contact previous health care providers to determine whether the information provided is accu-

rate. Obtain information from the caregiver after interviewing the patient. Provide privacy and ask questions in a nonjudgmental manner. Ask nonthreatening questions (e.g., social history) first to build trust, then progress to more probing questions, finishing with the history of the injury. Use this opportunity to look for clues about the caregiver's cognitive abilities. Inquire about
- social history
  - quality of past and present relationship
  - events in a typical day
  - available support systems for caregiver
  - financial arrangements
  - caregiver coping methods
  - other stressors
- caregiver health history
  - chronic conditions
  - recent changes in health status or illnesses
  - mental health history
  - medications/drugs
    - alcohol use
  - self-care limitations
- patient health history
  - health status
  - recent changes in health status
  - self-care limitations
  - previous injuries
  - events surrounding this injury
  - time between injury and seeking health care

B. Physical assessment is focused on indications of abuse (see box below). Bruises and skin injuries should be observed for
    - location
    - size
    - color
    - shape
    - different stages of healing

Patient Indicators of Abuse

- Injuries inconsistent with reported cause
- Unusual patterns of injury or repeated injuries
- Hematomas and bruises, especially over soft tissues
- Chafing or excoriation on ankles, wrists, or trunk (due to prolonged or inappropriate restraints)
- Fractures
- Burns
- Drug toxicity
- Malnutrition or dehydration

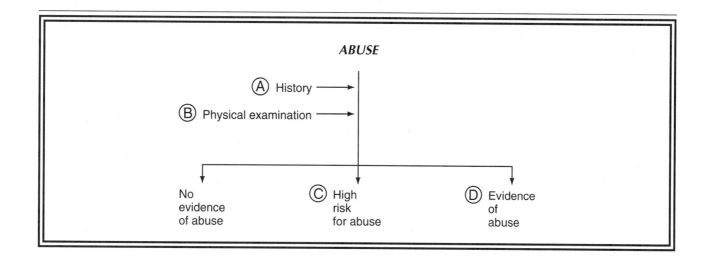

ABUSE

(A) History →

(B) Physical examination →

No evidence of abuse   (C) High risk for abuse   (D) Evidence of abuse

Determine the patient's
- functional status
- cognition
  - judgment
  - memory
- mood and affect
- hydration/nutritional status

Observe interactions between patient and caregiver and determine
- whether the patient is given an opportunity to speak
- whether there is an attitude of indifference or hostility toward the patient
- whether they communicate openly
- who makes the decisions
- whether the caregiver withholds affection or threatens nursing home placement

Laboratory tests may include
- electrolytes
- albumin
- protein
- CBC with differential
- sedimentation rate
- therapeutic drug levels

C. High-risk characteristics include
- a history of violence in the relationship
- a caregiver financially dependent on the patient
- a patient totally dependent on the caregiver
- inappropriate medications or polypharmacy
- a history of accidental injuries
- a patient having multiple physicians or changing physicians often
- limited informal support network
- a patient with alcohol or drug abuse
- a patient with complex disabilities due to Alzheimer's disease, cerebrovascular disease, etc.

Interventions appropriate in a high-risk situation are
- discussion of options for respite or assistance with care
- improvement of caregiver coping strategies
- listening to both caregiver and patient
- referral to a community agency for monitoring and state department of human services/adult protective services
- a protective custody order
- a petition for guardianship

D. When evidence of abuse is found,
- treat injuries
- report findings to Adult Protective Services
- contact social services for alternative care placement

For the patient's safety, it may be necessary to discuss other living arrangements, both short and long term. Hospitalization may be needed to treat injuries. Ask the patient about other family members or friends who could be caregivers. Explain other options such as
- use of a home health care agency
- foster care
- adult day care
- a retirement or nursing home

References

Beth Israel Hospital Elder Assessment Team. An elder abuse assessment team in an acute hospital setting. Gerontologist 1986; 26:115.

Fulmer T, Street S, Carr K. Abuse of the elderly: Screening and detection. J Emerg Nurs 1986; 11:131.

Haviland S, O'Brien J. Physical abuse and neglect of the elderly: Assessment and intervention. Orthop Nurs 1989; 8:11.

Quinn MJ, Tomita SK. Elder abuse and neglect. New York: Springer, 1986.

CAREGIVER STRESS

Barbara Harrison Nauss

Caregiver stress occurs when the caregiver-patient relationship becomes overwhelming for the caregiver. It may result from an increase in stressors or a decrease in coping. Most caregivers are female family members. The quality of the patient-caregiver relationship is influenced by
• the previous relationship
• the caregiver's willingness to assume the caregiver role
• financial need
• family obligation or pressure
• role conflict due to multiple roles the caregiver must manage
Spouse or same-age caregivers are more likely to suffer role entrenchment and isolation. Caregivers looking after mentally impaired elders for extended periods with inadequate social support are at greatest risk for stress and depression.

A. To elicit the history, interview the caregiver alone. The caregiver should be provided with the opportunity to discuss problems openly without promoting the patient's feelings of guilt concerning their personal and health care needs. Specific information to be determined is highlighted in Table 1.

B. Assess both patient and caregiver for
    • general appearance
      • hygiene
      • injury/lesions
      • affect
    • nonverbal communication
      • eye contact
      • body language
    • verbal communication
      • to each other
      • about each other
      • patterns of decision making
      • attention to needs
    To make appropriate referrals, physical examination of the patient may be required to determine
    • functional level
    • cognitive state
    Valuable data may be collected using the Burden Interview (see p. 305) or OARS Resource Scale (see p. 304). This information, in conjunction with assessment of physical care needs, will help to determine the ability of the caregiver to cope with the level of role stress identified and the need for interventions by health care providers.

C. If the caregiver is effectively coping with role stress,
    • listen actively
    • provide information about community services
    • discuss plans for
      • respite
      • change in patient condition
    • counsel on
      • normal effects of stress
      • early warning signs of coping problems
    • encourage him or her to ask for assistance with errands, chores, or caregiver tasks

D. When the caregiver appears at risk for not being able to cope with the caregiver role
    • encourage use of available support systems
    • arrange respite care
    • counsel on effective coping strategies
    • refer for
      • home health care
      • financial assistance
      • transportation
      • utilities
      • housing
      • food
    • fortify the support network
      • community volunteers
      • group meetings for caregivers
    • focus on the caregiver's well-being rather than trying to resolve an intractable patient problem

E. Ineffective coping with caregiver stress requires intervention to prevent abuse or neglect. Referrals can be made to
    • mental health specialists
    • a community agency for monitoring of home health care
    • social services to obtain assistance in obtaining auxiliary or alternative care

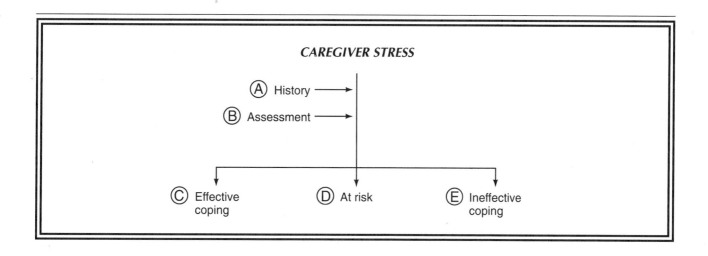

CAREGIVER STRESS

(A) History →

(B) Assessment →

(C) Effective coping   (D) At risk   (E) Ineffective coping

TABLE 1 Important Factors to Elicit in Determining Caregiver Stress

Topic	Respondent		Topic	Respondent	
	Patient	Caregiver		Patient	Caregiver
Social History			*Social History (cont'd)*		
• number and strength of other roles and risk of role conflict		X	• financial arrangements and resources	X	X
• spouse			• financial dependency on patient's income		X
• parent			• length of time in caregiving		X
• sibling			• caregiver self-esteem		X
• friend/companion					
• confidante			*Medical History*		
• job/career			• medical conditions	X	X
• reaction to role changes	X	X	• prognosis	X	X
• perception of caregiver role	X	X	• self-care/activities of daily living abilities	X	X
• availability of a confidante	X	X	• medication regimen	X	X
• relationship to caregiver	X	X	• psychotropic agents	X	X
• willingness to confront realities of situation		X	• medical/health care		
• quality of relationship prior to illness	X	X	• frequency	X	X
• length of time in relationship	X	X	• subspeciality care	X	X
• living arrangements	X	X	• primary care relationship	X	X
• other family members, friends, or community support systems	X	X	• perception of support	X	X
• frequency of contact	X	X	• case/care management	X	X
• type and frequency of assistance with caregiving activities		X	• cognitive status	X	X
• provision of respite		X	• mental health/psychiatric problems	X	X
• emotional reaction to patient's illness	X	X	*Environment*		
• leisure activities		X	• community/social or home health care		X
• religion/church participation	X	X	• assistive devices or equipment/aids	X	X
• receptiveness to and past seeking of counseling		X	• housing	X	X
			• utilities	X	X
			• transportation resources	X	X

References

Baillie V, Norbeck J, Barnes LE. Stress, social support and psychological distress of family caregivers of the elderly. Nurs Res 1988; 37:217.

Given C, Collins C, Given B. Sources of stress among families caring for relatives with Alzheimer's disease. Nurs Clin North Am 1988; 23:69.

Miller J. Coping with chronic illness. Philadelphia: FA Davis, 1983.

Zarit SH, Reever KE, Bach-Peterson J. Relatives of the impaired elderly: Correlates of feelings of burden. Gerontologist 1980; 20:649.

EXPLOITATION

Barbara Harrison Nauss

Exploitation is the misappropriation of assets or resources. It can range from the stealing of pain medication to inducing the signing over of a deed to a home. Exploitation can be difficult to detect, investigate, and prove. Indicators of exploitation may include a
- lack of amenities, especially when there are adequate finances
- caregiver, family member, or other individual who
  - expresses unusual interest in financial matters
  - attempts to isolate the patient from other family members and friends
  - spends inadequately on health care, possibly refusing services that would deplete the estate
  - fails to disclose finances or plans

A. Social history taking focuses on
- identification of resources
- people who have regular contact with the patient
- recent acquaintances
- family or significant others who may provide assistance
- financial data, specifically
  - income sources
  - checks coming to the house
  - bank accounts
    - independent
    - joint
  - documents of ownership
  - valuable property
  - financial relationships such as
    - power of attorney
    - trust
    - representative payee or joint tenancy
To assess loss, ask about
- food, clothing, or medications not provided
- strangers appearing with "deals," promises of assistance, or requests for help
- recent signing of documents
- accompaniment to the bank
- changes in bank accounts
- unexplained overdrafts or insufficient funds
- missing property from home or room
Validate any loss with another family member or friend.

B. Assessment focuses on
- general factors
  - discrepancy between caregiver and patient appearance
  - manner of communication between patient and caregiver
- cognition to
  - add credibility to the report of loss
  - counter possible attempts by a suspect to dismiss the allegations as related to patient dementia
- signs and symptoms of
  - neglect (see p. 300)
  - abuse (see p. 290)
- mood/affect
  - depression
Neuropsychological testing by a clinical psychologist may be indicated if there is no clear explanation for deficits in specific cognitive abilities.

C. If no loss can be validated, consider
- ongoing monitoring
- counseling
- reassurance
- referrals
  - social services
  - State Department of Human Services/Adult Protective Services
- assistance with financial and legal safeguards

D. If loss is validated or there is a high index of suspicion,
- report to an appropriate authority such as
  - police
  - State Department of Human Services/Adult Protective Services
- arrange a referral to establish financial and legal safeguards

References

Quinn MJ, Tomita S. Elder abuse and neglect. New York: Springer, 1986.
Thompson J, Pender S, Schmitt J. Retaining rights of impaired elderly. J Gerontol Nurs 1987; 13:20.
Weiler K. Financial abuse of the elderly: Recognizing and acting on it. J Gerontol Nurs. 1989; 15:10.

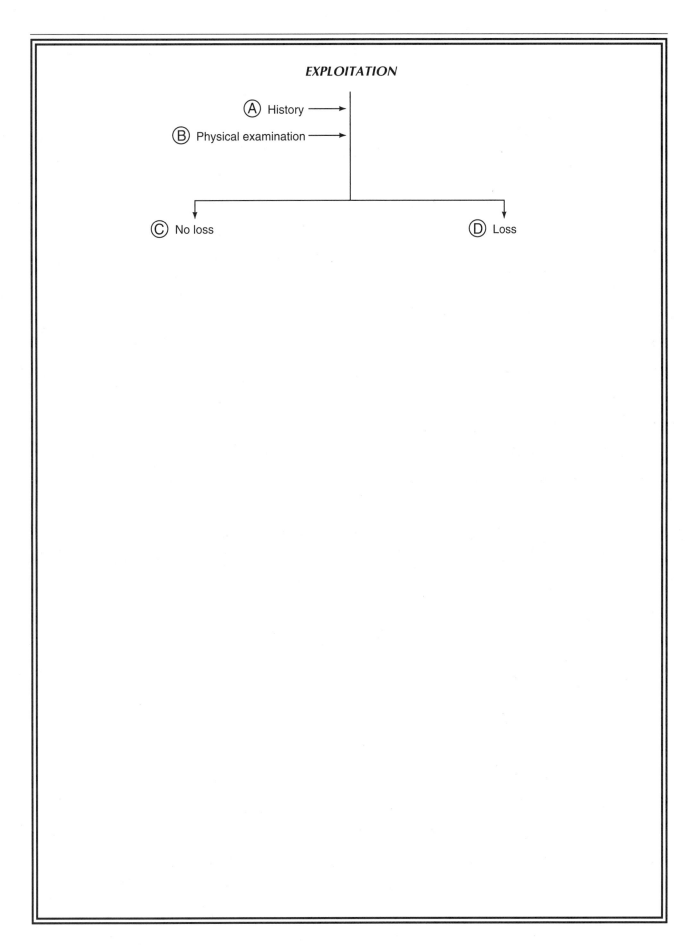

LONELINESS

Barbara Harrison Nauss

Loneliness is the unpleasant experience of deficient social relationships, in either quality or quantity, as a result of
• decreased social contact
• change in social needs
• perceived lack of support despite number and proximity of family and friends

Loneliness may be transient, situational, or chronic, setting the stage for depression, increased risk of suicide, and jeopardized psychological well-being. Situational loneliness may become chronic if ignored. Loneliness is nonproductive, resulting in expenditure of energy to protect against lonely feelings rather than deal with the feelings (see the box "Characteristics and Psychosocial Traits Correlating with Loneliness").

A. Social history includes questions about
  • support systems
  • depth of relationships
  • perceived support
  • property with emotional attachment, i.e., home
  • previous patterns of social contact
  • leisure activities: solitary or with others
  Ask about patterns of defense against loneliness, which may include
  • complaints about unfilled time
  • overplanning
  • expression of distorted self-esteem
  • somatic preoccupation
  • lack of planning
  • dependency on others
  • anxiety
  To assess self-evaluation of poor health, a strong indicator of loneliness, ask the patient to describe his or her health and listen for
  • negative comments
  • multiple physician visits
  • multiple somatic illness
  • history of polypharmacy (see Polypharmacy, p. 72)
  • inconsistent history
  • statements that "nothing helps"
  Attempt to quantify somatic complaints by obtaining information on frequency, intensity, and specificity. These complaints may represent attempts to gain attention and diminish loneliness. Assess mental health attributes (see the box "Mental Health Attributes of Loneliness"). Obtain a drug history, including
  • prescription
  • changes in medications
  • use of alcohol or illicit drugs
  • over-the-counter medications
  • overuse of medications

B. Evaluate mental status (see tools in Cognition/Perception section, pp. 268–272), which includes
  • cognition
  • signs and symptoms of depression
  • mood and affect
  • suicide risk (see Depression, p. 282)
  Assess
  • weight
  • vital signs
  • routine physical examination, targeting specific somatic complaints, such as
    • nausea
    • insomnia
    • decreased appetite
    • pain
    • fatigue (see p. 14)
    • headaches
    • constipation
  Laboratory tests may include electrolytes and glucose, protein and albumin, and/or therapeutic drug levels to rule out toxicity.

Characteristics and Psychosocial Traits Correlating with Loneliness

Characteristic	Psychosocial Trait
Female	Anxiety
Widowed	Hostility
Living alone	Dependency
Age in the 80s	Decreased self-esteem
Restricted mobility	Self-consciousness
Recent loss suffered	Introversion
Infrequent contact with family and friends	Lack of assertiveness
	External locus of control
Relatively infirm	Difficulty making friends
Lacking adequate transportation	Inability to participate in groups
Experiencing forced separation and/or role change	Inability to maintain friendships

Mental Health Attributes of Loneliness

Thoughts of
  being different
  being isolated
Feelings of sadness, depression, anger, loss of control
Actions such as avoiding social contacts, overeating or not eating, spending unusually long hours volunteering or with hobbies, neglecting personal appearance

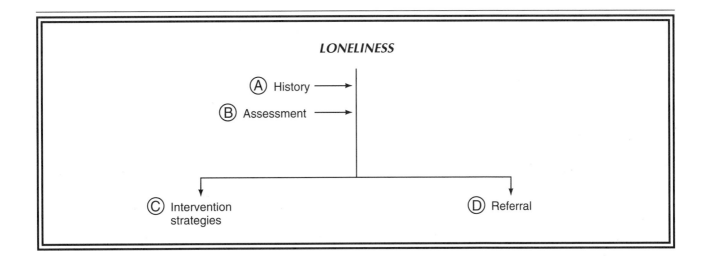

LONELINESS

- (A) History
- (B) Assessment
- (C) Intervention strategies
- (D) Referral

C. General interventions may include
- spending time with the patient
- developing a trust relationship
- encouraging the patient to verbalize loneliness
- expressing acceptance through touch and nonverbal behaviors

Specific interventions may be tailored to defense mechanisms and social conditions, such as
- exploring ways to enjoy leisure time
- discussing previous episodes of loneliness to encourage resolution
- validating perceptions of loss of control
- providing opportunities to make decisions, particularly about daily events
- encouraging patient to plan times for solitude
- exploring feelings of loneliness in a secure or therapeutic relationship
- examining degree of dependency, real or perceived
- encouraging independence and more appropriate attention-seeking behaviors
- reassuring patient with unsubstantiated somatic complaints
- encouraging focus on other interests
- redirecting discussion of worthlessness to other interests
- assisting to develop methods of coping

D. Depression, risk of suicide, and other emotional disorders require referral to mental health specialists.

Referral and follow-up of loneliness are essential because of the chronic nature of the problem with older adults. Referrals for addressing loneliness may include
- senior citizens centers
- recreational programs
- psychosocial counseling
- in-home assistance such as friendly visitors programs
- social services for transportation and senior community services
- nutrition sites
- volunteer activities
- telephone reassurance and contact projects
- involvement of family and friends, with permission

References

delaCruz LAD. On loneliness and the elderly. J Gerontol Nurs 1986; 12:22.

Replau LA. Preventing the harmful consequences of severe and persistent loneliness. Rockville, MD: National Institute of Mental Health, 1984.

Rodgers BL. Loneliness: Easing the pain of the hospitalized elderly. J Gerontol Nurs 1989; 15:16.

Ryan MD, Patterson J. Loneliness in the elderly. J Gerontol Nurs 1987; 13:6.

LOSSES AND GRIEF

Barbara Harrison Nauss

Aging people experience personal, social, and economic losses. The most damaging and significant losses are personal. Losses may be sudden and multiple. The emotional crises imposed by numerous losses can result in mental health problems. Grief from any loss is a painful emotion. Bereavement due to loss of a spouse has been associated with an increased risk of morbidity and mortality. Grief reactions may also result in multiple somatic complaints.

A. The history of loss should include
    • previous experiences with significant losses
    • coping methods
    • recent losses
    • available support systems
    • secondary losses
      • financial
      • role changes
    • spirituality (see section Spiritual Care on pp. 308–317)
    • religious affiliation and attendance
    Ask the family or friends to identify
    • inappropriate behavior
    • the patient's ability to discuss loss
    • any new plans, habits, or relationships
    Health history taking elicits
    • potential and actual health care needs
    • medications
      • sedatives
      • analgesics
      • antidepressants
      • polypharmacy (see p. 72)
      • overuse/abuse
    • alcohol use/abuse
    • psychiatric or emotional problems
      • depression (see p. 282)
      • suicide attempts or ideation
    • sleep disorders (see Sleep Pattern Disturbances, p. 82)
    • hormonal problems
    • thyroid dysfunction

B. Assessment is aimed at
    • identifying health problems that may reduce the patient's ability to cope
      • electrolyte imbalance
      • oxygenation and perfusion
      • drug toxicity
    • conditions that may mimic or prolong grief reactions
      • sleep disorders exhibited by
        • fatigue (see p. 17)
        • lethargy
        • inattention
        • confusion (see Confusion/Cognitive Changes/Dementia, p. 254)
    • thyroid dysfunction
    • drug toxicity
    • hormonal imbalance
    Determine the patient's
    • cognitive status (see tools on pp. 268–272)
    • mood/affect (see tools on p. 268)
      • depression (see p. 282)
      • suicide risk
    • weight
    • ability to perform activities of daily living (ADL) and instrumental ADL
    • ability to express feelings of sadness, loss, and anxiety
    Laboratory tests may include
    • electrolytes
    • glucose
    • albumin
    • protein
    • therapeutic drug levels
    • thyroid function tests, including TSH

C. Indicators that suggest progress in the resolution of grief and effective coping include the patient's ability to
    • recall the deceased with both good and bad memories
    • reach out to others who are grieving and offer comfort
    • reinvest in new relationships or revive old friendships and interests
    Effective coping strategies used by older adults may include
    • reaching out to or helping others
    • making new friends
    • joining groups
    • setting goals
    • maintaining independence
    • learning new skills
    • maintaining a sense of humor
    • sustaining family ties
    • avoiding isolation and self-pity
    • talking with the deceased
    • prayer and religious support (see pp. 308–317)

D. Ineffective coping may occur when part or all of the grief process becomes
    • excessive
    • prolonged
    • inhibited
    • delayed
    • disruptive to relationships
    Patients without support systems are at greatest risk for abnormal grief reactions. A patient with emotional or social withdrawal for 6 months or longer risks experiencing chronic grief. Because of emotional pain and

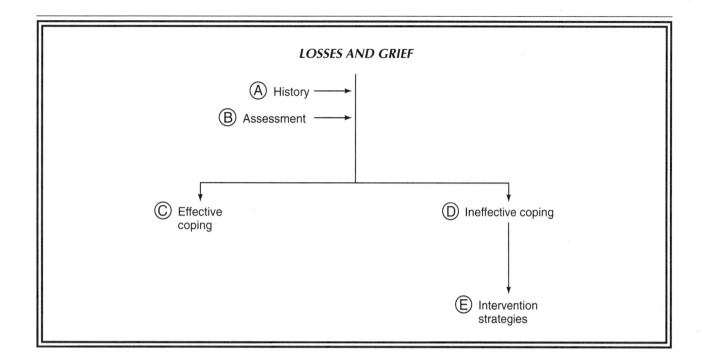

LOSSES AND GRIEF

A. History
B. Assessment
C. Effective coping
D. Ineffective coping
E. Intervention strategies

previous life focuses, the patient may become unable to reinvest in new relationships.

Common problems that may follow a significant loss include
- loneliness (see p. 296)
- social isolation
- anxiety (see p. 278)
- exacerbation of chronic health conditions
- medication overuse
- alcohol abuse (see Undiagnosed Alcohol Abuse, p. 274)
- mood disorder
- depression (see p. 282)
- suicide

The patient's ability to cope with loss depends on many factors, which vary with each person (see box below).

Factors Influencing Ability to Cope with Loss
• health status • number of recent losses • previous experience of loss • previous methods of coping • existence and use of a support system • belief in a power greater than oneself (see pp. 308–317)

E. Grieving older patients respond to the same strategies and interventions appropriate for any grieving patient. Assistance in the grief process may include
- attentive listening
- obtaining permission to involve family, friends, or spiritual supports
- review of and reassurance about the grief process
- encouraging use of previous effective coping strategies
- reminiscence therapy

Consider referrals
- for psychosocial counseling
- to a mental health specialist
- to a support group
- for grief counseling

References

Alexander J, Kiely J. Working with the bereaved. Geriatr Nurs 1986; March/April:85.

Garrett JE. Multiple losses in older adults. J Gerontol Nurs 1987; 13:8.

Gass KA. Coping strategies of widows. J Gerontol Nurs 1987; 13:29.

McCue J, ed. Medical care of the elderly. Lexington, MA: DC Heath, 1983.

NEGLECT

Barbara Harrison Nauss

Neglect consists of failure to provide the necessities of life such as food, clothing, shelter, hygiene, and medical care. The neglect victim is usually female, over age 75, living with a relative, and with a physical or mental impairment, or both. Victims may or may not be aware of their own neglect. They may
- be passive
- be compliant
- be socially isolated
- feel low self-esteem

Neglect may be active or passive depending on the intent of the caregiver (see the box).

A. If neglect is suspected, interview the patient first and alone to build trust and collect baseline information for comparison when interviewing the caregiver.
   Social history to be gathered includes
   - relationship to caregiver
   - name(s) of other caregiver(s)
   - living arrangements
   - monetary arrangements and finances
   - past and present nature of relationship with caregiver
     - presence of neglect and/or abuse
   - the length of time the patient has required caregiving
   - support systems
   - events in a typical day
   - coping patterns
   - stressors in the home
     - conflicting responsibilities such as jobs or child care
   - use of respite care
   - use of community services
   Patient health history taking determines
   - chronic conditions
   - recent illnesses or changes in condition
   - medications, prescribed and over the counter
     - adequacy
     - accuracy of administration by the caregiver
     - withholding of pain medication
     - frequent use of sedatives
     - refilling without re-evaluation
   - treatments
     - type
     - frequency
   - knowledge of home care skills

Caregiver Characteristics in Active Versus Passive Neglect	
Passive Neglect	*Active Neglect*
Ignorance	Indifference
Impairment	Deliberate withholding of care
Lack of support systems	Caregiver stress (see p. 292)
Lack of resources	

- health care provision
  - last visit
  - interval between visits
- assistive devices
- adequacy of supplies
- description of when and how daily care is provided
- home health care use or refusal
- reason for visits and precipitating events

If possible, contact previous health care providers to determine whether the information provided is accurate. Caregiver health history taking elicits
- ability to render care
- illnesses, chronic and acute
- medications
- alcohol or illicit drug use
- mental health problems
- self-care abilities
- mobility limitations
- sensory limitations
- limitations of energy level

During the interview, determine the caregiver's
- cognitive abilities
- experience in caring for elders or sick persons
- receptiveness to home health or respite care

B. Physical indicators of neglect may include
   - poor hygiene
   - weight loss
   - inappropriate dress
   - contractures
   - dehydration
   - anemia
   - skin breakdown
   - malnutrition
   - illness due to lack of medication
   - urinary tract infection

Sores about the ankles or wrists and under the armpits may indicate prolonged or inappropriate use of restraints. Look for subtle signs or the appearance of
- changes in cognitive abilities
  - confusion
- personality change
- passivity
- lethargy
- withdrawal
- communication problems
  - domination by the caregiver
  - poor quality

Laboratory work-up includes
- electrolytes and glucose
- CBC
- albumin and protein
- therapeutic drug levels
- sedimentation rate
- urinalysis

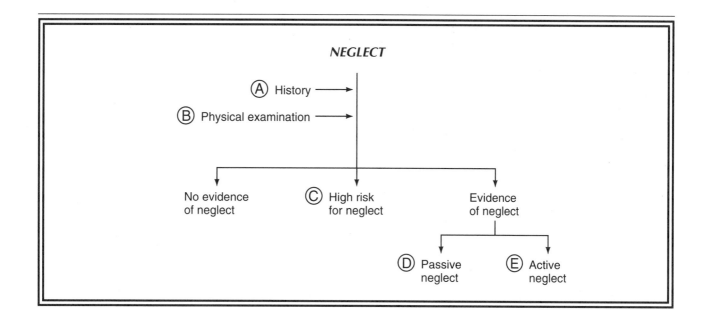

NEGLECT

A History →

B Physical examination →

No evidence of neglect

C High risk for neglect

Evidence of neglect

D Passive neglect

E Active neglect

A chest film and CT scan may also be warranted for pulmonary concerns and mental status evaluation.

C. High-risk situations occur in the presence of
- a history of patient and caregiver neglectful or abusive relationship
- patient resistance or hostility to assistance with care
- patient dementia

High-risk situations involve a caregiver with
- multiple or overwhelming responsibilities
- an attitude of indifference
- a passive personality
- previous dependency on the patient
- immaturity
- a habit of leaving the patient isolated for long portions of the day

Interventions in a high-risk situation include
- discussion of options for respite or assistance with care
- improvement of caregiver coping skills
- listening to both caregiver and patient
- exploration of alternatives for care
- referral to a community agency for monitoring

D. Neglect due to passive reasons may be amenable to
- education in patient care and the aging process
- support services
  - home health aide
  - transportation
  - counseling
  - respite care
  - chore/homemaker services
  - nursing care
- substance abuse programs
- assistance to increase communication effectiveness and stress relief

- referrals to community agencies for
  - monitoring
  - an advocacy group
  - an ombudsman program

E. Active neglect due to hostility, exploitation, or indifference requires more extensive and invasive intervention, including
- exploration of alternative living arrangements such as
  - nursing home
  - adult foster care
  - other family
  - hospitalization
- social service referral
- home health care monitoring
- referral to the State Department of Human Services/ Adult Protective Services for removal from home and placement and guardianship

References

Beth Israel Hospital Elder Assessment Team. An elder abuse assessment team in an acute hospital setting. Gerontologist 1986; 26:115.

Fulmer T, Street S, Carr K. Abuse of the elderly: Screening and detection. J Emerg Nurs 1986; 11:131.

Haviland S, O'Brien J. Physical abuse and neglect of the elderly: Assessment and intervention. Orthop Nurs 1989; 8:11.

McCue J, ed. Medical care of the elderly. Lexington, MA: DC Heath, 1983.

Quinn MJ, Tomita SK. Elder abuse and neglect. New York: Springer, 1986.

RETIREMENT

Barbara Harrison Nauss

Retirement is a major life change that may affect all aspects of an individual's life. Perceptions of retirement vary greatly and may be influenced by
- ideas about old age
- experiences with the retirement of others
- feelings of self-worth associated with work
- ability to plan financially for retirement
- interest in leisure activities

A. Social history provides information to determine the patient's ability to cope with retirement, such as
    - marital status
    - living/housing arrangements
    - employment history and its significance
    - family members
    - social support
    - financial resources
    - personal interests
    - sixual interest and activity
    - family and community roles
    Health history taking elicits details of
    - habits
      - alcohol intake
      - tobacco use
      - dietary
    - activity level and exercise
    - hospitalizations
    - chronic medical conditions
    - recent illnesses
    - medications, prescribed and over the counter
    - allergies
    - frequency of visits with health care providers

B. Health assessment includes
    - cancer screening
      - rectal
      - stool for occult blood
      - breast
      - mammography
      - prostate
      - Pap smear
      - pelvic
      - skin
    - cardiovascular screening
      - blood pressure
      - baseline electrocardiography
      - auscultation for bruits
      - palpation of peripheral pulses
    - neurological examination
    - sensory evaluation
      - visual acuity and fields
      - hearing acuity
    - vaccination update
      - annual influenza
      - tetanus-diphtheria
      - Pneumovax

C. Inadequate adjustment to retirement has been associated with psychological and physiologic problems. Help patients to plan interventions to improve their ability to cope with retirement (see box). Prepare patients for retirement changes through
    - anticipatory guidance
    - health teaching about normal aging changes
    - counseling
    - community referrals such as the American Association of Retired Persons (AARP)
    - psychosocial services for problem solving and resolution

---

Techniques for coping with retirement

- Financial
  - financial planning
  - investigation of benefits
  - application for Social Security and other benefits
- Social
  - develop interests
  - explore social networks
- Psychological
  - verbalize feelings
  - explore fears
  - discuss role changes
- Spiritual
  - life review
  - exploration of meaning

References

Futrell M, et al. Primary health care of the older adult. North Scituate, MA: Duxbury Press, 1980.

Neuhs H. Pre-retirement planning. AAOHN J 1986; 34:571.

Shaughnessy J. Pre-retirement planning and the role of the occupational health nurse. AAOHN J 1988; 36:70.

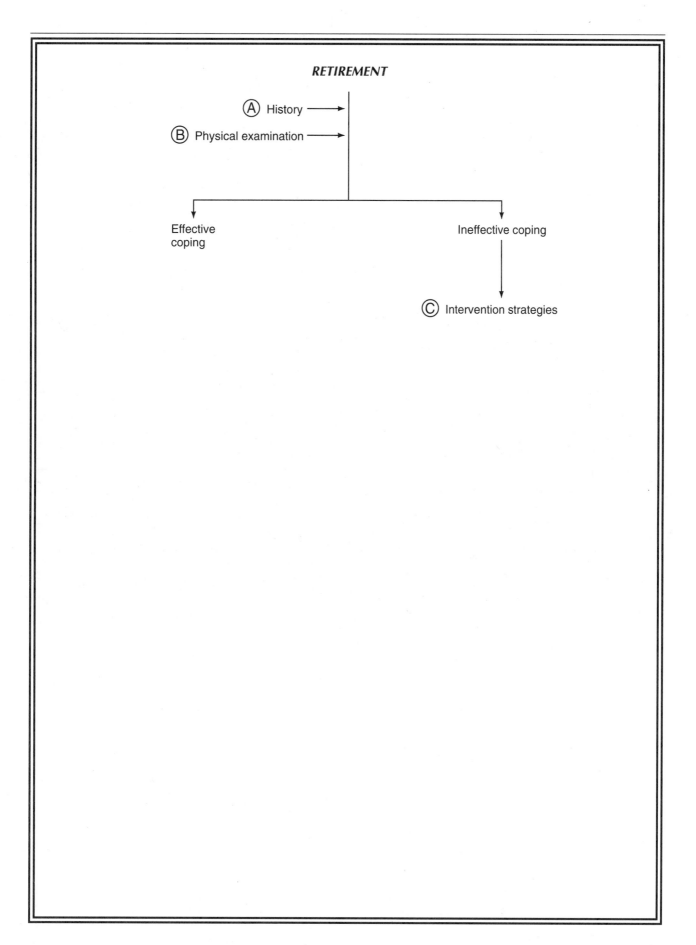

RETIREMENT

(A) History ⟶

(B) Physical examination ⟶

Effective
coping

Ineffective coping

(C) Intervention strategies

OARS Social Resource Scale (Combined Community and Institutional Version)

Now I'd like to ask you some questions about your family and friends.

Are you single, married, never married, widowed, divorced, or separated?

1 Single	3 Widowed	5 Separated
2 Married	4 Divorced	— Not answered

If you are married, does your spouse live here also?

   1 Yes   2 No   — Not answered

Who lives with you?
(Check yes or no for each of the following.)

Yes	No	
_____	_____	No one
_____	_____	Husband or wife
_____	_____	Children
_____	_____	Grandchildren
_____	_____	Parents
_____	_____	Grandparents
_____	_____	Brothers and sisters
_____	_____	Other relatives (does not include in-laws covered in the above categories)
_____	_____	Friends
_____	_____	Nonrelated paid help (includes free room)
_____	_____	Other (specify) _____

In the past year about how often did you leave here to visit your family and/or friends for weekends or holidays or to go on shopping trips or outings?*

1 Once a week or more
2 One to three times a month
3 Less than once a month or only on holidays
4 Never
— Not answered

How many people do you know well enough to visit with in their homes?

3 Five or more
2 Three to four
1 One to two
0 None
— Not answered

About how many times did you talk to someone—friends, relatives, or others—on the telephone in the past week (either you called them or they called you)? (If subject has no phone, question still applies.)

3 Once a day or more
2 Twice
1 Once
0 Not at all
— Not answered

How many times during the past week did you spend some time with someone who does not live with you, that is, you went to see them, or they came to visit you, or you went out to do things together?

How many times in the past week did you visit with someone, either with people who live here or people who visited you here?*

3 Once a day or more
2 Two to six
1 Once
0 Not at all
— Not answered

Do you have someone you can trust and confide in?

1 Yes
0 No
— Not answered

Do you find yourself feeling lonely quite often, sometimes, or almost never?

0 Quite often
1 Sometimes
2 Almost never
— Not answered

Do you see your relatives and friends as often as you want to, or are you somewhat unhappy about how little you see them?

1 As often as wants to
2 Somewhat unhappy about how little
— Not answered

Is there someone (outside this place*) who would give you any help at all if you were sick or disabled, for example, your husband or wife, a member of your family, or a friend?

1 Yes
0 No one willing and able to help
— Not answered

If yes, ask a and b.

a. Is there someone (outside this place*) who would take care of you as long as needed, or only for a short time, or only someone who would help you now and then (for example, taking you to the doctor or fixing lunch occasionally)?

1 Someone who would take care of subject indefinitely (as long as needed)
2 Someone who would take care of subject for a short time (a few weeks to six months)
3 Someone who would help subject now and then (e.g., taking him to the doctor or fixing lunch)
— Not answered

b. Who is this person?
Name _____
Relationship _____

Rating Scale

Rate the current social resources of the person being evaluated along the 6-point scale presented below. Circle the *one* number that best describes the person's present circumstances.

1. *Excellent Social Resources:* Social relationships are very satisfying and extensive; at least one person would take care of him (her) indefinitely.

2. *Good Social Resources:* Social relationships are fairly satisfying and adequate and at least one person would take care of him (her) indefinitely, *or*
Social relationships are very satisfying and extensive, and only short-term help is available.

3. *Mildly Socially Impaired:* Social relationships are unsatisfactory, of poor quality, few; but at least one person would take care of him (her) indefinitely, *or*
Social relationships are fairly satisfactory and adequate, and only short-term help is available.

4. *Moderately Socially Impaired:* Social relationships are unsatisfactory, of poor quality, few; and only short-term care is available, *or*
Social relationships are at least adequate or satisfactory, but help would only be available now and then.

5. *Severely Socially Impaired:* Social relationships are unsatisfactory, of poor quality, few; and help would be available only now and then, *or*
Social relationships are at least satisfactory or adequate, but help is not available even now and then.

6. *Totally Socially Impaired:* Social relationships are unsatisfactory, of poor quality, few; and help is not available even now and then.

*Applies to those living in institutions.
Adapted from Fillenbaum GG. Multidimensional functional assessment of older adults: The Duke Older American Resource and Services Procedures. Hillsdale NJ: L Erlbaum Associates, Inc., 1988; with permission.

The Burden Interview

Instructions: The following is a list of statements, which reflect how people sometimes feel when taking care of another person. After each statement, indicate how often you feel that way—never, rarely, sometimes, quite frequently, or nearly always. There are no right or wrong answers.

1. I feel resentful of other relatives who could but who do not do things for my spouse.

2. I feel that my spouse makes requests that I perceive to be over and above what she or he needs.

3. Because of my involvement with my spouse, I don't have enough time for myself.

4. I feel stressed between trying to give to my spouse as well as to other family responsibilities, job, and so on.

5. I feel embarrassed over my spouse's behavior.

6. I feel guilty about my interactions with my spouse.

7. I feel that I don't do as much for my spouse as I could or should.

8. I feel angry about my interactions with my spouse.

9. I feel that in the past I haven't done as much for my spouse as I could have or should have.

10. I feel nervous or depressed about my interactions with my spouse.

11. I feel that my spouse currently affects my relationships with other family members and friends in a negative way.

12. I feel resentful about my interactions with my spouse.

13. I am afraid of what the future holds for my spouse.

14. I feel pleased about my interactions with my spouse.

15. It's painful to watch my spouse age.

16. I feel useful in my interactions with my spouse.

17. I feel my spouse is dependent.

18. I feel strained in my interactions with my spouse.

19. I feel that my health has suffered because of my involvement with my spouse.

20. I feel that I am contributing to the well-being of my spouse.

21. I feel that the present situation with my spouse doesn't allow me as much privacy as I'd like.

22. I feel that my social life has suffered because of my involvement with my spouse.

23. I wish that my spouse and I had a better relationship.

24. I feel that my spouse doesn't appreciate what I do for him or her as much as I would like.

25. I feel uncomfortable when I have friends over.

26. I feel that my spouse tries to manipulate me.

27. I feel that my spouse seems to expect me to take care of him or her as if I were the only one he or she could depend on.

28. I feel that I don't have enough money to support my spouse in addition to the rest of our expenses.

29. I feel that I would like to be able to provide more money to support my spouse than I am able to now.

Interpretation: No norms for rating. Useful in estimating how much stress the caregiver is currently experiencing. Can be used before and after an intervention to indicate success or improvement in the caregiver's situation.
From Zarit SH, Reever KE, Bach-Peterson J. Relatives of the impaired elderly: Correlates of feelings of burden. Gerontologist 1980; 20:649; with permission.

Spiritual

GUILT

Mary L. Nowotny

Guilt is a feeling of knowing you have committed a crime or offense or violated a law or belief. Unresolved and painful past or present experiences for which forgiveness from God, others, or self is not received result in feelings of guilt. The box shown below identifies the characteristics of patients feeling guilty.

A. Elicit information from the patient and family or caregiver about
   - feelings of
     - guilt
     - remorse
   - acts of omission and commission
   - bitterness and revenge
   - anger toward God, self, or others
   - blaming others
   - stopping participation in religious practices
   - refusal to talk about spiritual beliefs
   - role relationships (see pp. 290–303)

B. Assess factors such as
   - general
     - posture
     - facial expression
   - cognitive level (see tools on pp. 268–272)
   - functional motor skills (see tools on pp. 28–31)
   - use of negative self-statements
   - mood
     - restricted affect
   - neurologic status
     - presence or absence of sensory impairment
   - physiologic changes, to rule out other conditions

C. When behaviors are exhibited that indicate feelings of guilt, interventions are needed to help the patient find forgiveness from God, others, or self. Strategies to help patients who are feeling guilty include:
   - help patients to give and receive forgiveness
   - listen
   - provide support
   - affirm their worth
   - use prayer
   - use scripture
   - promote communication toward God and others
   - give permission to express feelings

D. Consider referral to
   - clergy for increased spiritual guidance
   - counseling for feelings of guilt or displayed behaviors

Presentation of Patients Feeling Guilty

- hostility or aggression
- withdrawal
- anxiety
- anger
- dysthmia
- depression (see p. 282)
- grief (see Losses/Grief, p. 298)

References

Carson VB. Spiritual dimensions of nursing practice. Philadelphia: WB Saunders, 1989.

Peterson EA. The physical . . . the spiritual . . can you meet all of your patient's needs? J Gerontol Nurs 1985; 11:23.

Shelly J, Fish S. Spiritual care: The nurse's role. Downer's Grove, IL: InterVarsity Press, 1988.

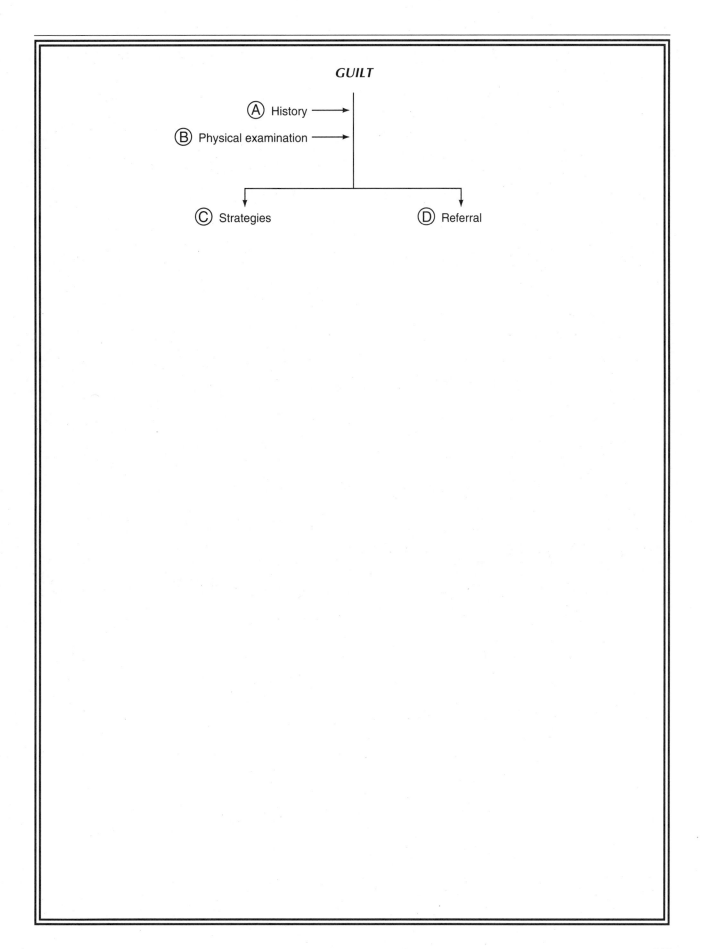

GUILT

Ⓐ History

Ⓑ Physical examination

Ⓒ Strategies

Ⓓ Referral

LOSS OF HOPE

Mary L. Nowotny

Hope can be defined as a dynamic expectation of achieving a possible future good that requires active involvement and relates to others or to a higher being. As the elderly are faced with the loss of friends, family members, health, and independence, they frequently experience feelings of loss of hope. The future may appear empty, with numerous obstacles to carrying out activities of daily living.

A. Ask questions to elicit information specified in Table 1. The Nowotny Hope Scale (see p. 318) may be used as a framework for assessment and interventions. Obtain a general health history about
  - chronic illnesses
  - medication and drug use
  - recent injuries or illnesses
  - recent losses (see Losses/Grief, p. 298)
  Determine past and present coping patterns.

B. Assess factors such as
  - general
    - appearance
    - hygiene
  - cognitive level (see tools on pp. 268–272)
  - functional motor skills (see tools on pp. 28–30)
  - use of negative self-statements
  - mood
    - presence of restricted affect
  - neurologic status
    - presence or absence of sensory impairment
  - physiologic changes, to rule out other conditions

C. When any of the behaviors that indicate a loss of hope are present, implement strategies that foster or reinforce hope (Table 2).

D. Counseling with a chaplain, priest, pastor, or rabbi may be needed for individuals exhibiting loss of hope. If patients continue to withdraw or exhibit depression, referral may be indicated to
  - a support group
    - grief support
    - new coping skills
  - a psychiatrist
  - a psychologic counselor
  - a physician
  - psychosocial counseling

TABLE 1 Assessment of Hope/Loss of Hope

Area	Definition	Indicators of Loss of Hope
Future is possible	A goal or an expectation that has not been met	• is overwhelmed by difficulty • finds it difficult to talk about the future • tends to speak only of the past or present
Active involvement	Setting a goal, planning or actively participating in a plan or event	• tends to be very passive or withdrawn • shows a lack of ambition of interest • shows a loss of gratification from roles and relationships
Comes from within	Inner readiness	• becomes pessimistic • shows lack of motivation • becomes discouraged with self
Spiritual beliefs (see tool on p. 320)	Dynamic and personal relationship with God or a higher being	• shows lack of faith • has stopped participating in religious practices • makes statements that God no longer cares • refused to talk about spiritual beliefs
Relates to others	Thoughts, feelings and actions that involve other individuals	• is discouraged with self and others • shows disbelief that others will help in times of distress • believes that if others try to help they will also fail • changes interactions with others
Confidence in outcome	Belief that hope will be fulfilled	• shows lack of confidence in own strength or capacity to achieve goals • fails to use previous satisfactions or successes

Text continued on page 312.

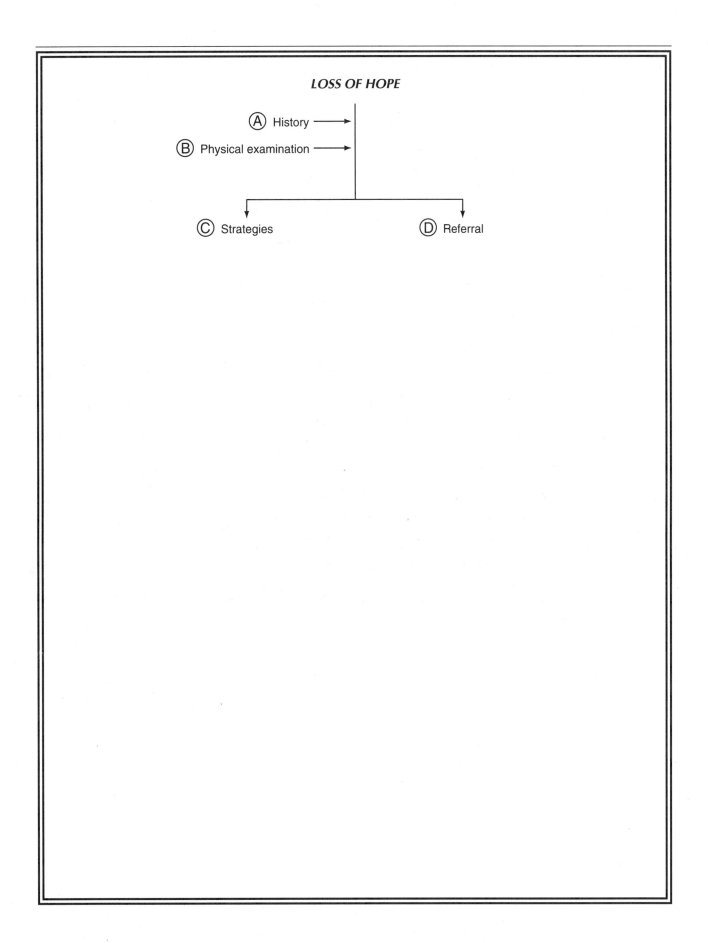

TABLE 2 Interventions in Dealing with Loss of Hope

Area	Interventions
Future is possible	• assist in looking forward to worthwhile aims • find ways to give as much control as possible over the situation • show patient how to have more control • be creative in assisting patient to accomplish own aims
Active involvement	• help to devise and revise aims • give support and guidance when aims need to be refocused • help to set short-term aims that are easily achievable • encourage discussion of hopes • share information on hope with patient and family/caregivers • assist to be independent in as many activities as possible • encourage laughter and humor • offer choices
Comes from within	• assist to identify and use own strengths • listen actively • stay with patient • assist patient to recognize own feelings • encourage discussion of feelings • encourage use of a diary to record feelings and experiences • encourage family members/caregivers to support patient
Spiritual	• determine importance of faith, prayer, religious practices, and relationship with God or some other higher being • create an environment in which patient feels comfortable to express spiritual beliefs • help patient renew spiritual self • arrange for a visit from a chaplain, priest, pastor, or rabbi as needed • support through reflection on meaning and purpose of life and death
Relates to others	• assess who is most significant to patient • talk to patient about significant people • involve family/caregivers • share hopes with family/caregivers • help patient reach out to others for support • assess support systems to determine strengths and weaknesses of relationships with family and friends • be available • be an advocate by creating conditions that foster caring relationships • encourage family/caregivers to allow patient to make decisions • use touch when appropriate • identify community resources • encourage closeness to foster a sense of belonging • become a source of hope • provide physical and emotional comfort
Confidence in outcome	• help patient maintain confidence • encourage family, friends, and caregivers to provide support • listen • identify strengths

References

Fischer K. Hope never ends: God's promise to the elderly. J Christian Nurs 1988; Fall:32.

Herth K. The relationship between level of hope and level of coping response and other variables in patients with cancer. Oncol Nurs Forum 1989; 16:67.

Miller J. Hope-inspiring strategies of the critically ill. Appl Nurs Res 1985; 2:23.

Miller J, Powers M. Development of an instrument to measure hope. Nurs Res 1988; 37:5.

Nowotny M. Assessment of hope in patients with cancer: Development of an instrument. Oncol Nurs Forum 1989; 16:57.

LACK OF LOVE AND RELATEDNESS

Mary L. Nowotny

Love and relatedness is the feeling of strong affection or close connection to family, friends, God, or a higher being. A lack of love and relatedness can result in feelings of
- isolation
- loneliness (see p. 296)
- anxiety (see p. 278)
- poor self-esteem
- helplessness (see p. 286)
- depression (see p. 282)
- suspiciousness (see p. 264)

A. Elicit information from the patient and family/caregivers about
- signs of
  - withdrawal
  - depression
- lack of
  - visitors
  - mail
  - phone calls
- expressions of feelings of
  - a loss of faith in God or a higher being (see the tool *Spiritual Perspective*, p. 320)
  - a lack of support from others
  - guilt feelings (see Guilt, p. 308)
  - aloneness and abandonment
  - fear of dependence
  - ambivalence or resentment toward God or a higher being
- refusal to
  - call on others for help when needed
  - participate in religious practices
  - talk about spiritual beliefs

B. Assess factors such as
- general
  - posture
  - appearance
- cognitive level (see tools on pp. 268–272)
- functional motor skills (see tools on pp. 28–30)
- use of negative self-statements
- mood
  - restricted affect
- withdrawal
- anxiety
- neurologic status
  - presence or absence of sensory impairment
- physiologic changes, to rule out other conditions

C. When behaviors are exhibited that indicate lack of love and relatedness, implement strategies to restore feelings of connectedness with family, friends, God, or a higher being. Interventions include
- listening
- encouraging sharing of
  - beliefs
  - feelings about family and God or a higher being
  - feelings of love toward others
- providing supportive atmosphere
- offering to
  - read scripture
  - pray with the patient
- supporting feelings of worth and dignity
- treating the patient with dignity and respect
- encouraging family and friends to share feelings of love
- discussing volunteer and community opportunities

D. Consider referral to
- clergy for
  - spiritual support
  - guidance
- psychosocial counseling
- psychiatric counseling
- social work for
  - community and volunteer activities
  - transportation
- support groups

References

Carson VB. Spiritual dimensions of nursing practice. Philadelphia: WB Saunders, 1989.

Shelly J, Fish S. Spiritual care: The nurse's role. Downer's Grove, IL: InterVarsity Press, 1988.

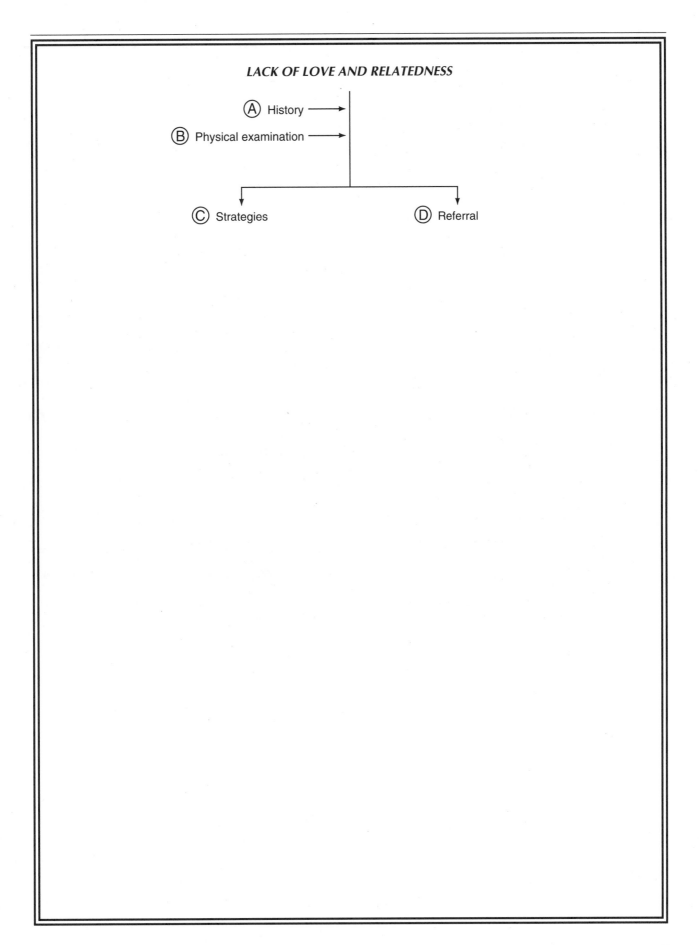

LACK OF LOVE AND RELATEDNESS

(A) History

(B) Physical examination

(C) Strategies

(D) Referral

LACK OF MEANING AND PURPOSE

Mary L. Nowotny

In later years it is common for life review to occur. Life review includes examination of accomplishments and failures in a search for meaning and purpose.

A. Elicit information from the patient and family or caregivers about
- expressions of
  - no reason to continue living
  - despair
  - emotional detachment from self and peers
  - not having lived according to a value system
  - discontentment with life
  - inability to make sense out of events and feelings
  - feelings of worthlessness
  - feelings of emptiness
- signs of pain and suffering
- spiritual aspects
  - decreased participation in religious practices
  - refusal to talk about spiritual beliefs

B. Assess factors such as
- general
  - appearance
  - hygiene
- cognitive level (see tools on pp. 268–272)
- functional motor skills (see tools on pp. 28–30)
- use of negative self-statements
- mood
  - restricted affect
  - depression
- neurologic status
  - presence or absence of sensory impairment (see section Sensory/Communication, pp. 118–142)
- physiologic changes, to rule out other conditions

C. When any of the behaviors that indicate a lack of meaning and purpose are exhibited, strategies are needed to restore meaning and purpose to living. Intervention strategies include:
- listen
- provide time for reminiscence
- encourage talk about past experiences
- encourage the showing of pictures and memorabilia
- encourage continued participation in current activities
- help the patient see meaning in present life
- help the patient restructure and revalue attitudes toward life and others
- encourage identification of positive aspects in past life
  - relationships
  - contributions to others
  - social activities and contributions

D. Consider referral to
- clergy for spiritual guidance
- psychosocial counseling for
  - life review
  - reminiscence

References

Brooke V. The spiritual well-being of the elderly. Geriatr Nurs 1987; 8(4):194.

Carson VB. Spiritual dimensions of nursing practice. Philadelphia: WB Saunders, 1989.

Shelly J, Fish S. Spiritual care: The nurse's role. Downer's Grove, IL: InterVarsity Press, 1988.

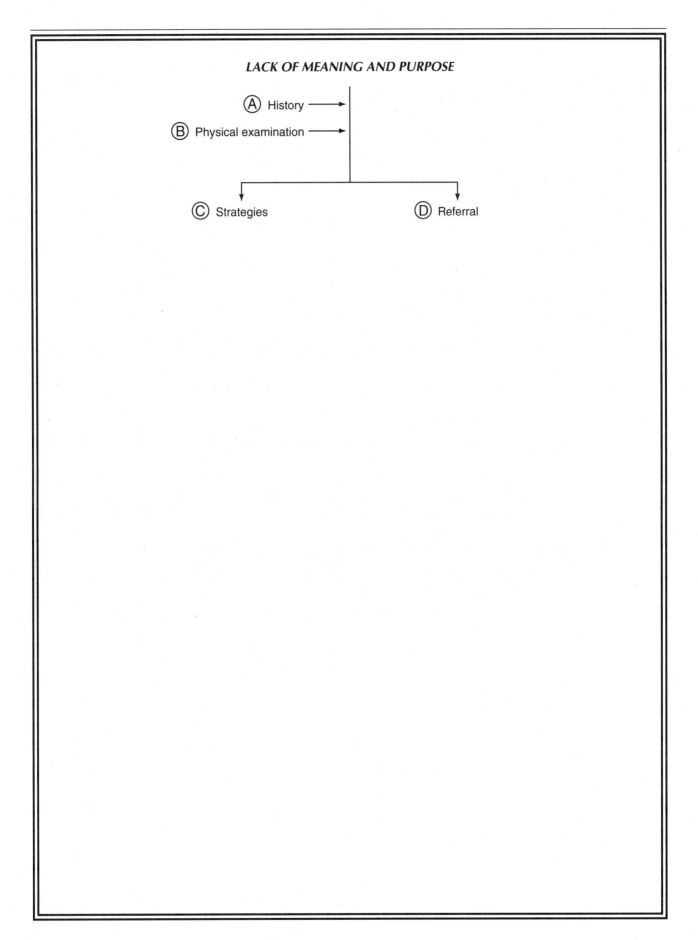

LACK OF MEANING AND PURPOSE

(A) History

(B) Physical examination

(C) Strategies

(D) Referral

Nowotny Hope Scale

Directions: Below are 29 statements which describe people's feelings after a stressful event. Please think of a significant event or situation where you felt stressed or pressured because of the necessary changes in your life. Imagine the event occurring right now. Place a check mark in the box to the right of the statement that *best* reflects your feelings about the statement. There are no right or wrong answers.

Key: SA = Strongly agree; A = Agree; D = Disagree; SD = Strongly disagree

Statement	SA	A	D	SD
1. I can take whatever happens and make the best of it.				
2. I have a positive outlook.				
3. I know I can make changes in my life.				
4. I think I can learn (or I have learned) to adapt to whatever limitations I have (or might have).				
5. I am ready to meet each new challenge.				
6. I feel the decisions I make get me what I expect.				
7. When faced with a challenge, I am ready to take action.				
8. I have confidence in my own ability.				
9. My family (or significant other) is always available to help me when I need them.				
10. I feel confident in those who want to help me.				
11. Sometimes I feel I am all alone.				
12. I share important decision making with my family (or significant other).				
13. I know I can go to my family or friends for help.				
14. In the future I plan to accomplish many things.				
15. I feel confident about the outcome of this event/situation.				
16. I see a light at the end of the tunnel.				
17. I know I can accomplish this task.				
18. I look forward to the future.				
19. My religious beliefs help me most when I feel discouraged.				
20. I use prayer to give me strength.				
21. I use scripture to give me strength.				
22. I like to do things rather than sit and wait for things to happen.				
23. I lack confidence in my ability.				
24. I have important goals I want to achieve within the next 10 to 15 years.				
25. I like to sit and wait for things to happen.				
26. I have difficulty in setting goals.				
27. I like to make my own decisions.				
28. I want to maintain control over my life and my body.				
29. I expect to be successful in those tasks that concern me most.				

Scoring of Nowotny Hope Scale

(This version of the Nowotny Hope Scale is for assessment.)

1. For total score:

Strongly agree	= 4
Agree	= 3
Disagree	= 2
Strongly disagree	= 1

   Except items 11, 23, 25, 26 are scored:

Strongly agree	= 1
Agree	= 2
Disagree	= 3
Strongly disagree	= 4

   Cutoff scores:

Hopeful	95–116
Moderately hopeful	73–94
Low hope	51–72
Hopeless	29–50

2. For subscales:

Confidence subscale	Items 1–8
Relates to Others subscale	Items 9–13
Future Is Possible subscale	Items 14–18
Spiritual Beliefs subscale	Items 19–21
Active Involvement subscale	Items 22–26
Comes from Within subscale	Items 27–29

Spiritual Perspective Clinical Scale

Directions: A spiritual perspective is that which relates one to a transcendent or non-physical realm, or to something greater than the self without disregarding the value of the individual. Please answer the following questions by marking an 'X' in the space above the group of words that best describes you.

1. In talking with others, how often do you typically mention spiritual matters?

Not at all	Less than once a year	About once a year	About once a month	About once a week	About once a day
1	2	3	4	5	6

2. How often do you engage in private prayer?

Not at all	Less than once a year	About once a year	About once a month	About once a week	About once a day
1	2	3	4	5	6

3. To what extent do you agree or disagree that having a spiritual perspective is an important part of your life?

Strongly disagree	Disagree	Disagree more than agree	Agree more than disagree	Agree	Strongly agree
1	2	3	4	5	6

4. To what extent do you agree or disagree that you seek spiritual guidance in making decisions at this time of your life?

Strongly disagree	Disagree	Disagree more than agree	Agree more than disagree	Agree	Strongly agree
1	2	3	4	5	6

5. To what extent do you agree or disagree that you feel a sense of connectedness to God or a higher power in your life?

Strongly disagree	Disagree	Disagree more than agree	Agree more than disagree	Agree	Strongly agree
1	2	3	4	5	6

6. To what extent do you agree or disagree that your spiritual perspective helps to answer questions about the meaning of life?

Strongly disagree	Disagree	Disagree more than agree	Agree more than disagree	Agree	Strongly agree
1	2	3	4	5	6

Please feel free to express any views you may have about your spiritual perspective that have not been addressed by these six questions.

_____

_____

Adapted by Reed from the Spiritual Perspective Scale, Pamela G. Reed, 1986; with permission.

Scoring Instructions for the Spiritual Perspective Clinical Scale

The SPCS is scored by calculating the arithmetic mean across all items, for a total score that ranges from 1.0 to 6.0. Responses to each item are selected using a 6-point Likert-type scale that is anchored with descriptive words for each of the six items. The instrument can be administered as a questionnaire or, better, in an interview format. The score may be compared with other scores previously reported in the literature based on Spiritual Perspective Scale data, even though this clinically-adapted instrument is being used here.

To interpret the score, in general, scores of 4.6 or above indicate a high level of spiritual perspective; scores between 3.0 and 4.5 indicate a middle range; and scores below 3.0 indicate a low level of spiritual perspective. Qualitative data (comments offered by the person) should be used in conjunction with the quantitative results to aid in interpreting the meaning of the score and the implications for intervention.

From Reed PG. Spirituality and mental health of older adults: Extant knowledge for nursing. Family and Community Health 1991; 14 (2):14.

INDEX

f indicates figure or illustration
t indicates table

Muscle strength—cont'd.
  testing, 67
Myoclonic seizure, 94t
Myoclonus, nocturnal, 82, 84t

N

Narcolepsy, 84t
Narcotics, 184, 213
Nardil; *see* Phenelzine
Nasal examination, 126
Neglect, 300—301
  caregiver characteristics in, 300
Neisseria gonorrhoeae, 240
Neurologic deficits in irritative voiding symptoms, 202
Neurologic status in trauma, 96
Neurologic system
  adverse effects of antidepressants on, 284
  in symptoms of dizziness, 140t
Neuromodulation, 112t
Neuromuscular system, 18
Neuropathic lesions of foot, 56t
Neuropathy, peripheral, 44t, 58
Nifedipine, 223
Nitrates in hoarseness, 128
Nitroglycerin (NTG), 222, 223
Nocturia, 203t
Nocturnal myoclonus, 82, 84t
Noise exposure in tinnitus, 124
Nongonococcal urethritis (NGU), 240t
Nonsteroidal anti-inflammatory drugs, 220
Nowotny hope scale, 318, 319
Numbness, foot, 58—59
Nursing approach to angry patients, 276
Nursing communication assessment, 146
Nutrition
  in burns, 88
  community services for, 102
  in diarrhea, 187t
  in edema, 11
  enteral, 154t
  in hemorrhoids, 192
  in hoarseness, 128
  in osteoporosis, 226
  supplementation, 154—155
  in weakness, 18
Nutritional assessment, 166
Nutritional defects requiring supplementation, 154—155

O

OARS Social Resource Scale, 304
Obesity in diverticular disease, 179
Occult blood in stool, 194
Oral examination, 174, 183
Oral history, components of, 182
Oral hygiene, 136, 174
  tools for, 172
Oral rinses, 174
Orthostatic hypotension, 3
Osler maneuver, 228
Osteoarthritis, 36
Osteoporosis, 224—227
  education for, 226
Otoscopic examination, 122, 124
Overflow urinary incontinence, 207t
  therapeutic options for, 209t
Overlapping toes, 54
Oxazepam, 278

P

Padding to relieve pressure, 106t
Pain
  assessment of, 38

back, 224—227
  low, 38—41
chest, 222—223
decreased sensation of, 138
dental, jaw, mouth, 176—177
foot, 58—59
joint, 36—37
management of, 37, 40, 139
  factors influencing, 39
  in osteoporosis, 226
  methods of, 112t
muscle, 34—35
rectal, 198—199
of voiding, 202—205
  definition and causes, 203t
Papanicolaou smear, 246
Papilloma, basal cell, 110t, 116t
Paraparesis, 44t
Parenteral nutrition, 155
Parkinson's dyskinesia, 44t
Parnate; *see* Tranylcypromine
Partial seizures, 94
Pelvic examination, 246
Pelvic muscles, exercises for, 216
Perceptual disturbances, 260—263
  therapeutic activities for, 262
Perineal excoriation, 190
Peripheral circulation, impaired, 230—231
Peripheral neuropathy, 44t, 58
Peripheral vascular disease, 58, 230
Personal loss, 298—299
  factors influencing ability to cope, 299
Phenelzine (Nardil)
  food and drug interaction information for, 78
  interactions of, 70t
Piles, 192—193
  teaching plan for patient with, 192
Pill rolling tremor, 49t
Plantar warts, 116t
Pneumonia, 108
Polypharmacy, 72—75
  patient teaching to prevent or reduce, 75t
Polysomnography, 85
Position sense, 2
Positioning to relieve pressure, 106t
Posthysterectomy hormone replacement regimen, 242t
Postvoid catheterized specimen, 202
Postvoid residual (PVR) determination, 208t
Potassium, 150
  interactions of, 70t
  urinalysis findings for, 203t
Potassium chloride, 220
Premarin (conjugated estrogen), 242t
Pressure, measures to relieve, 106t
Pressure sore, 106—107
  treatment for, 106t
Progestins, 242t
Prompted voiding, 210t
Propranolol, 223
Proprioception test, 2
Prostatic hypertrophy, 212t
Protein calorie malnutrition (PCM), 152
Proteus, 203t
Provera (medroxyprogesterone acetate), 242t
Provocative stress testing procedure for urinary tract assessment, 208t
Pruritus, 12
Pruritus ani, 196—197
Psychiatric pathophysiologic states associated with weakness, 18
Psychiatric disorder hallucinations, 262t
Psychoactive drugs, 276
  therapy, 252
Psychological changes in aggressive behavior, 250
Psychological methods of pain management, 112t

Psychosocial traits associated with loneliness, 296
Pupils, dilated, 24t
Purpose, lack of, 316–317
Purulent drainage, 12
Pus formation, 12
Pyelogram, intravenous (IVP), 217
Pyelogram, retrograde (RGPG), 217

Q

Questionnaire
  Cage, 274
  short portable mental status, 271

R

Radiography of back, 38
Range of motion, limited, 8–9
Rashes, 104–105
Receptive aphasia, 134t
Rectal bleeding, 194–195
Rectal itching, 196–197
Rectal pain, 198–199
Rectal skin, classification of changes in, 196
Regression, 276
Rehydration, 150
Relatedness, lack of, 314–315
Renal colic, 200
Renal stones, 202
Renal system, 18
Reorientation of patients with perceptual disturbances, 260
Respiratory alkalosis, 203t
Respiratory isolation, 108
Resting tremor, 49t
Restraint of patients, 250, 276, 277
Retinal detachment, 119
Retirement, 302–303
Retrograde pyelogram (RGPG), 217
Retrograde urethrogram (RGUG), 217
Rewarming, 24–26
Rheumatoid arthritis, 36
Rhinitis, 126t
Rigidity, 46–47
  hypothermia in, 24t
Rinne's test, 122, 123t
Roentgenographic urologic procedures, 217
Romberg test, 63
Rosenbaum Pocket Vision Screener, 118, 121f

S

Safety measures
  in burn management, 88
  in confusion, 254
  in coordination change, 4
  in decreased sensation, 138, 139
  in decreased sense of smell, 127
  home, 226
  in limited range of motion, 8
  in perceptual disorders, 263
  in prevention of falls, 90
  in wandering, 267
Saline depletion, symptoms of, 186
Salivary flow, 136
Scheduled toileting, 210t
Seborrheic eczema, 104t
Seborrheic keratosis, 110t
Seborrheic warts, 116t
Sedation, 80–81
Segmented urine culture in males, 204t
Seizures, 94–95
  classification of, 94t

Self-care
  index for, 29
  for vascular problems, 230
Self-catheterization, 218
Sensation, decreased, 138–139
  examination for, 138
Sense(s)
  adverse drug effects on, 74t
  of position, ways to test, 2
  of smell, conditions and medications associated with, 126
    decreased, 126–127
Sensory ataxia, 44t
Sensory system in symptoms of dizziness, 140t
Serosanguineous drainage, 12
Serum calcium, 225
Set test, the, 272
Sexual behavior, inappropriate, 256–257
Sexual dysfunction, 238–239
  contributors to, 238
  genitourinary examination in, 239
Sexuality
  counseling, 256, 257
  physiologic changes of, 238t
Sexually transmitted disease (STD), 240
Shingles, 108–109
Shivering, 24t
Short portable mental status questionnaire, 271
Shortness of breath, 232–233
Side effects
  antianxiety medications, 278
  antidepressants, 284
  commonly used drugs, 76
Skin
  cold, hypothermia in, 24t
  dry, 102–103
  rectal, classification of changes of, 196
  ulceration, 112–113
    in intervention for edema, 11
    precipitating factors for, 112t
    stages, 167
Skin cancer, 110–111
  differentiation of, 110t
Skin lesions, 112–113
  precipitating factors for, 112t
Skin tags, 114–115
Skin type, 100
Sleep
  dysfunctions associated with, 84t
  helpful hints for, 86
  non–rapid eye movement (NREM), 82, 84t
  rapid eye movement (REM), 82, 84t
  stages of and changes in elderly, 84t
Sleep apnea, 84t, 85
Sleep disturbance, 82–86
Sleep-wake schedule disorders, 84t
Slurred speech, 24t
Smell, sense of, decreased, 126–127
Smoking in decrease muscle strength, 32
Snellen's test, 119, 120f
Social resource scale, OARS, 304
Social services, 26; see also Community resources and services
Socks in foot care, 61
Somnambulism, 84t
Specimen, postvoid catheterized, 202
Speech
  assessment of, 132
  slurred, hypothermia in, 24t
Speech impairment, 132–135
  disorders in, 134t
Spiritual perspective clinical scale, 320–321
Splints, 45t
Sprue, 152
Squamous cell carcinoma, 110t
Stability, ways to test, 2

Stasis, venous, 234–235
Static tremor, 49t
Status epilepticus, 94, 95
Steroids, 256
Stool
  adverse drug effects on, 74
  false-positive occult blood test of, 194
Stress, caregiver, 292–293
  factors in, 292t
Stress management, 140
Stress urinary incontinence, 207t
  therapeutic options for, 209t
Structural factors contributing to falls, 90
Struvite stones, 203t
Suicide, 282, 285, 286
  alcohol abuse and, 274
  risk factors for, 284
Sun exposure, 100
Sundowner syndrome, 250, 254
Supplementation, nutritional, 155–156
  in osteoporosis, 226
Support systems, 7
Suppositories, 184
Suspiciousness, 264–265
Sway test, 2
Swelling, gum, 172t

T

Tables, Masters and Lasser, for weight and height, 161
Tactile senses, decreased, 138
Tagamet (cimetidine), interactions of, 70t
Tags, skin, 114–115
Tasks, Barthel index for independent performance of, 29
Taste, 136–137
Teeth, 170
Tegretol (carbamazepine), interactions of, 70t
Test(s)
  dexamethasone suppression, 16
  get up and go, 62
  hearing, 123t
  Marshall, 219
  for memory, 258
  Michigan Alcoholism Screening, 288
  muscle strength, 67
  proprioception, 2
  Rinne's, 122, 123t
  Romberg, 63
  set, 272
  Snellen's, 118, 120f
  stool occult blood, 194
  sway, 2
  vertebrobasilar, 2
  Weber's, 122, 123t
Thayer-Martin culture, 240
Theophylline
  in hoarseness, 128
  interactions of, 70t
Therapeutic communication, 250
Therapeutic diet, 156–157
Thermal sensation, decreased, 138
Thyroid disorders and dizziness, 141
Thyroid preparations, 228
Thyroid problems, 44t
Thyrotoxicosis, apathetic, 280t
Timolol, 223
Tinnitus, 124–125
  drugs that cause or aggravate, 124
Toenail deformities, 52–53
Toes, 54
Tongue blade, 94f
Tonic clonic seizure, 94t
Tonic seizure, 94t
Toothbrush, how to select, 170

Topical chemotherapy, 101
Total parenteral nutrition (TPN), 155
Toxic tremor, 50t
Tranquilizers, 184, 256
  concerns about, 278
Transdermal estradiol hormone replacement regimen, 242t
Tranylcypromine (Parnate)
  food and drug interaction information for, 78
  interactions of, 70t
Trauma, 96–97
  emergency care procedures for, 97
  parameter assessment and abnormal findings in, 96
Tremor, 48–51
  types, causes, and characteristics of, 50t-51t
Trichomonas vaginalis vaginitis, 244t
Tumors, skin, 110–111
  differentiation of, 110t

U

Ulcers
  mouth, 174–175
    characteristics of, 174t
  skin, 112–113
    in intervention for edema, 11
    precipitating factors for, 112t
    stages of, 167
Ultrasonography, 217
UPP (urethral pressure profile) , 219
Urethral discharge, 240–241
Urethral diverticulum, 212t
Urethral pressure profile (UPP), 219
Urethral strictures, acquired, 212t
Urethral swab, 240
Urethritis, 240, 241
  nongonococcal (NGU), 240t
Urethrogram, retrograde (RGUG), 217
Urge urinary incontinence, 207t
  therapeutic options for, 209t
Urgency of voiding, 202–205
  definition and causes, 203t
Uric acid stones, 203
Urinalysis, findings in, 203t
Urinary incontinence, 206–211
  behavioral techniques in, 210t
  indicators for urological referral in, 210
  lower urinary tract function assessment in, 208t
  pelvic muscle exercises for, 216
  roentgenographic urology procedures, 217
  self-catheterization in, 218
  therapeutic options for, 209t
  types of, 207t
  urodynamic studies, 219
Urinary retention, 212–213
  profile of, 212t
Urinary tract, lower, assessment procedures for, 208t
Urinary tract disorder, urinalysis findings in, 203t
Urinary tract infection, 202
Urine, adverse drug effects on, 74
Urine culture, segmented, in males, 204t
Urine reagent test strip, 202
Urodynamic studies, 219
Urologic procedures, roentgenographic, 217
Urticaria, 12

V

Vagina, postmenopausal changes in, 246
Vaginal bleeding, 244–245
  treatment for, 245
Vaginal cream, 246
Vaginal discharge, 244–245
  identification, 244t
  treatment for, 245